PSYCHIATRY IN MEDICAL PRACTICE

To my mother, who taught me how to care for people
at the time of their distress.

Psychiatry
in
Medical Practice

Edited by
R.G. PRIEST
M.D., F.R.C.P. (Edin.), F.R.C.Psych., D.P.M.
Professor of Psychiatry (University of London)
St. Mary's Hospital Medical School, St. Mary's Hospital
London W9

Contributors:

Dougal Mackay
Enid Balint
Robin Steel
Alan J. Cooper
Alistair M. Gordon
Henry R. Rollin
Robert J. Daly
Alexander Shapiro
Marian Leyshon
Anthony G. Carroll
J. Kenneth Binns

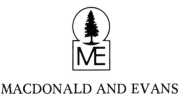

MACDONALD AND EVANS

MACDONALD & EVANS LTD.
Estover, Plymouth PL6 7PZ

First published 1982

© Macdonald and Evans 1982

ISBN: 0 7121 1672 9

Printed in Great Britain by
Butler & Tanner Ltd,
Frome and London.

Preface

When I left the cloistered environment of my medical school and started work as a family doctor I was reassured to find that on the whole my training had prepared me to diagnose and treat most of the serious medical problems that I came across. There was just one large area where I felt naked, and that was where my patients were persistently distressed but had no abnormal physical signs.

It only slowly dawned on me that a high proportion of my patients had psychological rather than physical problems. Even when I did realise that a patient had a psychiatric disorder I had no idea what to do about it. Thus it came about that a large part of my own motivation in taking my first psychiatric job was the prospect of relieving my own ignorance.

Today, undergraduate education in psychiatry has improved a great deal. All the same, it is still far from perfect, and I know that for many physicians psychiatry is a baffling subject. I believe that principles of diagnosis, classification, aetiology and so on are important parts of the subject, and should be taught to undergraduates in some detail, but that what the busy physician wants most of all is to know, when he has a patient with psychiatric problems, what to *do* about it. That is what this book aims to tell him.

The orientation is an essentially practical one. It makes no pretensions to substitute for standard psychiatric texts. Do not look within these pages for lists of pathognomonic symptoms of schizophrenia or solutions to complex problems in differential diagnosis. What the authors *have* aimed to do is to write as simply as possible about the treatment and management of the wide range of psychiatric problems that the non-psychiatric medical practitioner is likely to come across.

We have aimed to clarify what treatment the general physician can carry out himself, what can be done by his local psychiatrist and what can be done at a few super-specialist centres. The book

can be read as a whole as an up-to-date refresher course in practical
psychiatry — there will be few who do not learn a lot that is new.
Each chapter can be read independently of the rest for the same
purpose.

One of our hopes is that, as well as being used in this systematic
way, the book can be used as a help in day-to-day clinical problem
solving. Suppose you are trying to treat and manage a difficult
psychiatric case. It should not take too long to find the appropriate
chapter of this book that deals with the problem, e.g. ask yourself
what is the patient's classification: is the patient a child, a psychogeriatric patient, a case of a sexual disorder? Having located the
chapter, it should not then be too difficult to track down the
alternative methods of coping with the clinical situation and, where
relevant, see whether it is best to manage the patient yourself or
refer him for specialist advice.

This is what we hope. As far as we know, at the time of writing
this, the book is unique, so we have no precedent to guide us. If the
book fails in these goals do feel welcome to write to me, care of the
publishers, to let us know how future editions could be improved.

Finally, I should like to acknowledge the unfailing support I
received from Marilyn and the skilled dedication of Ursula, without
which this book would not have appeared.

June 1982   R.G.P.

Contents

Preface   v

ONE: Techniques of Behaviour Therapy   1
Dougal Mackay

TWO: Talking Treatments   73
Enid Balint

THREE: Useful Psychotropic Drugs   93
Robin Steel

FOUR: The Diagnosis and Management of Sexual Inadequacy   133
Alan J. Cooper

FIVE: Dealing with Common Forms of Drug Dependence   193
Alistair M. Gordon

SIX: Disturbances of Behaviour: A Consideration of Their Causes   239
and Management
Henry R. Rollin

SEVEN: Psychological Help for Physical Illness   273
Robert J. Daly

EIGHT: Coping with Mental Handicap   309
Alexander Shapiro and Marian Leyshon

NINE: Childhood Emotional Problems in Medical Practice   341
Anthony G. Carroll

TEN: Therapeutic Management of the Elderly   419
J. Kenneth Binns

APPENDIXES

ONE: Male/Female Sexual History Schedule   473

TWO: Rules for compulsory admission to hospital (reproduced
    from the Mental Health Act 1959 of England and Wales)   481

Index   489

Techniques of Behaviour Therapy

Dougal Mackay,

B.A., M.Sc., A.B.Ps.S.

District Psychologist, Bristol and Weston Health District

Techniques of Behaviour Therapy

INTRODUCTION

Although the term "behaviour therapy" was first used by Skinner in the 1950s to refer to operant conditioning work with psychotic patients, the establishment of the psychotherapy school of this name is usually associated with Wolpe (1958) and, in particular, Eysenck (1960). In contrast to other forms of psychological treatment which have their roots in clinical practice, behaviour therapy was regarded by its founders as the applied branch of a basic science. Thus Wolpe (1958) defined this approach as "the use of experimentally established principles of learning for the purpose of changing unadaptive behaviour". In other words, it was claimed that the "laws of behaviour" derived from the animal experiments of Pavlov and Skinner could provide the basis for the effective treatment of neurotic disorders. The assumption here is that the neurosis is nothing more than its symptoms and that once these have been eliminated there is no condition left to treat. However, as will be seen, behaviour therapy has become much more sophisticated in the last decade, both in terms of the ways in which problems are formulated and the sorts of interventions that are made. Nevertheless, the fundamental postulate, that abnormal behaviour patterns can be modified by direct means, remains unchanged.

The traditional behaviourist view of the nature, genesis and treatment of neurotic disorders is very different from that held by psychodynamically oriented psychotherapists. To them, maladaptive behaviour is merely an indication of a deep-seated, intrapsychic conflict which constitutes the core of the problem. Consequently they would argue that lasting change at the symptomatic level is unlikely to occur unless the patient has acquired some "insight" into his difficulties. Furthermore, in those cases where change is observed, they would predict that the old symptom would be replaced by a new one.

Symptom substitution is perhaps the most controversial issue in the whole field of psychotherapy. Partisan behaviour therapists such as Yates (1958) have denied the existence of the phenomenon, whereas Bookbinder (1962) has argued that, not only is the formation of a new symptom inevitable, but that the replacement may actually endanger the patients' lives. Although it might appear that this issue could be quickly resolved by the collection of appropriate empirical data, such a simple solution is not possible for a number of reasons. There is no general agreement as to what constitutes a "symptom", what form the substitute should take, or when it should emerge. Furthermore, even if an unambiguous symptom were to manifest itself shortly after a course of behaviour therapy, it would be unclear as to whether this constituted a replacement as such, a newly acquired form of maladaptive behaviour, or a longstanding but less severe difficulty which had previously been ignored. Finally, it has been argued by some behaviourists that substitute deviant behaviour is quite likely to occur if the antecedents and consequences of the original behaviour were not taken into account when modification was carried out. Thus there is no evidence that symptom substitution does occur and, even if there was, this would not necessarily invalidate the behaviourist model. For a fuller account of this complex issue, the reader is referred to Bandura (1969).

While psychotherapists have tended to accuse behaviour therapists of clinical naivety, behaviourists have retaliated by pointing to the unscientific nature of the psychodynamic models. Eysenck, in particular, has continually asserted that the psychotherapies are based on loosely formulated notions which have never been validated experimentally. Furthermore, he claims that there is no evidence to show that psychotherapy is any more effective than letting time take its course. His argument (Eysenck, 1952) is that since the "spontaneous remission" rate for untreated neurotics, two years after they present, is approximately 70 per cent, psychotherapists should demonstrate success rates in excess of this figure to justify the continued use of this very expensive treatment method. Fourteen years after his invitation to psychotherapists to demonstrate scientifically the efficacy of their approach, Eysenck reached the following conclusion:

"The writer must admit to being somewhat surprised at the uniformly negative results issuing from all this work. . . . [It] rather seems that psychologists and psychiatrists will have to acknowledge the fact that current psychotherapeutic procedures have not lived up to the hopes which greeted their emergence fifty years ago." (Eysenck, 1966).

More recently, however, this damning judgment has been challenged by psychotherapists and behaviour therapists alike. In his recent review of psychotherapy outcome studies, Shapiro (1979) points out that since the so-called "spontaneous remission" rate varies from study to study, the whole notion of a universally applicable baseline is untenable. He also states that since psychotherapists do not have the same target goals as general psychiatrists or behaviour therapists (i.e. symptom removal), the appropriateness of the outcome-criteria used by Eysenck and his colleagues is open to question. Others have argued that the question "How effective is psychotherapy?" is meaningless unless related to a particular type of psychotherapy. The term itself is used to refer to a wide range of counselling techniques administered by a variety of therapists working in diverse settings. Bergin (1971) reaches the conclusion that most types of brief psychotherapy are effective but that outcome depends to a large extent on the experience and expertise of the therapist. Finally, Shapiro and Shapiro (1977) make the point that, if the same rigid criteria are applied to evaluate behaviour therapy as have been employed in relation to psychotherapy studies, then there is very little difference between the approaches so far as efficacy is concerned.

In view of the differences in their background and basic assumptions, it was perhaps inevitable that behaviour therapists and psychotherapists should have expended so much energy on attempts to discredit each other's approach. However, in recent years, such antagonism has become much less noticeable and, indeed, a crossfertilisation process appears to be taking place. Behaviour therapists have come to recognize that such non-specific factors as the therapist-patient relationship play as important roles in their work as in other types of psychotherapy. Similarly, several psychotherapists have expressed dissatisfaction with the untestable set of propositions on which their approach was originally based and have advocated a closer relationship between psychodynamics and the basic sciences. For instance, Crown (1976) argues that "Psychoanalytic theory chiefly needs to reformulate its economic principle so as to replace outmoded 'energy' concepts with concepts expressed in terms of learning, information theory and contemporary neurophysiology".

This breaking down of barriers has had two main consequences. On the one hand, some clinicians now consider it legitimate to borrow techniques from a variety of schools and employ them on what the detached observer might regard as a relatively ad hoc basis. However, Rachman (1971) takes the view that "such an integration is theoretically undesirable because it would obscure the fundamental and important differences between the two approaches". Advances are unlikely to be made, theoretically or practically, should such a woolly, eclectic approach become widespread. A more interesting development has been the move towards the study of different types of reaction by different clients to different types of treatment (Goldstein and Stein, 1976). In the light of the recent outcome-research referred to earlier, it is no longer possible for any one school to claim that it should have the monopoly over the treatment of any particular condition. The major challenge facing clinical researchers in the future is not to determine whether, say, behaviour therapy is any more effective than psychotherapy, but to devise ways of matching client to both therapy and therapist.

THEORETICAL RATIONALE

As has already been intimated, behaviour therapists consider neurotic disorders to be maladaptive patterns of responding, which have been acquired as a result of traumatic or inappropriate learning experiences. Although it is obviously outside the scope of this chapter to consider this process in any depth, some knowledge of the ways in which learning principles have been utilised to account for the genesis of various psychiatric disorders is necessary, in order fully to appreciate the nature and goals of behaviour therapy. A more detailed account of the basic concepts, for those working in a health care setting, is provided elsewhere (Mackay, 1977).

Principles of learning
The two basic paradigms of (1) classical and (2) operant conditioning will be presented here together with a brief description of the processes involved in (3) vicarious learning (*see* p. 11).

1. Classical conditioning
The clearest illustrations of this procedure are the basic experiments carried out by Pavlov and his colleagues, relating to the salivatory reflex in dogs. In a typical study, a neutral stimulus (e.g. a musical tone) was presented at the same time as a potent stimulus (food) which previously had been shown to elicit a particular autonomic response (salivation). After a number of pairings of this sort, it was found that salivation, which formerly would only occur in the presence of food, could be elicited by the tone itself. Thus by presenting two stimuli close together in time, a new response was learned (*see* Fig. 1). The basic concepts in this experimental design are as follows.

Conditioned stimulus (C.S.) is the name given to a signal which is neutral with regard to the particular response in question before the experiment, but which will subsequently elicit it. In the above example, the tone is the conditioned stimulus.

A stimulus which is consistently followed by a specific autonomic reaction is referred to as the *unconditioned stimulus* (U.C.S.). This signifies that no additional response-eliciting properties are acquired as a result of this procedure.

In the example given, although food served as the U.C.S., this is not an unconditioned stimulus in the strictest sense of the word, since the sight of food as such could only have acquired its potency through prior association with taste. However, since this connection had been formed before the experiment in question, it is legitimate to refer to the visual presentation of the food as the U.C.S. Similarly, when the tone has acquired saliva-eliciting properties, it is possible

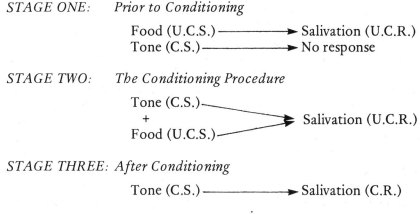

STAGE ONE: *Prior to Conditioning*

      Food (U.C.S.) ⟶ Salivation (U.C.R.)
      Tone (C.S.) ⟶ No response

STAGE TWO: *The Conditioning Procedure*

      Tone (C.S.)
      +   ⟶ Salivation (U.C.R.)
      Food (U.C.S.)

STAGE THREE: *After Conditioning*

      Tone (C.S.) ⟶ Salivation (C.R.)

FIG. 1. *The three stages in the classical conditioning paradigm*

to use it as a U.C.S. and pair it with a new neutral stimulus (e.g. green light) in a later classical conditioning experiment. The dog will then learn to respond to the light, although never at any stage have food and light been presented simultaneously. This procedure, of creating more and more remote links with the original U.C.S., is known as *higher order conditioning.*

The processes of salivation, stomach muscular contractions, pupil dilation and so on which follow the presentation of food are collectively referred to as the *unconditioned response* (U.C.R.). Once again the word "unconditioned" denotes the fact that no learning has occurred, so far as this particular stimulus and response are concerned, on this occasion.

Conditioned response (C.R.) is the name given to the newly acquired reaction to the previously neutral stimulus. Although the form the C.R. takes is very similar to the U.C.R., it is worth emphasising that, in the type of experiment described above, the two are not identical. Pavlov noted that, even after a large number of trials, the amount of saliva secreted in response to the C.S. was less than to the U.C.S. Furthermore, the muscular contractions of the stomach, which were such a marked feature of the U.C.R., were virtually absent from the C.R. For this reason it is customary to distinguish between the conditioned and unconditioned responses.

Classical conditioning would not occur at all were it not for the phenomenon of *stimulus generalisation*. Pavlov discovered that if he presented a tone which was similar but not identical to the C.S., salivation would be elicited even though the new stimulus had never been paired with food. As a rule, the greater the dissimilarity between the new stimulus and the C.S., the lower the amplitude of the response. If some degree of generalisation did not occur, then no learning of this sort could take place because of the impossibility of replicating environmental conditions. Potential sources of variation include temperature, humidity, appearance of the experimenter, activity level of the subject, and so on.

If the C.S. is presented on a number of occasions without the U.C.S., then *extinction* will occur. In other words, the amplitude of the C.R. will gradually diminish and eventually disappear. That the C.R. has not been lost altogether can be demonstrated by presenting the C.S. after a fairly lengthy time interval. The weakened version of the C.R. which will be observed is referred to as the *spontaneous recovery* process. Repeated presentations of the C.S. alone will once again lead to extinction. Its re-introduction following a delay will, as before, give rise to spontaneous recovery of the C.R., but its strength will have decreased still further. After a series of trials of this sort, the conditioned response will be extinguished completely. The process of learning, extinction and spontaneous recovery are illustrated in Fig. 2.

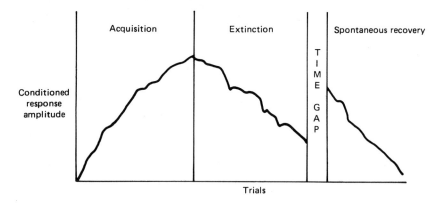

FIG. 2. *Learning and extinction curves in classical conditioning*

The effectiveness of a classical conditioning programme depends very much on the *timing* of the C.S. and U.C.S. The strongest C.R.s can be obtained by presenting the C.S. just before the U.C.S. with some degree of overlap (*delayed conditioning*). *Trace conditioning*, which is less effective, involves presenting and terminating the C.S. before the onset of the U.C.S. Whether any learning can take place if the U.C.S. precedes the C.S. (i.e. *backward conditioning*) is unclear, but this is certainly the least efficient procedure of all.

2. *Operant conditioning*

While classical conditioning can account for learning involving the autonomic nervous system, operant (or instrumental) conditioning is concerned primarily with voluntary behaviour. This means, in effect, that whereas the subject remains passive throughout the Pavlovian procedure, he has to make responses in the operant conditioning situation, otherwise learning of this sort will not take place. Most of the basic research in this area was carried out by Skinner (1953) who worked mainly with rats and pigeons because of the relative ease with which their environments can be controlled.

The fundamental principle underlying this model is that behaviour is governed by its consequences. A person does not behave in a totally random fashion when placed in a particular situation. Instead he carries out responses which, under similar circumstances in the past, produced favourable outcomes. Thus, according to Skinner, a person's behaviour can be predicted entirely from a knowledge of his previous experiences. The three types of consequence which influence the future probability of a particular response are positive reinforcement, negative reinforcement and punishment.

Positive reinforcement (reward) can be defined as the consequence of an action which will increase the likelihood of it being performed in the future. Skinner prefers to use operational definitions rather than to employ abstractions such as "drive reduction". For this reason he has been open to the charge of tautology. However, as Skinner points out, the fact that an outcome produced an increase in the frequency of a particular response would enable one to predict that it would produce similar results if applied to another type of behaviour. For example, if it can be demonstrated that a child will wash his hands in order to receive a sweet, it can be assumed that this reward will serve as an incentive for say, teeth-cleaning. Hence the circularity of the definition is more apparent than real.

Negative reinforcement is the term used to refer to the consequence of a response, but which does not involve the provision of a tangible reward. Instead, it is *the removal of an unpleasant stimulus* which leads to the strengthening of that behaviour. Thus a pigeon can be trained to peck a key, not in order to receive grain, but in order to avoid receiving a shock. The dutiful husband who is never late home may not be so concerned to be reunited with his family as he is to avoid the unpleasantness caused by a nagging wife! The two examples given refer to *avoidance* learning. Negative reinforcement is also involved in *escape* learning. The overstressed businessman who drinks heavily at the end of each working day, and the elderly person who moves from the town to the country to get away from the noise and the people, are both responding in order to escape from something unpleasant.

Punishment can be operationally defined as the consequence of a response which will lead to a decrease in the probability of its future occurrence. The disadvantage of controlling behaviour by this method is that the subject is not made aware of what constitutes appropriate ways of responding. However, although the application of positive reinforcement is necessary in order to train the subject to carry out a specific response, the simultaneous punishment of unwanted behaviour can facilitate the learning process.

One reason why punishment is often used in preference to positive or negative reinforcement is that the particular response one is wishing to increase may occur relatively infrequently. Consequently the change agent (e.g. parent, teacher) may choose to punish rather than reward since the latter approach will involve lengthy periods of inactivity on his part, which could prove frustrating. However, as Skinner pointed out, there is a more effective way of producing change through reinforcement than waiting for the performance of the target behaviour. *Shaping* involves reinforcing the subject for behaving in a way which approximates to the desired response. When the frequency of vague approximations has increased to an acceptable level, the criteria are raised so that only closer matches are reinforced. In this way the individual's behaviour is "shaped" until it corresponds to that desired by the change agent. For example, the father who shows pleasure when his infant first addresses him as "Dadoo" may grow accustomed to this form of address and smile only when the child makes sounds which bear a closer resemblance to the target response (e.g. "Dadda"). Ultimately only the word "Daddy" will produce a reaction. Here the father is unwittingly shaping the verbal behaviour of his child. This procedure enables the trainer to be actively involved in the modification of behaviour on a continuous basis without necessarily having to use punishment.

In operant conditioning, behaviour is controlled, not only by its consequences, but by the stimuli which set the occasion for its occurrence. The individual does not simply learn that carrying out a response will lead to positive reinforcement. He also learns that this will only occur under certain circumstances. For example, a child may swear in order to receive social reinforcement when he is with his peer group, but refrain from this behaviour in the presence of his parents. His behaviour can thus be said to be under *stimulus control.*

Although operant conditioning is usually thought of in relation to the skeletal musculature, it has proved possible to modify visceral responses directly by this procedure (Miller, 1969). In the early experiments in this area, rats were given the drug curare to exclude interference from muscular activity. Various autonomic responses were then shaped, using electrical stimulation to parts of the limbic system in the brain as the positive reinforcer. Thus, as a result of operant conditioning, rats could exert control over their heart rate, gastric acidity level, systolic blood pressure, and peripheral circulation without using skeletal muscles. This work formed the basis of biofeedback training, which will be discussed later in this chapter.

3. *Vicarious learning*

In both classical and operant conditioning, the individual has to be directly involved in the procedure for learning to take place. However it is clearly inconceivable that complex behaviour such as language and interpersonal skills could arise simply through the shaping of random sounds and movements. Some type of nonparticipatory learning is therefore required to explain how so much information can be assimilated in a relatively short space of time. Bandura (1969) maintains that imitation can account for much of human learning. He cites a number of experiments which demonstrate convincingly that subjects will learn a response after having had the opportunity to observe others (i.e. *models*) being rewarded for behaving in this way. The sudden emergence of a complete response following an observation experience cannot be accounted for in terms of conventional operant conditioning principles. According to Bandura, learning of this sort takes place through proximity of the stimuli which arise through perception of the model, and the images and thoughts to which these stimuli give rise. These images subsequently act as discriminative stimuli for the response in question in much the same way as external stimuli operate in instrumental conditioning.

Learning theory explanations of psychiatric disorders

Since psychiatrists such as Wolpe, Marks and Gelder were important early contributors to this field, it is perhaps not surprising that learning theory accounts of causation of psychiatric disorders are closely linked to the "medical model" approach to abnormal behaviour. By this is meant the assumption that it is meaningful to think in terms of syndromes, which have a particular aetiology and for which there is a specific cure. This way of conceptualising abnormalities is at its most useful when applied to infectious diseases and has a degree of validity in relation to so-called psychotic disorders but, some would argue (e.g. Mackay, 1975), contributes little to the understanding and management of what Szasz (1960) refers to as "problems of living". For example, in his review of the diagnostic literature on "depression", Kendell (1976) reaches the conclusion that there is some evidence to support the existence of a syndrome which can be referred to as psychotic or endogenous depression. However, no such clear-cut constellation of symptoms has emerged so far as neurotic or reactive depression is concerned. Nevertheless, rather than conclude that such a syndrome does not exist, Kendell encourages future diagnosticians to be more diligent.

In recent years, many behaviour therapists (e.g. Kanfer and Phillips, 1970) have argued that it is quite inappropriate for basic psychological principles to be used to support a schema which rests entirely on the questionable assumption that people can be meaningfully categorised on the basis of their responses alone. Instead they maintain that each individual case constitutes an object of scientific enquiry in its own right. A way of behaving which is common to any two patients may be being maintained by entirely different environmental circumstances. This notion will be developed further at a later stage. For present purposes, it is sufficient to point out that, although it is possible to provide broad, learning theory formulations of neurotic disorders, this is, to an extent, an artificial exercise. Nevertheless the discussion which follows should help to clarify some of the ways in which behaviourists have attempted to account for complex clinical problems in terms of the three types of learning presented above.

1. Phobias

The traditional behaviourist explanation of phobias is that they are acquired emotional responses which have become established through the process of classical conditioning. In other words, previously neutral stimuli develop anxiety-eliciting properties as the result of being paired with a noxious stimulus. Subsequently, through stimulus generalisation and higher order conditioning, a wide range of stimuli, which are not aversive in themselves, come to give rise to anxiety. The fact that the learning of this maladaptive response involves the autonomic nervous system can account for the fact that is is rarely fruitful to attempt to reason with a person who demonstrates phobic anxiety.

It would be wrong to conclude from this that the simple Pavlovian paradigm can, by itself, account for the genesis and persistence of phobias. This explanation has been challenged on a number of grounds as follows.

(a) Phobias comprise a non-arbitrary list of situations and objects. Fear of insects, heights, closed-in places, and wide open spaces are extremely common, whereas phobias concerning pencils or chairs are virtually non-existent. This is difficult to reconcile with the basic model outlined above, which implies that all stimuli have an equal chance of acquiring anxiety-eliciting properties. The notion of *preparedness* (Seligman, 1971) has been proposed to augment the classical conditioning paridigm and thereby preserve it. In brief, this states that certain stimuli possess properties which make them particularly likely to become phobic objects should they occur during a traumatic experience for an individual. Clearly this idea owes more to ethology than to learning theory.

(b) Phobias are persistent. One major problem for the classical conditioning model of neurosis is that the specific anxiety responses of phobic patients do not disappear, despite the fact that these phobic stimuli are no longer being paired with the U.C.S. As Taylor (1966) has pointed out, only a small percentage of people develop persistent neurotic reactions following acute trauma, such as a road accident. The extinction of the conditioned anxiety response is something which would have been predicted from the basic model. However the question as to why the fears of phobic patients do not weaken with time remains.

One crucial difference between the experimental setting devised by Pavlov and the everyday life situation of a neurotic patient is that there is far more scope for environmental control in the latter case. Whereas the dog is confined in a harness by the experimenter, the neurotic patient can avoid or escape from the situation, thus obstructing the extinction process. The negative reinforcement which is maintaining this behaviour is the reduction of anxiety (by avoidance of its cause). Thus classical conditioning can explain the genesis of phobias while operant conditioning can account for the fact that they persist. This formulation is known as the "two-factor" learning model (Mowrer, 1947).

(c) Phobias can increase in severity. Although a combined classical/operant model cannot explain why phobias do not always disappear with time, it can account for the fact that many phobias begin slowly, become stronger, and eventually reach panic proportions. Eysenck's (1976) theory of *incubation* is an attempt to account for this phenomenon. It has long been recognised, particularly in the Russian literature, that enhancement rather than extinction of the C.R. can occur. However it has proved difficult to explain why one should take place rather than the other. In brief, the conclusion Eysenck reaches is that conditioned responses which act as drives (e.g. pain avoidance), particularly where a strong stimulus is employed, will be subject to the law of incubation. It would seem to follow from this that the phobias which are likely to increase in severity are those which result from a particular traumatic experience.

(d) Individuals differ in their susceptibility to phobias. As mentioned above, most people do not develop incapacitating phobias following a traumatic experience. On the other hand, others seem to acquire them with remarkable ease. The basic model, by itself, cannot account for this. Although Pavlov proposed various physiological hypotheses to explain variations in conditionability, the most sophisticated theory of individual differences, which is relevant to this issue, is that of Eysenck (1957).

From the results of a number of factor analytic studies, Eysenck postulated that non-cognitive differences between people can be subsumed within two main dimensions of personality: *extraversion-introversion* and *neuroticism-stability.* A person who is high on neuroticism is considered to have a reactive and labile autonomic nervous system. Someone who is at the introverted end of the other dimension is regarded as possessing certain central nervous system characteristics which facilitate the conditioning process. The physiological make-up of a person is thought to be determined predominantly by hereditary factors. Thus an individual who inherits the type of nervous system which is characteristic of neurotic introverts is particularly likely to develop a phobia following a traumatic learning experience. Although Eysenck has accumulated a considerable amount of evidence to support his theory, the results from a number of studies (e.g. Davidson *et al.*, 1966) are directly contradictory to it.

(e) Many phobics do not undergo a traumatic experience. A large proportion of neurotic patients are unable to recollect any experience which might have led them to associate a particular object with anxiety. Although selective recall may be involved in some of these cases, it has to be conceded, particularly where such uncommon stimuli as snakes are concerned, that phobias can arise without any obvious C.S./U.C.S. pairings having taken place.

Two related explanations have been offered by behaviourists. The first is that a significant person in the patient's life (e.g. a parent) may have served as a model for phobic avoidance behaviour in the presence of a particular object (e.g. a cat). In this way, although the individual was never directly subjected to a traumatic conditioning experience, maladaptive behaviour has been instilled. Similarly, it has been proposed that a symbolic association between a stimulus and anxiety can be at least as effective as an "in vivo" pairing. Thus the experience of being told that an object or activity is unpleasant (e.g. "sex is painful") can, through repeated covert rehearsals, lead to subsequent avoidance at the behavioural level.

Thus, even so far as simple phobia is concerned, the classical conditioning paradigm, by itself, cannot fully account for all the facts. Concepts from ethology, physiology, and cognitive psychology have had to be used to support the simple model proposed by Watson and Wolpe. For a fuller account of the contemporary behaviourist position on the genesis of phobias, the reader is referred to the excellent review by Eysenck (1976).

2. Obsessive-compulsive disorders

The basic behaviourist explanation of obsessive-compulsive disorders is very similar to that of phobias and, consequently, is equally deficient as it stands. The rationale here is that the individual develops a specific fear (e.g. of dirt) in the manner described above but, rather than simply avoid the situation, he carries out an instrumental act (e.g. washing his hands ten times), which serves to reduce the anxiety. The fact that the performance of the ritual may not actually significantly influence the probability of occurrence of the noxious stimulus is neither here nor there. The wide range of superstitious behaviours which exist in every culture testifies to the fact that it is the belief in the effectiveness of the ritual which is important.

Although it is not necessary to repeat the various shortcomings of the phobia model referred to above, the non-arbitrary nature of the presenting compulsive acts requires some consideration here. In other words, whereas hand-washing is a frequently observed neurotic symptom, compulsive pencil-sharpening is relatively rare. One attempt to account for this phenomenon, in learning theory terms, is as follows.

> The frequency with which hand-washing is chosen as the obsessional ritual gives us some clue as to how such superstitious avoidance learning might take place. It is extremely common in our culture for parents to punish their children for getting dirty or coming into contact with possible sources of infection. Washing the hands is a sure way of avoiding or mollifying the parental ire under these conditions and, in the right personality (a neurotic introvert), could become a well-established way of relieving fear. (Gray, 1971.)

It follows from this that activities which, in childhood, are commonly associated with avoiding parental disapproval (e.g. washing; eating; going to the toilet) are particularly likely to be involved in the development of neurotic rituals.

The main weakness of explanations such as Gray's is that the ideational component of the disorder does not receive sufficient emphasis. Thus, so far as compulsive hand-washing is concerned, the ritual is usually secondary to ruminations about contamination. It is certainly possible to account for preoccupations about, say, dirt, by utilising the symbolic conditioning model outlined above and regarding obsessional thought patterns as the equivalent of avoidance and escape responses. However, where the focus of concern is more diffuse (e.g. causing death to significant others), the learning theory explanation becomes more than a little tortuous.

3. Depression

If learning theory is to be considered seriously as a viable model for understanding abnormal behaviour, then it has to be able to offer a satisfactory explanation of depression, the "common cold" of psychiatry. However, since behaviourists rely so heavily on observation and objectivity in their work, *depression* is a difficult condition for them to study. As Ferster (1965) points out, in order to determine whether motor retardation is due to depression or to the fact that the individual is moving slowly for some other reason, it is necessary to ask him. Nevertheless, a number of learning theory explanations have been offered, the most important of these being Seligman's (1975) model of "learned helplessness".

The fundamental concept in this model is controllability. On the basis of a variety of conditioning experiments, Seligman argues that, in addition to learning specific responses as a result of experience, people learn the probability of a particular outcome. They have an idea of how likely it is that a particular event will occur, both whether they make a response or do not. If these two probabilities are different, then the outcome can be considered to be controllable to a degree. However, if the probabilities are almost identical, then the individual will become aware that he has no influence over this particular outcome. The student whose essay marks do not reflect the amount of work he puts in, the husband who can find no way of reducing the nagging behaviour of his wife, and the pop star who is adulated no matter how badly he performs, are examples of people who are faced with response/outcome independence in at least one area of their lives. If this negative response set should generalise to other situations, then it can be said that *learned helplessness* has resulted.

From his experimental work, Seligman has been impressed by the fact that many of the features of learned helplessness (e.g. passivity, lack of aggression, weight loss, noradrenalin depletion) are regarded as symptoms of depression. Consequently he has put forward the proposal that depression arises when an individual becomes aware that he does not have a significant degree of control over one or more of the important areas in his life. Although there is no doubt that Seligman's theoretical statement and the high quality of the supporting experimental work have made a significant contribution to thinking about depression, it has been criticised by both academics and clinicians on a number of grounds. Some of the main points of contention are as follows.

(a) Do organisms actually stop responding when the outcome is uncontrollable? This basic assumption, upon which the whole model rests, is directly contradictory to the results obtained by Skinner

(1948) from his "superstitious behaviour" experiments. In these classic studies, grain was dropped at brief regular intervals in the proximity of food-deprived pigeons. Although the food reward was delivered on a fixed interval schedule, regardless of the behaviour of the subject, most of the pigeons developed a ritualistic pattern of behaviour (e.g. pecking; hopping) in this situation. The explanation given for this was that any response which the organism had been carrying out when the food was initially delivered was reinforced. This action sequence would therefore be more likely to be repeated and, in time, it would be followed by an additional food reward. After a number of trials of this sort, the organism would come to "believe" that the outcome was dependent on the emission of that response. The parallels with superstitious behaviour at the human level, and indeed with the compulsive rituals referred to above, are obvious. Seligman has responded to the assertion that these findings contradict his basic assumption, by claiming that the pigeons in Skinner's experiments were in fact engaging in involuntary species-specific behaviour rather than operant behaviour which had been reinforced. However, this issue has not been satisfactorily resolved.

(b) Not everyone develops "learned helplessness" when faced with obstacles. In Seligman's original experiments with dogs, helplessness occurred in two out of every three cases. Hiroto (1974), who carried out similar studies with humans, found that subjects varied enormously in terms of their susceptibility to the experimental procedure. Seligman has put forward a number of explanations of individual differences in responsivity, as below.

(i) A person who has had a lot of experience of controlling a particular outcome in the past will have difficulty in believing that its occurrence is no longer determined by his behaviour.

(ii) Physiological factors (e.g. hormone imbalance, drug withdrawal) can render a person more susceptible to helplessness at one time rather than another.

(iii) Someone who believes that events are determined by chance, destiny or the stars, i.e. an externaliser, is more susceptible to helplessness than a person who feels that he is primarily responsible for his successes and failures, i.e. an internaliser, (Hiroto, 1974). This "locus of control" dimension was originally proposed by Rotter (1966) as a personality trait.

(c) Is "learned helplessness" anything to do with depression? Many clinicians, while recognising the phenomenon which Seligman describes, would not label it as depression. "Helpless man" comes across as someone who is placid, apathetic and generally ineffectual. However the term depression is normally used clinically to refer to people who demonstrate more severe signs of disturbance than these. Furthermore, prior to committing the act, many successful suicides engage in aggressive outbursts, appear agitated rather than listless, and are able to function effectively in certain important areas of their life. Since there is no general agreement as to what constitutes reactive depression (Kendell, 1976), it is not possible to state categorically whether learned helplessness is an example of it or not. What can be said, however, is that many cases who have been reliably diagnosed as depressed do not behave in a helpless fashion.

Other behaviourists (e.g. Lewinsohn, 1975) have pointed out that a wide variety of environmental factors can trigger off a reduction in the frequency of adaptive responses. Removal of a source of positive reinforcements, e.g. death of a spouse, contact with a model of depressive behaviour, e.g. apathetic boss, traumatic events, e.g. exam failure, and stimuli associated with them, e.g. springtime, can lead to the occurrence of negative self-statements such as "I am worthless". Verbally labelling the affect in this way produces more intense negative feelings and less effective behaviour (Beck, 1970). Furthermore, this vicious circle is often maintained by removal of occupational and social responsibilities, i.e. negative reinforcement, and by concern and interest shown by significant people, i.e. positive reinforcement. The attraction of Lewinsohn's model is that it combines the advantages of simplicity, normally associated with a categorical system, and flexibility, which traditionally has been the hallmark of an ideographic approach. For this reason, much of the behavioural research currently being carried out in this area is based on this particular schema.

4. Sexual deviations

The learning theory explanation of abnormal sexual behaviour is based on the same "two factor" model (Mowrer, 1947) referred to in the section on phobias (pp. 12-15). In other words, the classical conditioning paradigm is used to account for the genesis of the learned response whereas an instrumental formulation is required to explain why extinction does not take place. Thus it is claimed that when a neutral object (e.g. underwear, same sex member) is present at the onset of sexual arousal, an association will be built up between the two events so that the sight of that object in the future will elicit a sexual response. This association would eventually weaken and disappear altogether were it not for the fact that the individual can voluntarily carry out his own conditioning trials, reinforcing the arousal on association.

The experiment of Rachman (1966) provides evidence to support the hypothesis that classical conditioning experiences can influence sexual orientation. Slides of fashion boots (C.S.) were presented immediately prior to slides of nude females (U.C.S.) which had been previously demonstrated to be arousing, so far as these subjects were concerned. Sexual arousal was measured by means of a penile plethysmograph (Bancroft *et al.*, 1966). All subjects eventually reached the criterion of five successive penile responses to the C.S. within sixty-five trials. Stimulus generalisation was demonstrated in every case to such objects as low-heeled shoes which had not been used in the experiment.

So far as the maintenance of the C.R. through instrumental conditioning is concerned, there is no equivalent supportive evidence. However, on the basis of their clinical findings, McGuire *et al.* (1965) put forward the notion that the voluntary activity of masturbation serves as an additional classical conditioning trial. These authors provide anecdotes about patients who, when trying to recall an exciting sexual experience, succeeded in conjuring up a relatively clear picture of the clothing their partner had been wearing, but had only a hazy recollection of the less tangible characteristics associated with that person. After a time, the fantasy consisted almost exclusively of the particular apparel which had been worn. Thus, through masturbation, repeated associations of clothing fantasies and sexual arousal gave rise to a fetish.

All of the qualifications of the basic phobia model apply equally well here. Thus Eysenck's notion of *incubation* can be employed to account for the insidious development of a particular type of sexual response. The quasi-ethological concept of *preparedness* can be adapted to explain why certain types of material, e.g. leather, silk, rubber, are more likely to become fetishistic objects than others, e.g. wool, cotton. Individual differences can be attributed to variability in terms of conditionability and autonomic lability, with neurotic introverts, once again, being particularly likely to develop sexual interest in specific objects.

Finally it must be emphasised that, so far as homosexuality is concerned, behaviourists do not maintain that conditioning plays a major role in every case. Feldman and MacCulloch (1971) make a distinction between *primary* and *secondary* homosexuality. A secondary homosexual is defined as someone who has been interested, to a degree, in members of the opposite sex at some stage in the past. It is conjectured that, in this case, attraction towards same sex members is the result of initial pleasurable experiences in a homosexual context, traumatic heterosexual ones, or a combination of the two. A primary homosexual, on the other hand, is someone who has never been attracted to members of the opposite sex. Feldman and Mac-Culloch take the view that, although social learning may play a part, the choice of sexual object in adulthood is probably mainly due to an imbalance of sex steroids in the developing brain. For a more detailed account of the behaviourist position on sexual deviations, the reader is referred to Mackay (1976).

Up until now, the discussion has centred on the need to embellish the basic paradigms in order to be able to account for a wide range of clinical phenomena. However, whether experimental work on conditioning has anything at all to do with the formation of abnormal behaviour patterns has been questioned (Breger and McGaugh, 1965). Since their argument is a long and involved one, it will only be possible here to outline their basic assertions.

(a) The results of early experiments on perception would seem to indicate that a stimulus is not simply "peripheral receptor stimulation" and that central processes are involved.

(b) The evidence would suggest that, even in simple animal experiments, subjects learn strategies rather than just "mechanical sequences of response".

(c) The terms stimulus, e.g. imagination of a scene, and response, e.g. relaxation, as used by clinicians bear little resemblance to their laboratory equivalents.

(d) It is dubious whether one can talk about universal "laws on learning" on the basis of results obtained with bar-pressing rats.

(e) The development of, say, agoraphobia, where the concept "outdoors" is the crucial feature, is much more readily explained in terms of cognitive processes rather than by reference to stimulus generalisation, which has been shown to operate strictly on the basis of physical similarity.

Since the publication of this important paper, behaviourists have paid much more attention to the role of cognitive processes in the formation of abnormal behaviour patterns. However, rather than reject the conditioning models, they have attempted to regard these unobservables as covert stimuli and responses. As a result, some of the allegations made by Breger and McGaugh can be accounted for, but perhaps the most critical one, that the clinical usage of the terms bears only an analogous relationship to the laboratory usage, carries even more weight now than before.

TREATMENT METHODS

While it is widely recognised that the psychodynamic school comprises a wide range of treatment approaches, e.g. Freudian or Jungian, which vary in terms of objectives, methods, and depth of focus, a common erroneous belief is that behaviour therapy is a homogeneous entity. The emergence of a variety of interest groups within this field in the last few years testifies to the fact that this is not so. Each of these groups can be located on a "hard-soft" dimension according to the degree to which they attempt to be faithful to the original experimental approach of Skinner. Essentially it is the demands made by different client populations and different work settings which have given rise to these splits within the behavioural movement, rather than fundamental differences of opinion regarding treatment philosophy. Thus while it would be appropriate to provide food rewards on a fixed ratio basis following specific responses emitted by a subnormal child, it would be difficult to carry out an equivalent programme with a professional person who is going through an existential crisis. It is possible to distinguish between four types of behaviour therapy which are presented here in ascending order of "hardness".

Firstly, there is the *behavioural counsellor*, working with relatively well-adjusted, articulate clients who are not characterised by crippling fears or significant response deficits. Instead they are attempting to develop more effective strategies for living. The aim of this form of treatment is to help the client to recognise the precise nature of the events which adversely affect him and to evolve plans for coping under these circumstances. At the same time, the counsellor attempts to make him aware of the effects of his own behaviour on those people who are contributing to his difficulties. Once again other possibilities are explored. Thus, as its name suggests, behavioural counselling involves talking about the interaction between the environment and the client's behaviour rather than an attempt to induce change by direct means.

Secondly, there is the *behavioural psychotherapist*, conducting an in-depth analysis of the client's problems and, on the basis of this, devising a treatment programme specifically for that individual. Although the individual need not be particularly intelligent or articulate, he must be prepared to take on some responsibility for change. Counselling plays an important role here as well, but techniques designed with that person in mind are the focal point of this type of intervention.

Thirdly, the term *behavioural technology* is used to mean the application of identical treatment "packages" to groups of people who happen to fall into a particular diagnostic category. This approach is used mainly by those engaged in research projects, the aim of which is to test out the efficacy of techniques rather than to provide the best help possible for the subjects who participate in the investigations. Many proponents of this approach have advocated automated procedures so that technique variables are not interfered with by patient/therapist variables (Elwood, 1975).

Fourthly, *behaviour modification*, which is often used interchangeably with behaviour therapy, is used here to refer to the application of operant conditioning principles to change the frequency of certain classes of behaviour. This can take place on an individual, small group or even ward basis. The techniques are very closely based on paradigms used in laboratory studies with animals. Not surprisingly, therefore, this approach lends itself easily to the collection of data.

A good example of a simple behaviour modification programme is the attempt by Isaacs *et al.* (1960) to reinstate speech in an adult, mute, catatonic patient. Since it had been observed that the sight of chewing gum produced a change in the facial expression of this patient, it was decided to use this stimulus as a positive reinforcer. During the initial stage of the programme, the patient was given a piece of chewing gum following any sort of eye movement. The standard shaping procedure was then introduced so that the reward was made contingent upon facial movements, lip movements, vocalisations and, finally, spoken words. By the end of the programme, the patient was able to utter a few words on appropriate occasions. Essentially, this procedure is identical to the one used by Skinner to train pigeons to peck a lever in order to obtain pellets of food.

Behaviour modification is used mainly to bring about improvements in the self-care and communication behaviour of handicapped children, chronic schizophrenics, psychogeriatrics and other institutionalised groups.

Since this chapter is concerned with the clinical uses of behavioural methods in a medical context, only behavioural psychotherapy and behaviour modification will be considered here.

Behavioural psychotherapy

Although behavioural psychotherapists are placed towards the "soft" end of the dimension referred to above and, although they are not averse to making use of concepts and methods usually associated with client-centred, psychodynamic or even humanistic psychotherapy, it would be wrong to conclude that these clinicians have abandoned learning theory altogether. Their whole approach rests on the belief that there is some degree of orderliness about behaviour. In other words it is assumed that thoughts, feelings and actions do not occur in a random fashion. They take place consistently in the presence of a specific pattern of environmental cues and are followed by certain outcomes which help to maintain them. So, in a general sense at least, behavioural psychotherapists would maintain that their *modus operandi* is very similar to that of experimental psychologists.

Similarly, although one critic has referred to behavioural psychotherapy as "the apotheosis of eclecticism" (Brown, 1975), it would be wrong to conclude that the practitioners of this approach see themselves as being virtually indistinguishable from the other psycho-therapies. Some of the propositions which their position does not espouse are as follows.

(a) "All psychiatric problems have their origins in the first five years of life" While it is an empirical fact that the majority of phobias begin in childhood, there are many examples where specific anxiety reactions have developed later in life. The same is considered to be true for other disorders.

(b) "Symptoms are caused by intrapsychic conflict" Although conflict is a commonly occurring noxious event, there are other potential U.C.S.s which can elicit anxiety.

(c) "Insight is necessary for change" There is no evidence to suggest that understanding why a particular problem is developed, even if it is possible, it is a prerequisite for change. However, awareness of stimulus-response connections can facilitate the deconditioning or reconditioning process.

(d) "Behavioural changes automatically follow cognitive changes" It does not follow that when a person learns to perceive himself, other significant people or a situation, differently, that his behaviour will alter accordingly.

Before looking at the techniques employed by behavioural psycho-therapists, it will be necessary to consider the assessment procedure in some detail.

Behavioural analysis

Although this is the most important and most complex aspect of this type of clinical work, relatively little space is usually devoted to it in behaviour therapy text books. Kanfer and Phillips (1970) and Hersen and Bellak (1976) are notable exceptions. Essentially the behavioural analysis involves the collection of data in order to set up and test out hypotheses in a systematic fashion. It is an on-going process which is terminated only when the therapeutic goals have been achieved. Thus any slowing down of progress or the emergence of new difficulties can lead to a drastic revision of the whole problem formulation at any stage during treatment. This assessment procedure differs in many important respects, outlined below, from the standard psychiatric interview.

(a) The aim of the exercise is to understand the behaviour of that particular individual rather than to classify him according to a certain taxonomy.

(*b*) The validity of self-report is never assumed and behavioural observations are carried out wherever possible.

(*c*) The relative importance of a piece of past information, e.g. parents' divorce, rests solely on its connection to the variables which are seen to be controlling the problem behaviour. Considering a traumatic incident in isolation can lead to too much emphasis being placed on it.

(*d*) The patient is encouraged to play an active role in the assessment process, e.g. setting up hypotheses, or testing them out.

The behavioural analysis comprises a set of questions aimed at teasing out precisely the nature of the interaction between the environment and the problem behaviour. The starting-off point is usually the presenting difficulty as it affects the individual at that particular point in time. Data from his past history is not collected until the therapist has formulated some hypotheses concerning the environmental factors which are maintaining that behaviour. This means that the importance of a particular past event can be quickly determined by relating it to the various hypotheses under consideration. At the same time, the collection of this material usually means that one hypothesis is strengthened at the expense of another. Thus there should be a purpose behind every question asked during the assessment interview.

Although it is customary to start from the present and work backwards, there are no universally accepted guidelines for carrying out a behavioural analysis. The approach which is described here is the one put forward by Mackay (1976) which is itself a modification of one of the original systems proposed by Kanfer and Phillips (1970). It can be broken down into six stages as follows.

1. *Obtain a precise description of the maladaptive behaviour.*
Whereas most clinicians are prepared to begin treatment with only the patient's self-report of his difficulties as a basis, the behavioural approach demands a very detailed picture of the presenting problem at the outset. It is important to emphasise right away that the term "behaviour" is being used here in the broad sense, as favoured by social learning theorists. As Mischel (1968) points out, "behaviour is often subtle and covert and not merely an overt act". Thus, the first task is to determine whether the problem manifests itself at the cognitive, affective or overt behavioural level, or whether only one or two are involved. Although it is customary to find that emotions, attitudes and actions are consistent with each other (Festinger, 1957), this is by no means always the case. The following three clinical examples should serve to illustrate this:

(a) the college lecturer who claimed he had a public-speaking phobia, although he had never missed a lecture, nor did he appear unduly autonomically "aroused" on a variety of psychophysiological measures obtained before and after the event;

(b) the patient who frequently cancelled his appointment at the last minute, and who appeared very agitated on the occasions he did attend, but denied feeling anxious about the sessions;

(c) the housewife who claimed that she dreaded intercourse, and was very tense throughout, but who never rejected the sexual overtures of her partner.

It will be apparent from these examples that the level (or levels) at which the problem is apparent has important implications for the measures to be taken and the techniques to be administered. It would obviously be inappropriate to use intercourse frequency counts to gauge the response to treatment of the patient with the sexual difficulty. Similarly, the lecturer would derive little benefit from a course of biofeedback. Thus there are very good reasons for obtaining a detailed description of the presenting problem.

In order to be able to assess the effectiveness of a particular treatment programme, it is advisable to obtain measures, of an appropriate sort, before treatment begins and at regular intervals during it. Cognitive assessment techniques range from simple self-report inventories (e.g. Geer, 1965) to the highly sophisticated repertory grid techniques (Fransella and Bannister, 1977). Measures of "arousal" include heart rate, skin conductance responsivity, and muscle tonus. Practical advice on how to record and interpret these and other psychophysiological measures is provided by Venables and Martin (1967).

Although these instruments can be extremely useful, behavioural psychotherapists prefer to record overt behaviour where possible, because this data is relatively objective and free from inference. Some of the most commonly used behavioural assessment methods are listed below in decreasing order of objectivity:

(a) direct observation, i.e. record of responses made in natural environment;

(b) structured role play, i.e. record of responses made in simulated social situation;

(c) diary, i.e. daily response frequency count carried out by the patient;

(d) behavioural ratings, i.e. global behavioural categorisation carried out by staff; e.g. "very restless";

(e) self-ratings, i.e. global behavioural categorisation carried out by patient;

(f) fantasy, i.e. patient's estimate of performance in hypothetical situations.

The whole field of behavioural assessment is comprehensively reviewed by Hersen and Bellak (1976).

2. Define the controlling stimuli

According to the basic principles of operant conditioning which were discussed earlier in this chapter, the individual does not behave in a psychological vacuum. Rather he learns to make a particular response in the presence of certain specific stimuli. The careful isolation of the environmental factors which influence the frequency and/or intensity of the response under investigation is the most critical aspect of the whole assessment procedure. It is a particularly difficult task to carry out because the stimuli themselves are often relatively intangible and usually interact with other variables. It is not made any easier by the fact that most patients are convinced that there is no pattern and that the panic attacks, or whatever, "just happen".

It is possible to divide up these antecedents into *object characteristics*, e.g. size and hairiness of the spider, *negativistic self-statements*, e.g. "this is not my day", *physiological disturbances*, e.g. hand tremor, and *situation variables*, e.g. presence of significant person. The following clinical examples should help to illustrate ways in which the occurrence of abnormal behaviour can be influenced by both covert and overt stimuli:

(a) the student who was unable to maintain an erection whenever he felt he was not in control of the situation (i.e. negativistic self-statement) and if the female in question remained passive throughout foreplay (i.e. object characteristic);

(b) the wife of the successful business executive who found it difficult to converse with people she felt to be her "superiors" (i.e. negativistic self-statement) particularly when her husband was present (situational variable);

(c) the female adolescent who avoided the company of attractive males (i.e. object characteristics) when her face felt flushed (i.e. physiological disturbance).

It will be apparent from these examples that a unit of behaviour can operate both as a response and as a significant stimulus. For example, a negativistic self-statement such as "this one is too difficult for me" is at the same time a reaction to a previous event and a cue for a subsequent response. This dual function of behavioural occurrences is the basis of the "vicious circle" phenomenon which is at the core of the vast majority of neurotic disorders.

3. *Determine the reinforcers.*

Having isolated the cues which trigger off abnormal behaviour, the next stage is to tease out the factors which help to maintain it. As pointed out in the section on operant conditioning principles, the outcome of a particular response influences the likelihood of its future recurrence under similar circumstances. Since the concepts of positive reinforcement, negative reinforcement and punishment have already been defined, it is only necessary here to consider their relevance to clinical work. The following examples should serve to illustrate the relevance of these concepts to psychiatric problems:

(a) the alcoholic who drinks in order to escape from feelings of low self-esteem (i.e. negative reinforcement) which follow a failure experience;

(b) the "crisis phobic" who constantly questions her husband about the Middle East situation since, by so doing, she is able to get him to pay attention to her (i.e. positive reinforcement);

(c) the emotionally undemonstrative housewife who is reluctant to show her husband any affection because he will be encouraged to demand more from her (i.e. punishment);

(d) the "agoraphobic" who avoids stressful situations by staying at home (i.e. negative reinforcement) and who, consequently, receives more visits from friends and relatives who carry out errands for her (positive reinforcement).

The last example is particularly important since it serves to demonstrate that a response can be maintained by more than one outcome. In fact, so far as the general psychiatric population is concerned, it is usual to find that the abnormal behaviour is followed by two or more significant events. In the case of hysteria, for instance, it has long been recognised that while the "primary gain" to the individual of having the symptom is avoidance or escape from a noxious stimulus, "secondary gain" (e.g. increased attention from others) is a likely consequence as well. It is essential to detect all the reinforcers which are operating in a particular case otherwise the problem formulation will be incomplete and the effectiveness of the eventual treatment programme will consequently be limited.

4. *Test out the hypotheses.*

It has been emphasised throughout that the behavioural analysis is not simply a data gathering exercise for the purpose of acquiring a highly detailed collection of facts, most of which are of dubious relevance to the problem. Every question is designed to elicit information which will enable the clinician to build up a number of hypotheses. Once the list of antecedents and consequences has been drawn up, the next task is to test out the validity of the various formulations. In other words the relative importance of the variables which are thought to be involved in the maintenance of the problem behaviour has to be determined. This can be done by:

(*a*) suggesting to the patient that he alters his environment in a specific way (e.g. stops seeing his girl-friend for a fixed period);

(*b*) suggesting to significant persons in the patient's social systems (e.g. parents) that they alter their behaviour in clearly specified ways for stipulated periods;

(*c*) asking the patient or informants how he behaved under similar stimulus conditions in the past.

This "soft data" is then looked at in the light of the various hypotheses which are under consideration. Usually, at this stage, one particular formulation emerges as the most likely explanation of the problem. This then will form the basis of the treatment programme for the particular individual concerned.

5. *Administer techniques and evaluate response.*
If the problem has been clearly formulated, then decisions as to which technique to employ should follow automatically. Procedural details will have to be worked out with the patient in due course but the broad outline of the treatment programme should be apparent. If this is not the case then more information is required.

Occasionally, however, after many hours of data gathering, the problem formulation remains incomplete. For instance, one hypothesis may seem to fit most of the data but certain events have occurred which would not have been predicted from it. Under these circumstances, the only course to take is to administer the techniques which seem most likely to be appropriate and modify the hypothesis in the light of the patient's response to treatment.

One of the advantages of the behavioural approach is that the degree to which the patient is benefiting from treatment is quickly apparent to both parties involved. Because the objective is to produce a clearly defined change in behaviour as opposed to attain a less tangible goal such as "increased awareness", failure has to be acknowledged on the occasions when it occurs. Thus the risks to the patient of being involved in a lengthy but ultimately fruitless course of therapy are much less here than with other psychotherapies. Where the patient is clearly not responding, a reformulation is attempted. Alternatively, the question of a different therapeutic approach should be discussed with the patient.

6. Re-evaluate the hypothesis periodically.
Even if the patient appears to be responding to a particular type of intervention, it does not follow that the behavioural analysis is complete. He may fail to progress beyond a certain point, relapse quite suddenly, or develop problems in other areas of his life. Under circumstances such as these, the therapist should look again at his original formulation and explore possible deficiencies in it. Only when the objectives have been achieved and the patient is functioning at least as well in other areas can treatment be terminated.

The behavioural analysis is clearly a difficult and demanding task for both therapist and patient. It is much more time-consuming than simply applying a technique which has been shown to be effective with people who fall into a particular diagnostic category. What is not yet clear is whether the more sophisticated approach is actually any more effective than behavioural technology. No properly controlled clinical trials have as yet been carried out. Certainly the approach outlined above has a certain face validity since it seems more capable of dealing with the unique features of each case. The likelihood of a totally inappropriate technique being applied is much less if this complex analysis is carried out. From the clinical viewpoint this is a major advantage since, if one type of intervention should prove to be ineffective, the patient's confidence in both therapy and therapist will drop significantly.

Treatment techniques
In contrast to the assessment procedure just described, the treatment techniques which the behavioural psychotherapist employs are relatively easy to administer. For this reason, many people who have had only limited experience of psychiatry have gravitated towards the behavioural approach. Although this is a development to be encouraged, the *ad hoc* administration of techniques is likely to prove ineffective in a certain proportion of cases with general disillusionment with behaviourism, for both patient and therapist, as a possible consequence. Thus some knowledge of the behavioural analysis procedure is desirable before setting out to implement the techniques described below.

One reason why behavioural assessment has come to play such an important role is because the number of techniques available has increased dramatically in the last few years. In the 1950s, when the choice was virtually between *systematic desensitisation* and *aversion therapy*, there was little point in carrying out a comprehensive analysis of the problem. Nowadays, the bewildering array of techniques available necessitates a system for organising data. Since it will not be possible to describe and discuss the complete range of methods, those which should be in the repertoire of anyone interested in using this approach will be examined in some detail.

So far as the categorisation of treatment methods is concerned, any attempt to group the techniques on the basis of postulated similarities regarding theoretical underpinnings (e.g. extinction training) is ultimately futile since every method can be construed, with varying degrees of tortuousness, in either classical or operant conditioning principles. It is less confusing therefore to think about the techniques in terms of what they do rather than what form they take. The three categories which are used here are:

(a) anxiety-reducing techniques;
(b) techniques for eliminating unwanted behaviour;
(c) techniques for promoting desired behaviour.

1. *Anxiety reducing techniques*
One of the earliest reports of direct deconditioning of anxiety reactions with human subjects was the celebrated case of "Little Peter", a young boy with a fear of rabbits (Jones, 1924). While Peter was eating a meal, the experimenter brought a caged rabbit into the room, but not close enough to cause the subject any distress. The cage was gradually brought closer until eventually the rabbit was released while Peter continued to eat. In this way, the fear response to the rabbit was extinguished by building up an association between the phobic stimulus and a non-anxiety response.

When behaviour therapy emerged in the 1950s, the first technique to be introduced was *systematic desensitisation*, which is essentially a more clinically sophisticated version of the early work on counter-conditioning. It was thought to be based on the principle that: "If a response antagonistic to anxiety can be made to occur in the presence of anxiety-evoking stimuli, so that it is accompanied by a complete or partial suppression of the anxiety response, the bond between the stimuli and the anxiety response will be weakened" (Wolpe, 1958). Although Wolpe suggested a number of responses which are incompatible with anxiety (e.g. assertion, sexual arousal), muscular relaxation has been the most extensively employed, principally because it is easy to carry out in the consulting room, and because it is a useful skill to develop in its own right.

There is no one universally accepted method for carrying out relaxation training. Although Jacobson's (1938) procedure was originally recommended, it is now generally recognised that it is not necessary to teach the person to relax every muscle completely. In his review of the literature on systematic desensitisation, Rachman (1967) reached the conclusion that the major contribution of relaxation to this treatment method was mental rather than physical. Consequently most practitioners have developed their own much briefer methods for inducing a state of calmness.

Before looking at one such approach (Sharpe and Lewis, 1977), the practical arrangements for carrying out this work need to be considered. It is generally thought to be advisable to carry out relaxation training in the consulting room itself rather than to adjourn to unfamiliar surroundings in mid-session. The room should be dimly lit (never in darkness) and located in a building which is relatively free from extraneous noise. Although it is advisable to use a couch or relaxation chair, a large cushion can prove satisfactory. Obviously it is essential to ensure that there are no interruptions either by visitors or telephone calls. Plenty of time should be put aside so that the therapist does not feel under pressure to rush through the exercise with a patient who is experiencing difficulty in relaxing.

The following extract is a typical example of the way in which relaxation training is carried out during the first stage of a desensitisation programme.

> For about five seconds, clench both fists tightly, as tightly as you can, and feel the tension. Now relax them completely. Note the difference between tension and relaxation in your hands and lower arms. Continue to let the muscles unwind for about a minute. . . . Push your head back hard against the couch, bed or arm-chair in order to tense your neck mucles. Keep in this position for about five seconds. Feel the tension. Now relax your neck and simply let your head rest back gently. Concentrate on the feeling of letting go for about a minute. . . . Raise your eyebrows as high as you can as though enquiring. Feel the tension in your forehead and scalp. Maintain this tension for about five seconds. Really feel the tension in your muscles. Now relax. Notice the difference between tension and relaxation. Continue the feeling of just letting go. Keep your eyes still, looking straight ahead. Carry on the feeling of unwinding for about a minute. . . . Clench your teeth together for about five seconds. Feel the tension in your jaw. Now relax the muscles by parting your teeth slightly to release all the tension in your jaw. Focus on the feeling of letting go for about a minute . . . .
>
> For the next two or three minutes, concentrate on relaxing all the major muscle groups: legs, buttocks, stomach muscles, chest, mouth, throat, eyes, forehead, neck, shoulders, arms and hands.
>
> Feel yourself sinking deeper into the chair, couch or bed as your body becomes heavier and more and more deeply relaxed.
>
> (Sharpe and Lewis, 1977)

As will be apparent from this example, one important aspect of the procedure is to help the patient to become aware of the difference between tension and relaxation in the different parts of his body. Clearly he has to be able to recognise tension before he can control it. The other point to note from this extract is the deliberately monotonous style employed. As well as being somewhat hypnotic, the repetitious nature of the material provides the patient with a simple conceptual structure which he can recall easily when attempting to relax himself in a real life setting.

It is by no means unusual for patients to feel uncomfortable during the first session. By the second or third occasion, however, a relatively deep state of relaxation is usually achieved. Rather than devote many therapy hours to this repetitious procedure, most clinicians encourage their patients to practise at home. A number of commercially available cassettes are now available for this purpose. Patients are also advised to get into the habit of monitoring their physiological state in a variety of everday stress situations, e.g. traffic jams, and to relax any muscle groups which are needlessly tense.

Although the vast majority of patients are able to relax themselves quite successfully with practice, a small number find it difficult to attain the necessary state of calmness. Even where motivation is not a problem, some people are reluctant to lie back and close their eyes for more than a few seconds when someone is watching them. This difficulty can be overcome by using hypnosis or a modified shaping procedure called "relaxation programming". Alternatively, drugs can be used to induce a state of relaxation (Brady, 1972). The most commonly used procedure with highly anxious patients is to slowly inject intravenously a 1% solution of methohexitone sodium (Brietal) until a subjective state of calmness is achieved. Should the patient fall asleep then the injection is stopped. Since this drug is a short-acting barbiturate, the patient will soon awaken and the procedure can be continued.

The second stage of systematic desensitisation is the creation of a hierarchy of anxiety-provoking stimuli. The patient is asked to rank in order clearly defined situations which cause him distress. This can be a relatively simple operation as in the case of a height phobic who is more anxious on the fourteenth floor than on the thirteenth, and so on. With less tangible phobias, the relative position of the items is not so self-evident. For instance, a physiotherapy student, who was treated by the author, produced the following list of feared situations which are arranged in descending order of difficulty:

1. undergoing a physiotherapy practical examination;
2. eating a meal in a formal restaurant;
3. writing out a cheque in front of a shop assistant;
4. pouring out cups of tea for friends;
5. having a snack in a cafe;
6. driving with a friend in the car;
7. sitting in the middle of a crowded cinema;
8. travelling by underground train during the rush hour;
9. travelling by bus during the rush hour;
10. eating at home with her family.

Once the patient is able to relax and a hierarchy has been obtained, systematic desensitisation proper can begin. If the patient has produced a number of hierarchies, it is recommended that the one which is causing the patient most distress should be dealt with first. If the patient is able to overcome the major difficulty in this way, he may be able to extinguish the other phobias by himself, with only minimal assistance from the therapist. However, if more than two relatively distinct hierarchies have been elicited, the therapist may feel that anxiety-management training (*see* pp. 36-7) will prove to be more cost-effective in the long term than systematic desensitisation.

In the first session of desensitisation proper, the patient is asked to relax in the usual fashion. When he is feeling calm, he is told to imagine a control situation, e.g. lying on a sunny beach. Once he has attained a clear image, he is asked to fantasise about the least anxiety-provoking situation in the hierarchy. Although there are no universally accepted guidelines, many clinicians (e.g. Morris, 1975) recommend that this item should be presented three to four times for a period of about five seconds each. This time duration is gradually increased to thirty seconds. Should the patient experience any anxiety whatsoever, he is told to raise his finger to draw the therapist's attention to this fact. In this event, he is instructed to stop thinking about this item and imagine the control situation once again. One of the difficulties here is that many patients, particularly those who are highly motivated, are reluctant to report feelings of anxiety lest they give the impression of being uncooperative. Consequently, the therapist should emphasise strongly at the outset how important it is that the patient should remain anxiety-free throughout, if the association is to be broken. In addition, the therapist should observe the patient's behaviour carefully at all times, ideally with the assistance of a psychophysiological device, such as an electromyograph or equipment for measuring skin resistance. There are now a number of portable, easy-to-use, low-cost instruments available commercially which are ideal for this purpose. The procedure is then repeated with the next item, and so on, until the patient experiences no anxiety while fantasising about the item at the top of the hierarchy.

Occasionally, where the jump from one item to the next one proves to be too large, an intervening stage will be required. Furthermore, once treatment is under way, the ordering of items may be found to be inaccurate, in which case the hierarchy will have to be reconstructed. Thus, although it is basically an extremely simple procedure to implement, the success or otherwise of a particular programme rests on the ability of the therapist to take the necessary steps to ensure that the patient is never exposed, for any length of time, to an item which elicits anxiety.

Although systematic desensitisation in imagination is particularly useful in cases where it is difficult to recreate the feared situation, e.g. thunderstorms, most therapists nowadays prefer to carry out *in vivo* counterconditioning (Sherman, 1972) wherever possible. In other words, the patient is exposed *in reality* to each item in the hierarchy, while accompanied by the therapist. Although relaxation training is still usually carried out at the beginning of treatment, clearly the patient cannot be as free from tension in the real-life setting as he would be if lying on the couch. In this situation, the feelings of comfort, security and trust that the patient develops for the therapist serve as the anti-anxiety agents.

In addition to its obvious uses within psychiatric treatment, desensitisation has much to contribute to the treatment of difficulties which arise in a general medical setting. Patients with specific fears of blood, injections, losing consciousness, choking and dialysis equipment have all been treated by the author using this technique. The same procedure can also be used to "immunise" patients against the development of a negative emotional reaction. Childbirth is one potentially traumatic event which is clearly recognised as such by the medical profession. Many antenatal clinics attempt, in an elementary fashion, to teach expectant mothers how to relax while, at the same time, gradually exposing them to the idea of giving birth. Behaviourists would argue that this attempt at psychoprophylaxis would be more effective it if were to be carried out in line with the formal procedure of systematic desensitisation. Other areas where preparatory desensitisation could conceivably play a role include preparing young children for hospital admission, patients for surgery, and old people for the eventual death of their spouse.

Like systematic desensitisation, *implosive therapy* involves the presentation in imagination of anxiety-evoking material in a controlled fashion. However, in this case, the patient is required to fantasise about very frightening situations for a prolonged period of time without undergoing any preparatory relaxation training. This technique, which has been developed by Stampfl (1970) is apparently based on the process of extinction. In other words, it is assumed that, through continuous presentation of the anxiety-producing stimulus (C.S.) in the absence of aversive occurrences (U.C.S.), the strength of the fear response (C.R.) will diminish.

Although this procedure can best be understood in learning theory terms, much of the original thinking about implosive therapy involved psychodynamic concepts. The hierarchy which patient and therapist develop proceeds from external events to intrapsychic processes. For instance, in the treatment of claustrophobia, the therapist may begin by describing a closed-in room in detail and then proceed to suggest to the patient that his father had trapped him there in order to castrate him.

At the outset, the rationale of this approach is carefully explained to the patient and it is emphasised that the extent to which he can get "carried away" will determine the effectiveness of the programme. The therapist then proceeds to suggest some scenes to him which approximate to the situation in which the fear was first learned. Postulated psychodynamic themes, such as oral and anal impulses, bodily injury, rejection, aggression and loss of control are introduced where appropriate. The session is not terminated until the patient has experienced a significant diminution of anxiety. Failure to do this can lead to the problem being exacerbated. Consequently, the therapist would be ill-advised to set aside less than an hour-and-a-half for a session.

Although the term *flooding* is often used interchangeably with implosion, there is a difference between the two so far as choice of scenes is concerned. Instead of moving from the external, e.g. a room full of spiders, to the internal, e.g. castration fears, the therapist who uses flooding restricts himself to the feared situation. In other words, scenes based on psychodynamic interpretations are not employed. It follows from this that flooding can be carried out *in vivo*, whereas implosive therapy necessitates the use of imaginal stimuli.

In his review of the field, Beech (1976) reaches the conclusion that "it is difficult to arrive at a sound and balanced view of the contribution which this method makes". He is referring here to the fact that although some patients have responded dramatically to the implosive therapy method, others have actually deteriorated. For instance, Wolpe (1969) used implosive therapy to treat a dentist who was unable to give injections to patients in case they died as a result. Treatment involved asking him to imagine a patient slumping forward dead after having received an injection. After a few sessions of this sort, he was able to inject patients while experiencing only mild anxiety. A less successful case of Wolpe's was that of a doctor with a fear of mentally disturbed patients. After taking up a psychiatric post, which involved being exposed extensively to "insanity", he became much more anxious about mental illness. Anecdotal evidence of this sort would seem to indicate that prolonged exposure to the feared situation does not always lead to the extinction of the conditioned response. Thus, as yet, not enough is known about procedural details and individual differences in responsivity to help the therapist to decide exactly how and when to use this method. Although implosive therapy is a potentially useful technique, it should be used with caution, particularly where the clinician has had little experience of working with highly anxious patients.

The major limitation of both the techniques described so far, systematic desensitisation and implosion, is that they can only be applied to specific problems. However, relatively few monophobias present in a medical setting. On the other hand, neurotic disturbances, where the anxiety response has generalised, i.e. "free-floating", account for a significant proportion of the cases referred to a psychiatrist. Although it is possible to elicit a hierarchy of stressful situations from every neurotic patient, few contemporary behavioural psychotherapists would apply systematic desensitisation or implosive therapy with patients who do not have a relatively discrete phobia. Instead they would apply *anxiety management training* (Suinn and Richardson, 1971). This involves training patients to control the autonomic concomitants of anxiety under increasingly stressful circumstances. Relaxation training, of the type described above in connection with systematic desensitisation (*see* p.000) is carried out in the first instance. Then the therapist presents a noxious stimulus, e.g. sudden loud noise, or describes a traumatic scene until the patient begins to demonstrate signs of tension. As soon as this occurs, the stress source is removed and the patient is instructed to relax himself again. As with desensitisation, a hierarchy of aversive items should be employed so that the patient is not swamped with anxiety he cannot control in the early stages of the programme.

There is no general agreement as to the most effective ways of teaching people to control themselves once they have been made anxious. Suinn and Richardson (1971) favour the use of a tape recording comprising relaxation instructions with peaceful background music. Others (e.g. Sharpe and Lewis, 1977) recommend the use of *biofeedback* devices for this purpose. In addition to measuring specific autonomic responses, e.g. palmar skin conductance or alpha activity on the electroencephalogram, these psychophysiological devices emit a visual or aural signal which corresponds to the individual's level of "arousal" at a particular point in time. Since knowledge of results is necessary for the development of skills, it is easy to argue the case for using instruments such as these to help patients to become more effective at handling visceral activity. Other uses of biofeedback procedures will be considered in the next section.

Although anxiety management training bears a superficial resemblance to systematic desensitisation, there are important differences so far as the postulated underlying principles are concerned. The discriminative stimuli here are considered to be the physiological manifestations of anxiety rather than the characteristics of a particular object. Thus the individual is trained to carry out anxiety-reducing responses whenever he experiences tension. At a practical level, the most important distinction is that here the patient is deliberately made anxious by the therapist whereas, in systematic desensitisation, care is taken to ensure that the patient remains relaxed throughout each session. Finally, the objectives of the two techniques are very different. The aim of systematic desensitisation is to eliminate the sources of anxiety, whereas anxiety management training is essentially a strategy to help the patient to cope with the various stresses he will be subjected to in the future.

In the discussion of behavioural analysis (*see* pp. 23-9), it was pointed out that the patient's covert reactions can be regarded as responses which are subject to the same principles of learning which govern overt behaviours. The importance of cognitive factors in anxiety neurosis has been emphasised by Meichenbaum (1975) who claims that they are at least as important as external stimuli in determining the occurrence of abnormal behaviour. Thus a negative self-statement, such as, "I won't be able to cope", whether expressed or merely thought, can act as a self-fulfilling prophecy. Meichenbaum is also impressed by the fact that one of the key findings to emerge from research into behavioural treatments for phobias is that, following progress, cognitive changes are generally reported: "Writers who have attempted to reduce phobic behaviour by means of desensitisation, modeling, flooding, and altering cognitions about internal reactions have all commented on the importance of the client's self-statements in the change process, even when no direct effort has been made to change these statements". Meichenbaum then goes on to outline ways in which the modification of self-statements can be achieved while carrying out one of the orthodox behavioural programmes outlined above. However, before going on to outline Meichenbaum's work and its derivatives, one of its forerunners will be described briefly.

Anxiety relief conditioning (Wolpe and Lazarus, 1966) involves presenting a noxious stimulus, e.g. electric shock, to the patient for a few seconds. The patient then emits a prearranged response, e.g. saying "Calm" aloud, and the aversive procedure is immediately terminated. This is repeated on a number of occasions. Eventually, so it is claimed, the patient should be able to reduce his anxiety level in virtually any situation by instructing himself to be calm, which sets the occasion for the anti-anxiety response. Incidentally, since it is not always appropriate to vocalise the relief word, e.g. in a committee meeting, an attempt is usually made to shape the response from a shout to a whisper and ultimately to a covert reaction.

Meichenbaum's strategies for inducing cognitive change are not only more sophisticated than this technique but are intended to augment existing (overt) behavioural techniques rather than to replace them. For instance, he has proposed a *coping-imagery* procedure which he considers to be a useful modification to systematic desensitisation. As each item in the hierarchy is presented, the patient is encouraged to imagine himself coping with anxiety by combining relaxation with appropriate self-instructions. It will be recalled that in orthodox desensitisation, there is no suggestion that the patient will experience anxiety outside the treatment situation. In other words, what Meichenbaum is suggesting is that "mastery" imagery be replaced by "coping" imagery. However, rather than alter the fundamental nature of systematic descensitisation in this way, many clinicians (e.g. Sharpe and Lewis, 1977) consider it more appropriate to combine the modification of self-statements with anxiety-management training, since both types of intervention are essentially coping strategies. It is this latter approach which will be considered here.

Before carrying out *positive self-talk training* (Sharpe and Lewis, 1977), it is essential to isolate the "doom-laden prophecies" which have previously governed the patient's behaviour in stress situations. The patient himself should be absolutely clear as to what constitutes a negative statement in his case and should fully appreciate the part they play in maintaining his problem behaviour. The therapist and patient then proceed to construct positive self-talk statements which are appropriate for that particular individual. Sharpe and Lewis (1977) have put forward three guidelines to bear in mind when drawing up these statements, and these are as follows.

(a) They must relate specifically to the anticipated difficulty. Simply waking up in the morning and saying "I am going to make a bit of an effort to-day" is insufficient. The patient must devise self-statements pertaining to each of the stressful situations he is likely to encounter, e.g. spiders, arguments, interviews.

(b) They must be realistic. It is just as inappropriate to say to oneself "I will feel perfectly relaxed throughout" as it is to say "I am going to lose control". The former self-statement will be invalidated as soon as the patient experiences an anticipatory twinge of anxiety, and he is then very likely to revert to his original self-defeating strategy. A more realistic statement might be "entering this situation is going to prove quite difficult for me but I will be able to cope".

(c) They must offer some practical advice. A coping strategy should not only serve as a form of reassurance but should provide a cue for appropriate action. Sharpe and Lewis (1977) recommend that the patient's self-statement should lead him to concentrate on some positive feature of the situation, e.g. "the spider's web glistening in the morning dew". Alternatively the statement could be related to the relaxation exercises. This is an obvious way of combining positive self-talk with anxiety-management training so that the individual learns to cope by controlling both types of internal stimuli.

The following example of a positive self-talk statement meets all three requirements. "It is likely that I will experience some anxiety when I go into the room but, provided that I concentrate on keeping my breathing rate slow and regular, I will be able to cope". By itself, positive self-talk can achieve very little. However, when combined with anxiety-management training, it provides the individual with a comprehensive strategy for coping with stress.

Many of the techniques described so far are ideal for use with patients who experience anxiety in impersonal situations. However, for those who feel anxious when interacting with others, e.g. at interviews or parties, the ability to sit in the corner breathing deeply while uttering, subvocally, coping statements falls some way short of their target. In most cases of this sort, the goal is to be able to express one's opinions and feelings in an effective fashion. *Assertiveness training* is a behavioural technique which is particularly useful with patients who experience anxiety in interpersonal situations. It is particularly useful with patients who are:

(*a*) unable to stand up for themselves when others seem to be taking advantage of them, e.g. being short-changed;

(*b*) unable to express affection or hostility towards significant people in their lives; and

(*c*) frustrated by their inability to influence the behaviour of others, e.g. employees; committees.

Like systematic desensitisation, assertiveness training is based on the model of counterconditioning. In other words, it is assumed that carrying out a new response in a situation which previously elicited anxiety will lead to the weakening of the past association. This technique has an additional advantage in that appropriate assertive behaviour is usually rewarded by others. This, in turn, engenders feelings of self-confidence and reduces social anxiety still further. The most sophisticated procedure for improving performance in social situations is the "personal effectiveness" approach (Liberman *et al.*, 1975). This involves the following stages:

(*a*) *Goal-targetting.* The patient is encouraged to specify, as precisely as possible, his short-term objectives. Care should be taken to ensure that he is not too ambitious, thus increasing the probability of a failure experience.

(*b*) *Behaviour rehearsal (dry-run).* The patient selects one particular situation, related to his objectives, which he would like to work on. Parts are allocated to staff or other patients to enable the patient to demonstrate how he would approach the task. Ideally the role-play should be videotaped but, if that is not possible, a sound recording should be made.

(*c*) *Feedback.* At the end of the scene, those present analyse the patient's behaviour (both verbal and non-verbal) in some detail,

using the recording to help illustrate their points. Particu
should be given to the positive features of the performar

(d) *Modelling alternative behaviour.* If the performance is
deficient in some important respects, another member of the group
is asked to take over the patient's role in order to demonstrate a
different way of dealing with the situation. The model's behaviour
is then analysed carefully and the patient is encouraged to imitate
those aspects of it which are considered to be particularly effective.

(e) *Behaviour rehearsal (re-run).* The situation is repeated with
the patient playing his own part once again. If necessary, additional
modelling and role play sequences are carried out until the patient's
performance is considered to be satisfactory.

(f) *Homework assignment.* The patient agrees to set up an *in
vivo* situation for himself before the next session, which will involve
utilising the assertion skills he has been practising.

The personal effectiveness approach works best with people who
simply require to develop a strategy for handling specific social situations. However, many patients with assertion difficulties are anxious
about becoming involved in personal confrontations. In such cases,
it is more appropriate to desensitise the patient to situations involving
emotional demonstration using assertion, rather than relaxation, as
the anti-anxiety response (Palmer, 1973; Mackay, 1977). If necessary,
personal effectiveness training can be carried out subsequently.

Of the anxiety-reducing methods described in this section, the
most widely used are systematic desensitisation, anxiety-management
training combined with positive self-talk and assertiveness training.
Systematic desensitisation is the treatment of choice if the patient
presents with one or two fairly well-circumscribed phobias. If the
problem is more diffuse then training in cognitive and autonomic
control should be carried out. However, if the behaviour of others is
one of the key precipitants of anxiety then assertiveness should be
carried out either as an alternative or as an addition to one of the
other programmes.

2. *Techniques for eliminating unwanted behaviour*
Many patients seek help in order to break habits which are intrinsically rewarding in the short term but which are ultimately self-
defeating. The obsessive-compulsive patient, who has to wash himself
in a ritualistic fashion, the exhibitionist who feels compelled to ex-
pose himself, the obese person who goes on regular "binges" of
over-indulgence, and the alcoholic who spends most of his money
on liquor are common examples of people who are unable to exert
sufficient control over their own behaviour. As always, it is essential

to carry out a full behavioural analysis before implementing any of the techniques to be described here. Thus, for instance, if the patient engages in the unwanted behaviour when under stress, then it will probably be appropriate to administer one of the anxiety-reducing techniques in the first instance. In some cases, this may well be sufficient and a direct attack on the presenting problem may not be necessary. One additional point needs to be made at this stage. It is usually unwise to attempt to suppress one response without teaching the individual a more appropriate way of behaving in order to produce a similar outcome. The behavioural analysis should reveal the nature of the relevant reinforcers.

Although *aversion therapy* is the best known of the behavioural techniques for eliminating unwanted behaviour, it is currently used much more selectively than it was in the 1960s, following claims that it is needlessly cruel, unethical, simplistic, theoretically unsound, and not very effective in any case. Many of these allegations are based on emotional rather than rational grounds and, in the opinion of this author, the case against aversion therapy has been overstated. Although aversive procedures have been administered incompletely and inappropriately in the past, they still have a useful, though limited, contribution to make to the treatment of behaviour disorders. Essentially, aversion therapy involves pairing the unwanted behaviour, or the cues associated with it, with a noxious stimulus, thus rendering the former less attractive to the individual in the future. Although this sounds very straightforward, there are in fact many different ways of replacing approach behaviour with avoidance behaviour. Before examining these, the nature of the noxious stimuli used in aversive procedures requires some consideration.

The two main types of noxious stimuli which have been widely used are chemicals which produce unpleasant effects and electric shock. Injections of emetine and apomorphine, which give rise to nauseous sensations and vomiting, were used in most of the early studies in this area. Nowadays chemical agents are rarely employed. They act in an unpredictable fashion, the number of trials is obviously limited, the procedure is very unpleasant for all concerned, and the drugs themselves produce unwanted side-effects. Many of these problems can be overcome by using electric shock. With electrical aversion, the onset, intensity and duration of the stimulus can be more easily controlled. Furthermore, the patient recovers quickly from the experience which means that a number of trials can be conducted in any one session. Incidentally, it is now generally recognised that, in order to produce optimal effects, the shock should be delivered at a high level of intensity (rather than gradually increased) and that the duration should be relatively brief, e.g. 0.05 seconds.

So far as the procedures themselves are concerned, it will be useful to divide them up into three groups on the basis of the learning paradigm to which they are most closely related.

(a) Classical conditioning. The majority of studies based on the Pavlovian procedure have been carried out with alcoholics. Of these, the work of Lemere and Voegtlin (1950) is perhaps the best known. They treated over 4,000 alcoholics by pairing the taste, sight and smell of the patient's preferred drink (C.S.) with an emetic drug (U.C.S.) which elicited nausea and vomiting (U.C.R.). The rationale here is that an association should build up so that the presentation of alcohol by itself should produce this reaction. Although about half of the patients treated remained abstinent for at least two years following treatment, it cannot be concluded that these impressive results are due specifically to classical conditioning. Like most other studies on aversion therapy, this one lacks the necessary controls and other refinements which would permit the various components of the treatment "package" to be properly evaluated. In any case, as Franks (1963) points out, most of the work in this area bears little resemblance to the classical conditioning paradigm as originally conceived. A close examination of the literature on Pavlovian conditioning reveals that the time interval between the onset of the C.S. and U.C.S. is of critical importance. However, in many of the aversion therapy studies Franks refers to, the C.S. is presented too early in some cases and actually after the U.C.S., i.e. backward conditioning, in others. Thus it is unlikely that the results obtained from studies involving chemical aversion owe very much to principles of learning. Finally, the logic of using classical conditioning procedures to eliminate operant behaviour has been questioned (Sandler, 1975).

(b) Punishment. As stated earlier, one of the major differences between classical and operant conditioning is that, in the latter case, the individual has to make a voluntary response: otherwise no learning will take place. Once he has carried out that particular response, the probability of its recurrence under similar circumstances depends on the outcome. One obvious way to reduce the frequency of a behaviour pattern is to make a noxious stimulus contingent upon its occurrence. This is the basis of punishment training.

One of the earliest examples of response-contingent shock procedures is that described by Meyer and Crisp (1964). Two overweight women were exposed to their most preferred foods for increased periods of time. Any approach responses were immediately followed by shock. The treatment regime was gradually faded out so long as they were losing weight. It was immediately reinstated following a relapse. The results were mixed. One patient made significant progress which she maintained for two years whereas no demonstrable change was observed with the other one.

A similar procedure was employed with alcoholics by Vogler *et al.* (1970). Drinks were served to patients in a simulated bar situation. Each drinking response was immediately followed by an electric shock which was maintained until the individual spat out the drink. Although this is essentially a punishment procedure, some escape conditioning is involved as well, in that the spitting out response is being negatively reinforced.

Sandler's (1975) recommendations for a maximally effective programme of this kind are as follows.

(*i*) The aversive stimulus should immediately follow the response which is to be eliminated;

(*ii*) It should be presented each time the behaviour is observed and should never be administered in its absence;

(*iii*) Treatment should be continued until the problem has completely disappeared rather than after a predetermined number of trials. The best termination criterion of all is "the appearance of adaptive behaviour under circumstances in which the problem behaviour had previously occurred" (Sandler, 1975).

(*iv*) Care should be taken to ensure that the aversive stimulus is something which the individual himself would actually avoid, rather than an event which the therapist considers to be unpleasant.

(*c*) *Anticipatory avoidance conditioning.* Another way of using aversive stimuli to bring about a reduction in the frequency of a particular response is to negatively reinforce the individual for *not* carrying it out. In other words, rather than punish the individual for carrying out the unwanted behaviour, he is given an incentive (i.e. the removal of an unpleasant future occurrence) for abstaining. The best example of the clinical usage of the anticipatory avoidance paradigm is the work of Feldman and MacCulloch (1970) with homosexuals. Male slides were projected on to a screen for eight seconds, during which time the patient had the option of pressing a switch or not. If he did not do so, then he received a shock when the slide was removed. If he pressed the switch, then, on most occasions, the slide was removed and no shock was administered. The patients were asked to look at the slides so long as they found them attractive rather than to concentrate on shock-avoidance. There are other intricacies in Feldman and MacCulloch's design, all apparently derived from learning theory principles, which need not concern us here. The crucial component, so far as these authors are concerned, is the anticipatory avoidance procedure. As was pointed out earlier, however, most behavioural techniques can be accounted for in terms of classical or operant conditioning. Thus Rachman and Teasdale (1969) claim that the Feldman and MacCulloch work can be accounted for in terms of classical conditioning with the male slides serving as the C.S. and the shock as the U.C.S. This argument has been examined by Wilson and Davison (1974) who reach the conclusion that "it is reasonable to suggest that aversion-relief is the critical ingredient in the Feldman and MacCulloch package and that the presumed importance of conditioned aversion to homosexual stimuli is irrelevant".

Many behavioural psychotherapists, while recognising the appropriateness of implementing aversive procedures in certain cases, are reluctant to administer crude noxious stimuli such as electric shocks. Similarly, many patients who are highly motivated to change their behaviour, are unwilling to subject themselves to such a traumatic experience. Under these circumstances, a cognitive aversion treatment method, known as *covert sensitisation* (Cautela, 1967) should be employed. Here the patient is asked to imagine a scene, e.g. his favourite bar, which normally sets the occasion for the maladaptive behaviour, e.g. drinking whisky. The therapist describes the situation as vividly as possible, having obtained details of the physical lay-out from the patient beforehand. Suddenly aversive stimuli, of a physical and social nature, are introduced into the fantasy. These negative features are strongly emphasised until it is clear that the patient is experiencing intense discomfort. At this stage, an escape route is suggested to the patient and the beneficial aspects of leaving the bar-room are pointed out. The following passage is an abbreviated version of the fantasy scene used by the author to help treat an alcoholic.

"You walk into 'The George and Dragon' and sit on your usual bar stool. Bill serves you a large scotch on the rocks. You listen to the ice clinking against the glass and gaze at the golden liquid. You turn around to see who else is in the bar. You say 'Hello' to Fred who is checking the racing results in the evening paper. You raise your glass and have a sip. As you do so you suddenly feel unwell. Your stomach seems to have turned to acid. You can feel the colour disappearing from your face. Your hands are trembling violently. All conversation stops in the bar as everyone turns to look at you with horror in their faces. 'You can't be sick here', you think. But the vomit begins to rise in your gorge. You try to choke it back but you cannot. It's pouring out of your mouth, all over your tie — the green one your wife bought for you. The puke is green and lumpy, and you can see partially digested pieces of vegetables you had for lunch dripping down into your whisky. Your mother has just come into the bar and you can see the disgust on her face. You retch again and more vomit spills out of your mouth, this time on to the sleeves of your jacket. You stagger to your feet and as you set off for the door so you begin to feel better. Your head starts to clear. The stains gradually disappear from your clothing. You open the door and gulp in the fresh air. Your head clears completely. Your stomach feels much more settled. It's a beautiful day. The birds are singing and the sun is shining. You decide to go for a walk. A pretty girl smiles at you as she walks past. You cannot remember ever having felt so good."

For this approach to be effective, the client must be highly motivated and fully co-operative as far as setting up and imagining the scenes is concerned. A variety of scenes should be used, involving different drinking places and beverages, to ensure that the necessary degree of generalisation takes place. The aversive stimuli and incentives for escape must be appropriate for the individual concerned.

Although covert sensitisation is used by many clinicians, there are few rigorous scientific reports of its usage in the literature, presumably because the procedure, by its very nature, is difficult to objectify. It is a very useful clinical tool, since no special equipment is required, the patient can listen alone to tape-recordings and anecdotal reports suggest that it can be very effective after only a few sessions. Thus although there have been no properly controlled studies comparing the effectiveness of aversion therapy with that of covert sensitisation, most behavioural psychotherapists prefer to use the latter approach on those occasions when a disincentive type of intervention is required. It is, however, usually employed in conjunction with other techniques as part of the general treatment programme which has evolved from the behavioural analysis.

Earlier in this chapter, it was pointed out that the ritualistic behaviour of obsessive-compulsive patients can usefully be regarded as an avoidance or escape response sequence, which is negatively reinforced by anxiety reduction. It would seem to follow from this that if the underlying anxiety can be eliminated, then it should be relatively easy to extinguish the deviant behaviour. This is the rationale which underlies the *ritual prevention* treatment for compulsive behaviour (Meyer *et al.*, 1974). The patient is supervised on a continuous basis to ensure that he does not engage in the ritualistic behaviour, e.g. hand-washing. At the same time, systematic desensitisation or flooding is carried out in an endeavour to extinguish the anxiety response, e.g. fear of contamination, which is involved in the maintenance of the compulsive act.

As yet there are few systematic reports concerning the efficacy of this treatment approach but the results obtained so far are very encouraging. Meyer *et al.* (1974) treated fifteen severely handicapped obsessional patients on an in-patient basis. Prolonged exposure to the source of imagined "contamination" was carried out in combination with response prevention. As a result, three patients were left with no symptoms, seven were judged to be much improved, and five were considered to have improved to a degree. Many writers have pointed out that the stimuli which control the ritualistic behaviour are often only present in the individual's home environment. In such cases, although it may be useful to admit the patient to hospital in the early stages of treatment, some domiciliary work will have to be carried out if the patient is to maintain any progress made.

Although ritual prevention, used in combination with flooding, can be effective in eliminating compulsive acts, it is only of limited value with patients whose main problem is obsessional ruminations. Since this is essentially a cognitive disorder, it follows that the most appropriate technique is likely to be one which attacks the self-defeating thinking patterns directly. *Thought-stopping* is one such method. In this procedure, the patient is asked to concentrate on his anxiety-producing thoughts. The therapist then suddenly shouts "stop", administers an electric shock or creates some other form of disturbance. This procedure is repeated several times until the patient is able to report that his ruminations have been interrupted on a number of successive trials. The patient is then encouraged to interrupt his thoughts using a similar strategy. Once he is able to do this, he is trained to control his thoughts in a less obtrusive manner. Thus, for example, he may say the word "stop", whisper it, and ultimately think it. If, at any stage in this part of the procedure, he should fail to interrupt his ruminations, then it will be necessary for him to practise more at the earlier stages.

Rimm and Masters (1974) have developed a *covert assertion* programme which is very similar to the method described except that a more positive anti-anxiety statement, such as "Screw you", is recommended as an alternative to the more conservative self-command usually employed in covert sensitisation. Since assertion is a powerful anti-anxiety response, this would seem to be a useful modification to the original procedure.

Since behavioural psychotherapists encourage their patients to take on some responsibility for behavioural change, it is not surprising to find that, in recent years, considerable attention has been paid to developing *self-control* methods for the elimination of maladaptive responses. A wide range of problem behaviours, including obesity, cigarette smoking, drinking, gambling, compulsive rituals, and temper tantrums have been treated successfully by helping patients to help themselves.

Here, as always, the behavioural analysis plays a critical role so far as the setting up of individualised programmes is concerned (Kanfer and Koroly, 1972). It is essential to:

(i) identify the circumstances under which the behaviour occurs, e.g. coffee-break; watching television;

(ii) divide the behavioural sequence into discrete responses, e.g. removing cigarette packet from hand-bag; opening matchbox;

(iii) isolate the reinforcers, e.g. feeling of calm.

Having collected this information, the therapist can discuss with the patient ways of interrupting the sequence. In the example of the cigarette smoker, she might be advised to avoid coffee breaks, keep her cigarettes in her coat pocket, and practise relaxation in order to achieve the feeling of calm. She would probably also be advised to self-administer aversive stimuli, such as keeping the ash-trays full of stale butts, inhaling cigarette smoke for prolonged periods, and paying a fine for every packet purchased. As far as the last is concerned, an effective way of carrying out the fine is to make the patient contribute to the funds of a political party to which she is ideologically opposed! In addition, the patient is instructed to administer self-reward, e.g. buying a new record, when certain specific targets have been reached.

This approach is particularly relevant to the work of medical practitioners who are attempting to modify the health habits of certain "at risk" patients, but have relatively little time to devote to them. The work of Meyer and Henderson (1974) is of particular interest here. These workers demonstrated that self-control is more effective than any other method in helping patients, who were considered likely to develop cardio-vascular disorders, to regulate their life style accordingly.

Finally, although self-control training may appear to be just common sense, it must be emphasised that the effectiveness of this mode of intervention depends very much on the skills of the patient and therapist in isolating relevant precipitants and consequences of the behaviour, and developing effective ways of interrupting the sequence.

3. Techniques for promoting desired behaviour

At the beginning of the last section, it was emphasised that it is rarely advisable to eliminate one particular pattern of behaviour without helping the individual to respond in an alternative fashion which will achieve the same outcome. Although in some cases advice (e.g. change job) is sufficient, a more structured type of intervention is usually required with those who present in a medical setting. The reason for the behavioural deficit has important implications for the kind of programme which will be implemented. If the individual is capable of carrying out a more adaptive response but does not "choose" to do so, then clearly the focal point of treatment should be reinforcement process. On the other hand, if he does not have more adaptive responses in his repertoire, then a specific training programme is required. In this section, two techniques which concentrate on the consequences of behaviour, i.e. self-reinforcement and marital contract therapy, and two which involve the development of new responses, i.e. social skills training and masturbatory fantasy retraining, will be described.

Unlike the pigeons in the Skinner box, most of the responses emitted by an adult human being during the course of an ordinary day do not have immediate external consequences. The fact that he continues to be active, under these circumstances, would suggest some form of covert reinforcement is taking place. In other words, he cognitively "pats himself of the back" following the accomplishment of each task. There is considerable variation between people regarding the type of operant regime they have devised for themselves. Some administer rewards (e.g. telling themselves "I did well") following a relatively modest accomplishment, whereas others adopt such high performance criteria that self-praise is a relatively rare occurrence. According to Lewinsohn (1975), individuals who abstain from rewarding themselves are predisposed to become depressed. Similarly, the low self-esteem which is a characteristic of so many alcoholics and drug-abusers can also be usefully seen in this light. Consequently, the kind of internal environment the individual creates for himself has important implications for his overt behaviour.

Self-reinforcement training (S.R.), as its name suggests, involves teaching the individual to reward himself for carrying out specified behaviours which are within his capabilities. The therapist's first task is to make the patient aware of the four components of self-reinforcement systems (Jackson, 1972). These are as outlined below.

(a) Establish standard of acceptable performance. Since objective reference points are usually lacking, most individuals rely on their appraisal of the performance of peer group members or on their recollection of their previous level of competence when setting up standards. In the light of the vast experimental literature on perceptual and memory processes, it is clear that there is plenty of scope for distortion here. Thus there is evidence to indicate that severely depressed patients are apt to compare themselves unfavourably with others when there is no justification for so doing (Loeb *et al.*, 1967). Where the performance *is* actually lower than the standard set, the therapist has to point out to the patient that the tests he is using are too severe in view of his age, experiences, general condition or whatever. Finally, it is essential that the therapist should ensure that the criteria for acceptable performance are described precisely at the out-

set. Depressed patients, in particular, often raise their goals in the light of their own performance, thus placing themselves in a "can't win" situation.

(b) Perform the task. The task itself should be broken down into its various components, each of which should be tackled separately. For instance, a depressed patient who is unemployed might be advised to seek vocational guidance, scan the job vacancies, telephone for details, complete several application forms, undergo social skills training to work on interview performance, and finally present himself for job interviews.

(c) Appraise performance relative to the standards. If an acceptable level of performance has been precisely defined, the comparison between the actual and the ideal is usually a straightforward matter.

(d) Apply or withdraw reinforcement as appropriate. Before the task is carried out, the therapist and patient should decide what rewards the latter should give himself if he reaches or surpasses the goal. In addition, it may be thought useful to include a "penalty clause" in the event of the individual failing to reach the target. This latter option should be used with caution, particularly with patients who are severely depressed. The appropriate consequences should follow the completion of the task as soon as possible. Although the ultimate aim of this treatment approach is to train the patient to practice self-reinforcement using covert means, explicit rewards should be used initially: "An element of self-reinforcement training that appears critical is initially requiring the person to administer a tangible reinforcer such as points or tokens to themselves simultaneously with a positive verbalisation. This step encourages the person to engage deliberately and overtly in the act of self-evaluation and self-reinforcement and provides a means of recording these behaviours" (Jackson, 1972).

As yet, there have been few controlled studies of S.R. as a technique in its own right. Rehm and Marston (1968) successfully treated males with "minimal dating" problems by encouraging them to reinforce themselves with approval following the performance of progressively more difficult tasks in heterosexual situations. Marston (1969) describes an approach for helping students, with unrealistically high standards, to increase their work output. Jackson (1972) demonstrates how S.R. can be employed in the treatment of depression. Sexual deviations and eating disturbances have also been treated in this way. The main reason why so little work has been done in this area is because S.R. by itself, although effective with people who have minor problems such as study difficulties, has little to offer patients who present in a medical setting. It can however play a useful role when used in conjunction with other, more powerful behavioural techniques.

Marital contract therapy is another form of intervention which is concerned with modifying the reinforcement mechanism so that adaptive behaviour is more likely to be rewarded in the future. Although it is mostly used with married couples, it can be applied to any small-group situation where members are concerned to change each other's behaviour. However, in the interests of clarity, only the two-person relationship will be considered here. The aim of contract therapy is to teach the couple to use positive reinforcement, instead of coercion and punishment, in order to change each other's way of behaving. This is achieved by asking both partners to draw up lists of changes they would like to see in the other person. These requests must be described precisely. For instance, it is not sufficient to suggest that one's partner should help more with the housework or keep the house tidier. Specific details (e.g. washing the breakfast dishes; removing underwear from the bedroom floor) are required. When both parties have compiled their lists, an agreement is then negotiated so that the wife will receive a specified reward for carrying out the husband's requests and vice versa.

A distinction can be made between the *contingency contract* model proposed by Stuart (1969) and the *independent consequences* arrangement favoured by Patterson and Hops (1972). In Stuart's model, the two contracts are inextricably bound up with each other so that one person's programme can be jeopardised by the non-cooperation of the other person. To prevent such an occurrence, Patterson and Hops (1972) have put forward a contract system which keeps the two programmes separate. By making a distinction between rewards and behaviour change requests, these workers have demonstrated that it is possible for one person to comply with the wishes of his/her partner and receive an agreed reward while the other person is not participating in the reciprocal programme. The intricacies of this technique are discussed in more detail elsewhere (Mackay, 1976).

The behaviour therapy literature on interpersonal difficulties, makes it apparent that the distinction between assertiveness training (*see* pp. 39-40) and *social skills training* (S.S.T.) is by no means a clear one. The difference is basically one of emphasis. Assertiveness training is used principally with patients who are anxious about standing up for themselves or expressing their views in public. The assumption is that such patients have the necessary skills in their repertoire and will be able to demonstrate them once they feel less anxious about doing so. Although it is derived from Wolpe's counterconditioning model, modelling, practice and feedback are also used in assertion therapy to help the patient evolve strategies of behaviour for expressing his thoughts and feelings appropriately.

Social skills training (S.S.T.) programmes are designed to teach "social inadequates" more effective ways of behaving in inter-personal settings, although "social phobics" can apparently benefit as well (Trower *et al.*, 1978). This treatment method is much more closely linked to skills theory and the experimental research carried out into social interactions (e.g. Argyle, 1975) than is assertion therapy. This means that in S.S.T. there is much more emphasis on modifying specific responses, e.g. eye contact, directly, rather than evolving more global strategies. An additional difference is that, instead of concentrating on "output" skills, social skills trainers also help to teach "perceiver" skills, e.g. reading signals from body posture, and "receiver" skills, e.g. acknowledging the other person's message.

S.S.T. is usually carried out in a group setting, not only for time-economy reasons, but because this arrangement facilitates the simulation of social situations. Clearly it is outside the scope of this chapter to discuss such practical details as patient selection, optimal size of groups, the therapists' roles, and treatment termination. The interested reader is referred to Johnson (1973) for advice as to how to conduct group therapy along behavioural lines. As in the case of assertiveness training, the basic treatment components are model-ling, behaviour rehearsal, feedback and homework assignments. In addition, a wide range of exercises are now available to help patients to acquire specific communication skills (*see* Trower *et al.*, 1978).

Although S.S.T. is currently very popular in behaviour therapy circles, the results obtained from various outcome studies are dis-appointing. As far as out-patients are concerned, S.S.T. can bring about improved social functioning and symptomatic improvement but is no more effective than systematic desensitisation. The evidence from in-patient studies is even less encouraging. Although S.S.T. can increase the interpersonal effectiveness of acute and chronic schizophrenics and other disturbed patients, there are no reports in the literature of long-term clinical improvement resulting from this type of intervention (Marzilier, 1978).

In the opinion of this author, the main reason for these disappoint-ing results is that there has been a tendency for S.S.T. to be over-prescribed. Any psychiatric patient who is lonely or socially gauche is a potential candidate for this approach. In many of these cases, however, a full behavioural analysis would reveal that S.S.T. should be applied following a course of, say, anxiety-management training or assertion therapy. Thus although S.S.T. is a potentially useful technique, it is usually best administered in conjunction with other techniques as part of a comprehensive behavioural package.

A rather different technique for increasing the frequency of desired behaviour is *masturbatory fantasy retraining*. As its name might suggest, this procedure is used exclusively with patients who have sexual difficulties. More specifically, its purpose is to increase sexual responsivity to members of the opposite sex. For this purpose two variations of this form of retraining are currently employed, of which the better known is the method developed by Marquis (1970). Here the patient is instructed to masturbate, using his usual fantasy, until the point just prior to ejaculatory inevitability. He is then encouraged to switch to a heterosexual fantasy so that it will coincide with orgasm. In this way an association is built up between heterosexual stimuli and the height of sexual arousal. After he has been successful on several consecutive occasions, he is requested to switch fantasies at increasingly earlier stages until heterosexual images are being employed at the outset. If, at any stage, the patient feels that his level of arousal is diminishing, he should switch back to the original fantasy and change once again once he is more highly aroused. Marquis (1970) has found this technique to be effective with a wide range of sexual deviants.

The other masturbatory retraining method to be considered here is the one proposed by Annon (1973). Here, instead of replacing one fantasy with another, the original fantasy is gradually modified until a more adaptive erotic image has been obtained. One of the cases he describes is that of an orgasmic dysfunctional girl who typically used multi-rape fantasies when masturbating. In the early stages of treatment, it was suggested that she use the fantasy of large groups of men engaged in non-aggressive activities. She was then instructed to imagine small groups of men, two men, and finally her partner approaching her in a more acceptable manner. Once again, this technique is usually implemented in conjunction with other behavioural methods.

Summary
Behavioural psychotherapy is a form of treatment which is loosely based on the conditioning paradigms of Pavlov and Skinner. Although terms such as stimulus, response, reinforcement and generalisation are used by practitioners of this approach, they bear only a superficial resemblance, for the most part, to the equivalent terms employed by experimental psychologists. Self-statements, e.g. "Provided I concentrate on relaxing I can cope", social behaviour, e.g. introducing oneself to a stranger, and self-reinforcement, e.g. "I did well', seem

very far removed from the flashing lights, bar presses, and food deliveries of the operant conditioning laboratory. Nevertheless, behavioural psychotherapists and experimental psychologists are in agreement about the broad principles concerning the orderliness of behaviour. Furthermore the hypothesis building and testing of the behavioural assessment procedure are close to the ideals of all concerned with learning principles.

The key features of the approach are as follows.

(a) Each patient requires his own individualised programme. Although diagnosis can serve as a useful shorthand, it is only of limited value so far as treatment decisions are concerned.

(b) The therapist and patient make a contract at the outset to achieve certain objectives. These can be changed at any time but, in the event, both parties must be fully aware of any alterations to their agreement.

(c) The patient must take on some responsibility for decisions regarding objectives, hypothesis testing, treatment decisions, and the proper implementation of techniques. The fact that he may be unable to abandon the "sick role" in the initial stages, does not automatically signify that a behavioural approach is inappropriate. It is possible to employ conditioning principles, with the knowledge of the patient, to help him to co-operate more fully.

(d) The focal point of treatment is the present and immediate future. Past history and long-term goals are of only marginal relevance to the work of the behavioural psychotherapist. He is much more concerned to isolate carefully the stimuli which are currently maintaining the maladaptive behaviour than to explore possible causes and hypothesise about the distant future.

(e) Although behavioural psychotherapists are particularly interested in intervening at the level of overt behaviour, they are capable of working at the cognitive level and will choose to do so where appropriate. Furthermore, it is generally assumed that cognitive and affective changes follow behavioural gains.

Behaviour modification

The term "behaviour modification" is currently employed in two different ways. Sometimes it is used as a synonym for behaviour therapy. In other words it is thought to subsume all types of behavioural intervention and indeed any technique, e.g. hypnosis, which can be conceptualised in learning theory terms (Watson, 1962). Presumably one reason why "modification" is preferred by some to "therapy" is on account of the medical model connotations of the latter term. However others (e.g. Kiernan, 1975) prefers to reserve the use of behaviour modification to refer to the application of

Skinnerian principles, in their purest form, with human subjects. The term is used here in its least inclusive sense.

Behaviour modification differs from the behavioural psycho-therapy approach in the following ways.

(a) Although cognitive processes and language are by no means excluded from this work, the emphasis is much more on stimuli and responses which can be objectively described. Consequently the assessment tools used are based on observation rather than on self-reports by patients.

(b) Treatment techniques are closely based on the operant con-ditioning paradigms of Skinner and, to a lesser extent, on the experimental designs utilised by Bandura and others in studies of imitation learning. Thus the classical conditioning model, from which such techniques as systematic desensitisation, flooding and aversion therapy were derived, does not play a part here.

(c) Behaviour modifiers argue that change is more likely to occur through environmental alterations rather than as a result of brief therapy sessions in a setting far removed from everyday situations. As Ullman and Krasner (1965) point out, "all behaviour modifica-tion boils down to procedures utilising systematic environmental contingencies to alter the subjects' response to stimuli". Conse-quently the patient-therapist relationship is considered to be of much less importance here.

(d) So far as its applications in a medical setting are concerned, behaviour modification is usually carried out with patients who are mentally handicapped or psychotic, and who have spent a number of years in institutions. Operant conditioning programmes for eating disorders and biofeedback courses for psychosomatic disturbances are obvious exceptions.

(e) The nature of the contract between the change agent (thera-pist) and the patient is something which is not dealt with at length in the behaviour modification literature. By and large, it is the staff members who stipulate the programme targets although, in more re-cent studies, different goals have been set for each individual patient, according to his specific requirements. Nevertheless, statements such as "minor resistances following the implementation of contin-gent reinforcement procedures come as no surprise" (Kazdin and Bootzin, 1973) illustrate the fact that the patient undergoing be-haviour modification has much less responsibility for making decisions regarding the aims, design and methodology of his pro-gramme than his opposite number in behavioural psychotherapy.

Since the principles of operant conditioning and imitation have already been considered, it will only be necessary to describe some of the ways in which they have been applied by behaviour modifiers.

The various studies in this area can be usefully considered under the following three headings:

1. simple operant programmes;
2. ward management schemes;
3. biofeedback procedures.

1. *Simple operant programmes*

One of the classic examples of response shaping with human subjects is a treatment programme devised by Lovaas (1966) to induce speech in autistic children. The positive reinforcements used in this study were sweets and social approval. In the first stage of the programme, the patients were rewarded following the emission of any sound whatsoever. In the next stage, they were rewarded only for making a sound in response to a verbal signal provided by a staff member. When this had been mastered, successive approximations to the words uttered by the change agent were reinforced. As progress continued to be made, objects corresponding to these words were introduced while the rewards themselves were faded out. As before, only good approximations were rewarded. By the end of the programme, these children were able to form short sentences by chaining various responses together. Clearly, in this example, both modelling and response shaping were involved.

An example of an operant conditioning programme which involves the establishment of response "chains" in addition to shaping is provided by Watson (1973) in a study involving mentally retarded and autistic children. Many everyday behavioural sequences comprise a series of discrete responses which are closely interlinked. For example, the act of dressing oneself can be divided up into the following five components: putting on firstly, underpants, secondly, trousers, thirdly, shirt, fourthly, socks and lastly shoes. In a "chaining programme", the behaviour modifier works initially with the final response in the sequence, which is the one which is usually followed by reinforcement in the natural setting. Thus, in this example, he would dress the child but leave him to put on his shoes. Practical assistance, verbal cues, shaping procedures and social approval would be used until the response had been learned. The patient would then be trained to perform the preceding response. Each link in the chain would then be dealt with in their temporal sequence until the complete exercise could be carried out on command. Chaining procedures are very effective so far as teaching self-help skills to uncommunicative patients are concerned.

A quite different example of behaviour modification through the implementation of simple operant procedures is the *anorexia nervosa* case described by Bachrach *et al.* (1965). The patient was a 37-year-old divorcee who weighed forty-seven pounds at the beginning of the programme. A behavioural analysis revealed that one potentially powerful reinforcer for eating behaviour was having people read to her. She was then removed from her pleasant hospital room and placed in a "barren experimental box". When food was presented, movements associated with eating, e.g. spearing a piece of meat, were reinforced by the therapist talking about something she was interested in. Successive approximations to each of the required responses were reinforced in the manner described above. Once she started to consume food, access to radio and television was provided as an additional incentive. As time went on, more and more food had to be eaten until eventually she had to consume everything on her plate before receiving her reward. By the end of her stay in hospital, her weight had doubled, she took greater interest in her appearance, and interacted more frequently with other patients.

One reason why this study is quoted so frequently is because the authors took care to ensure that the eating response they had shaped up would generalise to the outside world. Specific instructions were given to members of the patient's family who agreed to supervise her following discharge. In brief, they were told to make meal time an enjoyable social occasion and not be overconcerned about her eating behaviour. Weight-gain was to be reinforced by compliments while any other forms of maladaptive behaviour were to be ignored. As a result of this programme, the patient was able to get a job and lead a relatively normal life, although she remained thin.

2. Ward management schemes
For many institutionalised patients, contact with nurses and doctors is a highly reinforcing event. However, in view of the low staff/patient ratio in most establishments, this type of reward is in short supply. One way of getting attention from the staff is to behave in a disturbed fashion. Ayllon and his co-workers in a series of investigations into the behaviour of psychotics in closed wards (e.g. Ayllon and Michael, 1959. Ayllon and Haughton, 1962), observed that "undesirable" responses, e.g. excessive washing, hoarding, feeding disturbances, were usually socially reinforced by the nursing staff whereas "desirable" behaviours were typically ignored. Consequently they implemented a change in ward management policy, so that only desirable behaviour would be followed by a reward. The positive reinforcers used in studies of this kind were mainly social approval, conversation, food and cigarettes. At the same time, steps were taken to ensure that undesirable behaviour would not be reinforced in the future. Thus, at meal times, for example, patients were not persuaded or helped to enter the canteen and failure to do so unaided, within a stipulated period, meant that they would forgo the meal. Those

who did manage to go into the dining room by themselves, within the time limit, were reinforced immediately with social approval.

Despite the apparently sound rationale underlying this approach, the early studies were not particularly effective in changing behaviour. These disappointing results were attributed to the fact that many of the reinforcers were relatively intangible and, furthermore, could not always be administered immediately after the performance of the target behaviour. Consequently, tokens, i.e. plastic discs, which could be exchanged later for desired objects and activities were introduced in order to bridge the gap between the activity and the reward. The additional advantages in using tokens are as follows.

(a) Tokens are not subject to satiation to the same extent as, say, food rewards, since they can be exchanged for a wide variety of reinforcers.

(b) The amount of reward the patient receives can be varied according to the level of his performance.

(c) The fact that the patient decides which primary rewards he will receive means that he plays a more active role in this type of scheme than in more orthodox operant programmes. The opportunity for autonomy within the structured system is presumed to be an additional therapeutic component of this type of treatment approach.

(d) The notion of receiving tokens for tasks accomplished is analogous to the way in which rewards are administered in real life. Consequently the system itself can play a useful role in the rehabilitation of the patient.

The classic series of experiments into *token economy* procedures are those reported by Ayllon and Azrin (1965). In each of the studies, tokens earned could be exchanged for the opportunity to engage in recreational activities, permission to leave the ward for specific periods, interviews with staff members, privileges relating to privacy, and a variety of articles which could not normally be exchanged in the hospital. In some studies, tokens were made contingent on desired behaviour, e.g. dressing, feeding, making the bed wheareas, in others, the number of tokens awarded depended on the standard of work during a six-hour stint on a job assignment. So far as the latter research is concerned, it was demonstrated that patients would work harder on non-preferred tasks which they were "paid" for than when carrying out tasks which they found intrinsically rewarding, but for which tokens were no longer given. The over-all findings were that the frequency of target behaviours increased when they were followed by tokens but that when the incentives were withdrawn there was a significant decrease in the response rate. Although this work is extremely interesting from the scientific point of view, the fact that the patients' behaviour returned to approximately base-line level following procedural alterations would suggest that its clinical applicability is limited.

More recently, attempts have been made to modify the original token-economy procedure in an attempt to increase the amount of transfer from the experimental to the natural setting. In a later publication (1968) Ayllon and Azrin, with this issue in mind, have proposed the *Relevance of Behaviour Rule.* They advise change agents to "teach only those behaviours that will continue to be reinforced after training". However, as Kazdin and Bootzin (1973) point out, this rule is not easy to follow as it sounds. In the real life setting, failure to carry out socially appropriate behaviour, e.g. self-care skills, is likely to be punished whereas its performance may not be positively reinforced. At the same time, rewards may be provided following deviant behaviour which had been effectively suppressed in the hospital setting. In view of the fact that the Relevance of Behaviour Rule is insufficient by itself, Kazdin and Bootzin (1973) have put forward several practical suggestions to help increase the amount of generalisation from ward to home. Their major recommendations are as follows:

(a) *Social reinforcement/fading out of tokens.* Following hospital discharge, social reinforcement can help to maintain the desirable behaviour, at least in structured situations, e.g. in school, at home. One way of increasing the reward value of praise is to pair it with token delivery and then gradually fade out the latter. The major limitation of social rewards is that they are relatively unlikely to be administered in everyday situations over which the therapist has no control, e.g. shops, parties.

(b) *Stimulus variation.* Although it is useful to deliver reinforcement in a restricted setting in the early stages of the programme, it is essential to carry out this work in a variety of settings with different therapists before formal treatment is terminated.

(c) *Levelled token economies.* With this system (Lloyd and Abel, 1970), the patient is initially rewarded for carrying out minimal responses in a situation where few reinforcers are available. After he has been performing well at this level for a prolonged period, he progresses to the next stage. Here it is more difficult to obtain reinforcers but they are more plentiful and varied. He works though the various levels in this way until he is able to perform highly desirable behaviours, e.g. work in the community, without receiving tokens. Although this would appear to be a potentially useful procedure for aiding generalisation, it remains to be properly evaluated.

(d) Training the patient's relatives. There are now a number of reports, e.g. Henderson and Scoles (1970), which suggest that family members can be effectively trained to manage the behaviour of the patient by means of operant principles in the home setting.

(e) Self-reinforcement. Although supportive research data is lacking, Kazdin and Bootzin can see long-term advantages in allowing patients to reinforce themselves in token economy regimes once the target behaviour is well established. However they concede that this could present problems with mentally retarded patients who are likely to experience difficulty in delaying gratification until the performance criteria have been met.

(f) Delay of reinforcement. In token-economy systems, it is possible to increase both the interval between the response and the token and between the token and the back-up reinforcer. Since reinforcement is very often delayed in the real-life setting, it is likely that training the patient to cope with reward postponement will increase his resistance to extinction. Again this hypothesis requires experimental verification.

Although there is no doubt that the behaviour of a large percentage of institutionalised patients can be significantly improved through the implementation of a ward management scheme, the evidence that these gains can transfer to the extra-treatment situation is less convincing. Clearly it is important to design programmes which include features pertinent to generalisation. Of the suggestions outlined above, it would seem probable that the co-operation of members of the patients' various social systems, e.g. family, work group, is the single most important factor so far as long-term efficacy is concerned.

3. Biofeedback procedures.

As pointed out earlier in this chapter, biofeedback is the name given to a variety of techniques aimed at bringing some aspect of physiological functioning under voluntary control. By this is meant that, when certain cues are present, the individual learns that changing one or more aspects of his bodily functioning in a specified direction will be followed by a desirable outcome. Thus, although visceral rather than skeletal responses are involved here, principles of operant conditioning would seem to apply. The finding (Miller, 1969) that autonomic responses can be controlled by direct means is of theoretical as well as of clinical significance since, before that time, it had been assumed that classical conditioning was concerned purely with the autonomic system, whereas operant conditioning dealt exclusively with the central nervous system. Not only has this work cast some doubts on the validity of the distinction between the two types of conditioning, but it has also raised the issue of whether psychosomatic and hysterical disorders can be clearly differentiated on aetiological grounds. These issues are discussed at length by Miller (*ibid*).

The main difference between the use of biofeedback techniques in behavioural psychotherapy and in behaviour modification is that, in the former, the aim is to produce a generalised state of calmness whereas in the latter, the main objective is to bring one or more specific responses under control. Therefore in this section, no mention will be made of the various studies which have demonstrated that control of, say, alpha activity can give rise to a relaxed state. Only the use of operant techniques to modify a particular response which is, in itself, a source of discomfort, will be considered here. Of the many disorders which have been treated in this way, the following four have been selected because of their potential clinical utility:

(*a*) tension headaches;
(*b*) epilepsy;
(*c*) essential hypertension;
(*d*) cardiac arrhythmia.

(*a*) *Tension headaches.* On the assumption that tension headaches are related to increased activity in the frontalis muscle group, Budzynski *et al.* (1970) devised a programme which involved providing electromyographic (E.M.G.) feedback from this specific area. The signal was a musical tone, the pitch of which was related to the degree of activity. After two preliminary relaxation sessions without feedback, the auditory signal was switched on and the patient was instructed to keep the tone as low as possible, i.e. corresponding to low E.M.G. level. The first patients who were treated in this way were also advised to practise relaxation at home. It was found that there was a steady decrease in E.M.G. level and activity over the training period. However tension headaches were only eliminated completely in two patients. One patient experienced less severe symptoms while the remaining two relapsed shortly after treatment termination.

In her recent review of research in this area, Philips (1977) makes the important point that the degree of muscle tension, subjectively expressed pain, and pain-motivated behaviour do not interrelate in a consistent manner. For instance, there is no evidence to support the common-sense prediction that the E.M.G. level of the frontalis muscle is higher during a headache period than during a control period. Similarly, in the experiment that she describes in depth, although the reduction in muscular activity which followed biofeedback training was accompanied by a drop in reported pain levels, more medication was actually taken by patients at this time. Results such as these suggest that there is more involved in tension headaches than simply a physiological abnormality. Consequently there is a need to develop other types of intervention to be used in conjunction with E.M.G. feed-back.

(b) Epilepsy. Since epileptic fits are typically preceded by an abnormal E.E.G. pattern, one obvious application of biofeedback is to train patients to exercise control over brain activity, thereby reducing the frequency of seizures. In an early study in this area, Miller (1969) reported that the provision of feed-back, whenever paroxysmal spikes occurred, led to a reduction in the frequency of abnormal E.E.G. responses. However no data was provided in this study concerning the clinical effects of this training or the degree of transfer to situations outside the laboratory.

A rather different approach is that described by Sterman (1973). Rather than teach patients to recognise and deal with E.E.G. abnormalities, he advocates training in order to maximise the occurrence of an optimal *sensorimotor rhythm.* Auditory feedback is provided whenever a rhythm of between twelve and fourteen Hertz is recorded over the sensorimotor cortex. The patient is instructed to increase the frequency of the signal which he has been told corresponds to brain activity. This study is particularly interesting from the methodological point of view since attempts were made to use patients as their own controls in an endeavour to determine the efficacy of the biofeedback procedure as such. The results demonstrated convincingly that decreases in seizure frequency were associated with the experimental trials, while the base-line rate returned after a few weeks without training. Despite these encouraging results, ways of improving generalisability will have to be developed if self-control of E.E.G. activity is to be used clinically as a treatment for seizure disorders.

(c) Essential hypertension. The most celebrated study in this area is the one carried out by Benson *et al.* (1971). Base-line sessions were conducted initially with each patient until stable levels of systolic blood pressure were recorded over five consecutive sessions. The experimental procedure, which involved providing patients with both auditory and visual feedback on a beat-to-beat basis, was then implemented in an endeavour to bring about a decrease in blood pressure. Treatment was discontinued when no further reduction took place over five consecutive sessions. Although five of the seven patients demonstrated significant decreases in systolic blood pressure, only two were able to reach normal limits. However, since no follow-

up data were provided, it is difficult to assess the clinical utility of biofeedback techniques in relation to hypertension at this stage.

(d) Cardiac arrhythmias. Much of the work in this area has been carried out by Engel and his associates (e.g. Engel, 1977; Weiss and Engel, 1971). The procedure they employ in all their cardiac conditioning studies is as follows. One of two lights is switched on to indicate to the patient whether heart acceleration or deceleration is required. A third light comes on when the patient is performing correctly and is switched off during a period when he is functioning badly. The criteria for good performance are established, for each individual patient, during the base-line period which immediately precedes the training period.

A wide variety of cardiac arrhythmias, e.g. premature ventricular contractions (P.V.C.), atrial fibrillation, atrial and ventricular tachycardia, have been treated by these workers by means of heart rate control training. It is difficult to summarise this work because it comprises a series of case reports rather than controlled treatment trials. Some of the most interesting findings are as follows. Patients with atrial fibrillation, through learning ventricular control, were able to synchronise the generation of impulses through the atrioventricular node. One patient learnt to produce or inhibit ventricular ectopic beats by altering his heart rate. As a result of direct feedback, a patient with Wolff-Parkinson-Whyte syndrome learned to produce both normally conducted beats and abnormally conducted beats on request. This ability was still present ten weeks after the termination of training.

The nearest to a controlled study in this area is the work carried out with eight P.V.C. patients (Weiss and Engel, 1971). Five patients demonstrated decreases in P.V.C. rate, although one could not maintain this progress whenever feedback was withdrawn. However no consistent patterns emerged between patient response and phase of treatment, e.g. slowing or speeding of heart rate or keeping the heart rate within a range. Consequently no overall conclusions regarding the relative contributions of the various treatment components can be drawn.

Although biofeedback is one of the most exciting areas of behaviour modification, it suffers from the same limitations as token economy systems and, indeed, operant conditioning programmes in general. Unless it can be shown that transfer of training can take place from the ward or laboratory setting to the home situation then its clinical utility will be restricted. Furthermore, even if these procedures can be made more sophisticated to facilitate generalisation, biofeedback techniques will never be the treatment of choice until it can be demonstrated that they compare favourably with more orthodox medical treatments as far as cost-effectiveness is concerned. Consequently the advice given in an editorial of the *British Medical Journal* (1974), that "clinicians should keep a keen but critical watch on this research", is as appropriate now as when it was first delivered.

Summary

Operant conditioning programmes, ward management schemes and biofeedback techniques have, as was suggested at the beginning of this section, many features in common. It will be useful, at this stage, to re-examine briefly the five characteristics of behaviour modification procedures in the light of the material reviewed.

(a) The focal point of these treatment methods is behaviour which can be precisely defined and reliably measured. Whether the response under consideration is a drop in systolic blood pressure or a fork being lifted to mouth, objectivity is given particular emphasis.

(b) Patients are reinforced for carrying out specific responses under particular stimulus conditions in keeping with operant conditioning principles. However it should be noted that, in all cases, the patients are told what they have to do in order to receive rewards. This is an important departure from the experimental work with infra-human subjects. Nevertheless behaviour modifiers are clearly more faithful to basic operant principles than behavioural psychotherapists.

(c) Although it is likely that the patient-therapist relationship in the anorexia study (Bacharach *et al.*, 1965) was of some therapeutic significance, most of the studies referred to place the emphasis on the environmental changes rather than on non-specific factors associated with patient communication.

(d) Although the patients used in these studies are not all institutionalised, they are all helpless to a degree and require assistance from an external agent in order to ascertain what changes are required and how these goals can be achieved.

(e) It follows from this that the change agent (therapist) determines which responses will be modified and how change will be effected. The only exception here is those token-economy programmes where the individual can choose to work for extrinsic or intrinsic reinforcers. Otherwise the therapist is totally in control of the programme.

CONCLUSIONS

Behaviour therapy has made considerable progress since the early writings of Wolpe and Eysenck. Not only have a wide variety of techniques emerged, but the process of assessment and problem formulation has become much more sophisticated. At the same time the gulf between the "experimentally established principles of learning" (Wolpe, 1968) and clinical practice appears to be widening. Nowadays the pragmatic practitioner, faced with a challenging problem, is more likely to improvise or "invent" a new technique which would appear to be appropriate for his patient, rather than to consult the literature on the bar-pressing behaviour of pigeons in order to develop one from first principles. However, the fact that behaviour therapists are not so concerned as formerly to explain all their interventions in stimulus-response terms does not mean that they have abandoned their beliefs in the importance of objectivity, openness to refutation, and other scientific principles (Popper, 1963). For example, the fact that the validity of the statements of Eysenck and others, that behaviour therapy is significantly more effective than any other kind of psychotherapy, has been challenged (e.g. Shapiro, 1979) testifies to the fact that a weakening of the theoretical foundations of the approach has not led to intellectual apathy or a diminution of experimental zeal.

So far as the future is concerned, the goals of behaviour therapists should not be solely to produce more and more techniques. As has been emphasised throughout this chapter, the difficult task is not finding and implementing a procedure to do a particular job but deciding which type of intervention to carry out. What is required most of all, therefore, is the development of a research strategy which will meet both the needs of the clinician for flexibility and the objectivity requirements of the research worker. In this regard, the approach of Lewinsohn (1975) seems to be particularly promising.

One clinical research area which has been relatively neglected until now is the relationship of the *behaviour of the therapist* to the type of change which occurs. Many behaviour therapists will admit (privately, at least) that often a patient gets better "before he is supposed to". Rather than regard such an occurrence with embarrassment, clinicians should be encouraged to explore the factors responsible for non-predicted improvement and attempt to utilise them in their future work. Research with large groups of therapists could help to clarify whether it is possible to make generalisations concerning certain features of the interaction process between patient and therapist.

Behaviour therapists must also concentrate more on developing strategies for increasing the involvement of patients throughout the treatment process. In both behavioural psychotherapy and behaviour modification programmes, the most intricately designed methodology will prove ineffective if the patient's attitudes to his problems are not in accord with those of the change agent (therapist). Thus, the patient who is convinced he is "ill" and needs "proper treatment" is as unlikely to participate fully in an anxiety-management training programme as he is in a token-economy system. It is surprising, in view of the extensive psychological literature on attitude change, that behaviour therapists have not yet developed standard induction courses for patients prior to undergoing treatment. It is likely that such a development would significantly increase the cost-effectiveness of the whole approach.

Finally, at a time when there is comparatively little rivalry between behaviour therapy and the other approaches, there is a need for combined treatment research programmes to determine which kinds of problems and, indeed, patients, each school works best with. Behaviour therapy, like psychotherapy and chemotherapy, has its limitations, and it is in the interests of all parties concerned that these should be clearly recognised. As a result, the likelihood of patients undergoing time-consuming programmes which fail to meet their needs will be significantly reduced.

REFERENCES

Annon, J. S. (1973): "The therapeutic use of masturbation in the treatment of sexual disorders", in R. D. Rubin, J. P. Brady and J. D. Henderson (Eds.), *Advances in Behavior Therapy Vol. 4*, Academic Press, New York.

Argyle, M. (1975): *Bodily Communication,* Methuen, London.

Ayllon, T. and Azrin, N. H. (1965): "The measurement and reinforcement of behavior of psychotics", *J. exp. Anal. Behav.,* 8, 375-383.

Ayllon, T. and Azrin, N. H. (1968): *The Token Economy: A Motivational System for Therapy and Rehabilitation*, Appleton-Century-Crofts, New York.

Ayllon, T. and Haughton, E. (1962): "Control of the behaviour of schizophrenic patients by food", *J. exp. Anal. Behav.,* 5, 343-352.

Ayllon, T. and Michael, J. (1959): "The psychiatric nurse as a behavioral engineer", *J. exp. Anal. Behav.,* 3, 323-334.

Bachrach, A. J., Erwin, W. J. and Mohr, J. P. (1965): "The control of eating behavior of an anorexic by operant conditioning techniques", in L. P. Ullmann and L. Krasner (Eds.), *Case Studies in Behavior Modification,* Holt, Rinehart and Winston, New York.

Bancroft, J., Jones, G. J. and Pullan, B. R. (1966): "A simple transducer for measuring penile erection, with comments on its use in the treatment of sexual disorders", *Behav. Res. Ther.,* **4,** 239-241.

Bandura, A. (1969): *Principles of Behavior Modification,* Holt, Rinehart and Winston, New York.

Beck, A. (1970): "Cognitive therapy: Nature and relation to behavior therapy", *Behav. Ther.,* **1,** 184-200.

Beech, H. R. (1976): "Behaviour modification", Ch. in H. J. Eysenck and G. D. Wilson (Eds.), *A Textbook of Human Psychology,* Medical and Technical Publishers, MTP Press, Lancaster, England.

Benson, H., Shapiro, C., Tursky, B. and Schwartz, G. E. (1971): "Decreased systolic blood pressure through operant conditioning techniques in patients with essential hypertension", *Science,* **173,** 740-742.

Bergin, A. E. (1971): "The evaluation of therapeutic outcomes", in A. E. Bergin and S. I. Garfield (Eds.), *Handbook of Psychotherapy and Behavior Change,* Wiley, New York.

Bookbinder, L. (1962): "Simple conditioning versus the dynamic approach to symptom and symptom substitution: a reply to Yates", *Psychol. Rev.,* **10,** 71-77.

Brady, J. P. (1972): "Systematic desensitization", in W. S. Agras (Ed.), *Behavior Modification: Principles and Clinical Applications,* Little, Brown, Boston.

Breger, L. and McGaugh, J. (1965): "Critique and reformulation of 'learning theory' approaches to psychotherapy and neurosis", *Psychol. Bull.,* **63,** 338-358.

British Medical Journal (1974): Editorial, *Brit. Med. J.* 17th August, 427-428.

Brown, P. T. (1975): "What is behavioural psychotherapy?", in D. Bannister (Ed.) *Issues and Approaches in the Psychological Therapies,* Wiley, London.

Budzynski, T., Stoyva, J. and Adler, C. (1970): "Feed-back-induced muscle relaxation: application to tension headache", *J. Behav. Ther. & Exp. Psychiat.,* **1,** 205-211.

Cautela, J. R. (1967): "Covert sensitization", *Psychol. Rep.,* **20,** 459-468.

Crown, S. (1976): "Psychoanalytic psychotherapy", in D. Bannister (Ed.) *Issues and Approaches in the Psychological Therapies,* Wiley, London.

Davidson, P. O., Payne, R. W. and Sloane, R. B. (1966): "Cortical inhibition, drive level and conditioning", *J. abnorm. soc. Psychol.*, **71**, 310-314.

Elwood, D. L. (1975): "Automation methods", Ch. 14 in F. H. Kanfer and A. P. Goldstein (Eds.) *Helping People Change*, Pergamon, New York.

Engel, B. T. (1977): "Operant conditioning of cardiovascular function: a behavioural analysis", Ch.4 in S. Rachman (Ed.), *Contributions to Medical Psychology Vol. 1.*, Pergamon, Oxford.

Eysenck, H. J. (1952): "The effects of psychotherapy: an evaluation", *J. consult. Psychol.*, **16**, 319-324.

Eysenck, H. J. (1957): *Dynamics of Anxiety and Hysteria*, Routledge and Kegan Paul, London.

Eysenck, H. J. (1960): "The effects of psychotherapy" in H. J. Eysenck (Ed.) *Handbook of Abnormal Psychology*, Pitmans, London.

Eysenck, H. J. (1966): *The Effects of Psychotherapy: an evaluation*, International Science Press, New York.

Eysenck, H. J. (1976): "The learning theory model of neurosis – a new approach", *Behav. Res. Ther.*, **14**, 251-267.

Feldman, M. P. and MacCulloch, M. J. (1971): *Homosexual Behaviour: Therapy and Assessment*, Pergamon, Oxford.

Ferster, C. B. (1965): "Classification of behavioral pathology", in L. P. Ullman and L. Krasner (Eds.), *Research in Behavior Modification*, Holt, Rinehart and Winston, New York.

Festinger, L. (1957): *A Theory of Cognitive Dissonance*, Row, Peterson, Evanston, Illinois.

Franks, C. M. (1963): "Behavior therapy: the principles of conditioning and the treatment of the alcoholic", *Q. J. Stud. Alcohol*, **24**, 511-529.

Fransella, F. and Bannister, D. (1977): *A Manual for the Repertory Grid Technique*, Academic Press, London.

Geer, J. H. (1965): "The development of a scale to measure fear", *Behav. Res. Ther.*, **3**, 45-53.

Goldstein, A. P. and Stein, N. (1976): *Prescriptive Psychotherapies*, Pergamon, New York.

Gray, J. (1971): *The Psychology of Fear and Stress*, World University Library, Weidenfeld & Nicholson, London.

Henderson, J. D. and Scoles, P. E. (1970): "Conditioning techniques in a community-based operant environment for psychotic men", *Behav. Ther.*, **1**, 245-251.

Hersen, M. and Bellack, A. S. (Eds.) (1976): *Behavioral Assessment: A Practical Handbook*, Pergamon, New York.

Hiroto, D. S. (1974): "Locus of control and learned helplessness", *J. exp. Psychol.*, **102**, 187-193.

Isaacs, W., Thomas, J. and Goldiamond, I. (1960): "Application of

operant conditioning to reinstate verbal behaviour in psychotics",
J. Speech Hearing Disord., **25**, 8-12.

Jackson, B. (1972):"Treatment of depression by self-reinforcement,
Behav. Ther., **3**, 298-307.

Jacobson, E. (1938): *Progressive Relaxation,* Chicago University
Press, Chicago.

Johnson, W. G. (1975): "Group therapy: a behavioral perspective",
Behav. Ther., **6**, 30-38.

Jones, M. C. (1924): "A laboratory study of fear: the case of
Peter", *Pedagog. Semin.,* **31**, 308-315.

Kanfer, F. H. and Karoly, P. (1972): "Self-control: A behavioral
excursion into the lion's den", *Behav. Ther.,* **3**, 398-416.

Kanfer, F. H. and Phillips, J. S. (1970): *Learning Foundations of
Behavior Therapy,* Wiley, New York.

Kazdin, A. E. and Bootzin, R. R. (1973): "The token economy: An
examination of issues", in R. D. Rubin, J. P. Brady, and J. D.
Henderson (Eds.) *Advances in Behavior Therapy Vol. 4,* Academic
Press, New York.

Kendell, R. E. (1976): "The classification of depression: a review of
contemporary confusion", *Brit. J. Psychiat.,* **129**, 15-28.

Kiernan, C. (1975): "Behavior Modification", in D. Bannister (Ed.),
Issues and Approaches in the Psychological Therapies, Wiley,
London.

Lemere, F., and Voegtlin, W. L. (1950): "An evaluation of the
aversive treatment of alcoholism", *Q. J. Stud. Alcohol.,* **11**,
199-204.

Lewinsohn, P. M. (1975): "The behavioural study and treatment of
depression", in M. Hersen, R. Eisler and P. Miller (Eds.), *Progress
in Behaviour Modification, Vol. 1.,* Academic Press, New York.

Liberman, R. P., King, L. W., De Risi, W. and McCann, M. (1975):
Personal Effectiveness, Research Press, Champaign, Illinois.

Lloyd, K. E. and Abel, L. (1970): "Performance on a token
economy psychiatric ward: A two year summary", *Behav. Res.
Ther.,* **8**, 1-9.

Loeb, A., Beck, A. T., Diggory, J. C. and Tuthill, R. (1967):
"Expectancy, level of aspiration, performance and self-evaluation
in depression". *Proceedings of the 75th annual convention of the
American Psychological Association,* **2**, 193-194.

Lovaas, O. I. (1966): "A program for the establishment of speech in
psychotic children", in J. K. Wing (Ed.), *Early Childhood
Autism,* Pergamon, Oxford.

McGuire, R. J., Carlisle, J. M. and Young, B. G. (1965): "Sexual
deviations as conditioned behaviour: a hypothesis", *Behav. Res.
Ther.,* **2**, 185-190.

Mackay, D. (1975): *Clinical Psychology: Theory and Therapy,* Methuen, London.

Mackay, D. (1976): "Modification of sexual behaviour", in S. Crown (Ed.), *Psychosexual Problems,* Academic Press, London.

Mackay, D. (1977): "Learning", in J. C. Coleman (Ed.) *Introductory Psychology,* Routledge and Kegan Paul, London.

Marquis, J. N. (1970): "Orgasmic conditioning: changing sexual object choice through controlling masturbation fantasies", *J. Behav. Ther. & Exp. Psychiat.,* 1, 263-271.

Marston, A. R. (1969): "Dealing with low self-confidence", *Educ. Res.,* 63, 134-138.

Marzillier, J. (1978): "Outcome studies of skills training: a review", in *Social Skills and Mental Health,* Methuen, London.

Meichenbaum, D. (1975): "Self-instructional methods", in F. H. Kanfer and A. P. Goldstein (Eds.), *Helping People Change,* Pergamon, New York.

Meyer, V. and Crisp, A. (1964): "Aversion therapy in two cases of obesity", *Behav. Res. Ther.,* 2, 143-147.

Meyer, V., Levi, R. and Schnurer, A. (1974): "The behavioural treatment of obsessive-compulsive disorders", in H. R. Beech (Ed.), *Obsessional States,* Methuen, London.

Meyer, A. J. and Henderson, J. B. (1974): "Multiple risk factor reduction in the prevention of cardiovascular disease", *Prevent. Med.,* 3, 225-236.

Miller, N. E. (1969): "Learning of visceral and glandular responses", *Science,* 163, 434-445.

Mischel, W. (1968): *Personality and Assessment,* Wiley, New York.

Morris, R. J. (1975): "Fear reduction methods", in F. H. Kanfer and A. P. Goldstein (Eds.), *Helping People Change,* Pergamon, Oxford.

Mowrer, O. H. (1947): "On the dual nature of learning — a reinterpretation of 'conditioning' and 'problem solving' ", *Harvard educ. Rev.,* 17, 102-148.

Palmer, R. D. (1973): "Desensitization of the fear of expressing one's own inhibited aggression: bioenergetic assertive techniques for behavior therapists", in R. D. Rubin, J. P. Brady and J. D. Henderson (Eds.), *Advances in Behavior Therapy Vol. 4,* Academic Press, New York.

Patterson, G. R. and Hops, H. (1972): "Coercion, a game for two: Intervention techniques for marital conflict", in R. E. Ulrich and P. Mountjoy (Eds.), *The Experimental Analysis of Social Behavior,* Appleton-Century-Crofts, New York.

Philips, C. (1977): "A psychological analysis of tension headache", Ch. 5 in S. Rachman (Ed.), *Contributions to Medical Psychology,*

Vol. 1, Pergamon, Oxford.

Popper, K. R. (1965): *Conjectures and Refutations: The Growth of Scientific Knowledge*, Routledge and Kegan Paul.

Rachman, S. (1966): "Sexual fetishism: an experimental analogue", *Psychol. Rec., 16*, 293-296.

Rachman, S. (1967): "Systematic desensitization", *Psychol. Bull., 67*, 93-103.

Rachman, S. (1971): *The Effects of Psychotherapy*, Pergamon, Oxford.

Rachman, S. and Teasdale, J. (1969): *Aversion Therapy and Behaviour Disorders*, Routledge and Kegan Paul, London.

Rehm, L. P. and Marston, A. R. (1968) "Reduction of social anxiety through modification of self-reinforcement: An instigation therapy technique", *J. Consult. Clin. Psychol., 32*, 565-574.

Rotter, J. B. (1966): "Generalised expectancies for internal vs. external control of reinforcement", *Psychol. Mon., 80*, 1-28.

Sandler, J. (1975): "Aversion methods", in F. H. Kanfer and A. P. Goldstein (Eds.), *Helping People Change*, Pergamon, New York.

Seligman, M. E. P. (1971): "Phobias and preparedness", *Behav. Ther., 2*, 307-320.

Seligman, M. E. P. (1975): *Helplessness: On Depression, Development and Death*, Freeman and Co., San Francisco.

Shapiro, D. A. (1979): "Effective psychotherapy: issues and prospects", in N. S. Sutherland (Ed.), *Tutorial Essays in Psychology, Vol. III*, Erlbaum, Hillsdale, New Jersey.

Shapiro, D. A. and Shapiro, D. (1977): "The 'double standard' in evaluation of psychotherapies", *Bull. B.P.S., 30*, 209-210.

Sharpe, R. and Lewis, D. (1977). *Fight your Phobia and Win*, Behavioural Press, London.

Sherman, A. R. (1972): "Real-life exposure as a primary therapeutic factor in the desensitization treatment of fear", *J. abnorm. Psychol., 79*, 19-28.

Skinner, B. F. (1948): "Superstition in the pigeon", *J. Exp. Psychol., 38*, 168-172.

Skinner, B. F. (1953): *Science and Human Behavior*, Macmillan, New York.

Stampfl, T. G. (1970): "Implosive therapy: An emphasis on covert stimulation", in D. J. Levis (Ed.), *Learning Approaches to Therapeutic Behavior Change*, Aldine, Chicago.

Sterman, M. B. (1973): "Neurophysiological and clinical studies of sensorimotor E.E.G. biofeedback training: Some effects on epilepsy", in L. Birk (Ed.), *Biofeedback: Behavioral Medicine*, Grune and Stratton Inc., New York.

Stuart, R. B. (1969): "Operant interpersonal treatment for marital discord", *J. Consult. Clin. Psychol., 33*, 675-682.

Suinn, R. M. and Richardson, F. (1971): "Anxiety management training: A non-specific behavior therapy program for anxiety control", *Behav. Ther.*, **2**, 498-510.

Szasz, T. "The myth of mental illness", *Amer. Psychol.*, **15**, 113-118.

Taylor, F. K. (1966): *Psychopathology: Its Causes and Symptoms*, Butterworth, New York.

Trower, P., Bryant, B., and Argyle, M. (1978): *Social Skills and Mental Health*, Methuen, London.

Ullmann, L. P. and Krasner, L. (Eds.) (1965): *Case Studies in Behavior Modification*, Holt, Rinehart and Winston, New York.

Venables, P. H. and Martin, I. (Eds.) (1967): *A Manual of Psychophysiological Methods*, North Holland Publishing Co., London.

Vogler, R. E., Lunde, S. E., Johnson, G. R. and Martin, P. L. (1970): "Electrical aversion conditioning with chronic alcoholics", *J. Consult. Clin. Psychol.*, **34**, 302-307.

Watson, R. I. (1962): "The experimental tradition and clinical psychology", in A. J. Bachrach (Ed.), *Experimental Foundations of Clinical Psychology*, Basic Books, New York.

Watson, L. S. (1973): *Child Behavior Modification: A Manual for Teachers, Nurses and Parents*, Pergamon, New York.

Weiss, T. and Engel, B. T. (1971): "Operant conditioning of heart rate in patients with premature ventricular contractions", *Psychosom. Med.*, **33**, 301-321.

Wilson, G. T. and Davison, G. C. (1974): "Behavior therapy and homosexuality: A critical perspective", *Behav. Ther.*, **5**, 16-28.

Wolpe, J. (1958): *Psychotherapy by Reciprocal Inhibition*, Stanford University Press, Stanford, California.

Wolpe, J. and Lazarus, A. A. (1966): *Behavior Therapy Techniques*, Pergamon, New York.

Yates, A. J. (1958): "The application of learning theory to the treatment of tics", *J. abnorm. soc. Psychol.*, **56**, 175-182.

FURTHER READING

Goldstein, A. and Foa, E.B.: *Handbook of Behavioral Interventions. A Clinical Guide*, Wiley, New York, 1980.

Hersen, M. and Bellack, A.S. *Behavioral Assessment: A Practical Handbook*, Pergamon, New York, 1976.

Kanfer, F. H. and Goldstein, A. P., (Eds.) *Helping People Change*, Pergamon, New York, 1980.

Kanfer, F. H. and Phillips, J. S. *Learning Foundations of Behavior Therapy*, Wiley, New York, 1970.

Stern, R., *Behavioral Techniques. A Therapist's Manual*, Academic Press, London 1978.

Talking Treatments

Enid Balint

B.Sc. (Hon)

Seminar Leader, Postgraduate G.P. Training Courses,
Training Analyst, Institute of Psychoanalysis, London.

Talking Treatments

INTRODUCTION: THE NATURE OF TALKING TREATMENTS

What are the facts about talking treatments? Have they a right to a place in medicine? Have any so-called psychotherapeutic methods a scientific basis and, if so, can they be taught? What are the methods and who should teach and practise them? This chapter can only briefly examine some of these questions, all of which aim to help doctors decide on the right treatment for some of their patients.

We can start our discussion of these questions with the work of a well known physician, Breuer, in the 1880s. Breuer, a doctor with a high reputation, was treating hysterical patients; Freud was a friend of his, although much younger and only just qualifying as a doctor. Breuer described to Freud the treatment of a particular hysterical patient known as Fräulein Anna O., a treatment involving listening to her talk and described more fully below, so that later when Freud became interested in the study of hysteria and found the currently recommended methods of treatment, such as hydrotherapy, massage, rest cures and so on were not very effective, his thoughts gradually turned to the remarkable success which Breuer had reported with Fräulein Anna O. Later Breuer, together with Freud, described this work in *Studies on Hysteria.* This book is usually regarded as the starting-point of psychoanalysis. It is interesting to ask ourselves to what extent, and in what ways, did the procedures and findings described in these studies pave the way to the practice of all talking treatments as they exist today and influence medicine as a whole.

Perhaps one of Freud's most outstanding achievements was his invention of the first instrument for the examination of the human mind — a systematic method for exploring the unconscious. One could say that Breuer came across it, but Freud started systematically examining it and continued to do so, together with his colleagues, all his life. He, perhaps, was not the first to explore the nature of the human mind, or the existence of the unconscious, but he did discover a method for exploring it and he described his method and proposed a structure of the mind based on his findings, which is still used. His work enables us to trace the development of the means he discovered for this exploration, and the structure and dynamics of the mind on which his theories are based. At that time, what he described was primarily a one-person psychology but gradually psychoanalysts have, on the basis of his findings, developed theories of two- and three- and multi-person psychology and nowadays many analysts think of their work partly as a basis for the study of human relationships, rather than entirely as a study of the human mind and its structure.

Breuer's patient, Anna O., herself, demonstrated how to overcome some of the obstacles in the way of doctors who wished to undertake this work and she herself invented the title of her cure. She referred to it as a "talking cure" and also as "chimney-sweeping".

Breuer, and Freud too, had experimented with hypnosis and hypnotic suggestion, but with Anna O. only very slight use of these methods was necessary. This patient produced streams of verbal material and all Breuer had to do, he said, was to sit by and listen to them without interrupting her. Freud describes how he, too, gradually gave up hypnosis and contented himself with listening and occasionally putting his patient into a state of concentration with the use of pressure on her forehead. Many of us now find that if we learn to wait and to listen, the patient, if he wants us to do so, will concentrate without any encouragement and will talk in a way which is important to him, even if we ourselves do not understand the meaning of what he says right at the beginning. We have also found that patients will do so in many different professional settings.

A talking treatment should perhaps also be called a listening treatment, because listening — or a certain kind of listening — is necessary before a patient is able to embark on talking in a way that would be likely to be useful to him. In my view, this kind of talking-cum-listening should not be labelled psychotherapy (although it is difficult to avoid doing so when writing about it) as this suggests to the reader that it is a speciality and not an integral part of medicine, which I consider it to be.

In medicine as a whole, patients have to learn how much, and what sort of, help they may expect from their doctors and how much anxiety and suffering they must bear on their own. Doctors, too, need to know how much they must bear on their own and how much help they can expect from their colleagues, from specialists and others, and how much increased understanding of their patients' illnesses, or their patients as whole people with or without illnesses, they can acquire by listening. In my view, the acquisition of the skill to listen can in some cases ease the doctor's load of suffering, i.e. make his responsibility for the patient less arduous. This only applies to doctors who feel dissatisfaction with their work with particular kinds of patients and look around for ways of easing that dissatisfaction.

There seems little doubt that a considerable proportion of the complaints about which patients consult their doctors are not solely related to physical illnesses, but originate also from emotional problems and conflicts. For our purpose, it is irrelevant to establish the exact proportion of those patients who have emotional as well as, or rather than, organic illnesses. The figures vary in the literature available. It may be worth recording that as far as I know the lowest figure given speaks of about 10 per cent of all patients. It is interesting here to quote from an article in *Pravda* (Vel'vovskii, 1973), where it is stated that on an average, 20 per cent of those that were admitted to a clinic by doctors of different specialities would not have received much help unless they had also consulted a "psychotherapist doctor"; and a further 30 per cent were in need of his advice in the course of treatment. This was a result of a study of a sample of patients carried out in a poly-clinic which serves the workers in a factory in Russia. It is a rather surprising source of information and it would seem that, if it is true, there cannot possibly be enough psychotherapists or psychiatrists to meet the need and that perhaps other doctors must develop skills, so as to be able to listen in the right way in order to diagnose where an emotional problem exists as well as, or rather than, an organic one in a patient who shows that he is suffering, but finds it difficult to say exactly where his pain comes from. Even if treatment cannot follow, the skill to make a diagnosis alone is a considerable one which is largely based on a skill to listen and to talk with the patient; the diagnostic stage can be therapeutic in itself.

Before going further, I want now to consider a particular use of talking treatments in medicine, that used in Balint Groups, as described by Loch (Loch and Dantigraber, 1976). Following this it should be possible to examine the different settings in which the treatments can take place.

Loch says that the aim of Balint Groups — where doctors are helped to rethink their ways of relating to their patients and to listen to them in a different way — is to enable a suffering individual (the patient) to understand part of the situation in which he finds himself. By helping patients to understand the situation in which they are "imprisoned", which is caused by the simultaneous activity of contradictory tendencies in themselves, they can regain a basic feeling of well-being or of "at one-ness with themselves". Loch quotes

Hampshire as saying that man has to understand himself and be understood in order to be free, in order to extend his active life (Hampshire, 1972). Loch thinks that the kind of work that is done in talking treatments enables a patient to become active again, to find his way.

Here is an example from my own work in this field.

Recently in a training group for young doctors (i.e. a Balint Group) one doctor discussed a patient, Mr. F., aged 34. He was a married man, with a son aged 18 months, and a tool-maker by trade. The general practitioner presented the patient at the seminar because the patient had been off work for some months and the doctor felt that he was making no headway in getting him back. The patient appeared to be depressed and the doctor was rather angry with the patient's employers for making him do such exacting work. He talked with the patient and prescribed appropriate drugs.

In the discussion in the seminar it was thought that the doctor had strong ambitions for the patient. The doctor thought, however, that the man should leave his job and take an easier one because he was harassed and overstrained. The patient had not said this, but the doctor had inferred it. He did not know, nor did the other doctors in the seminar, what the patient wanted for himself and what, if any, conflicts he had about his work and what contradictory tendencies. The group gave plentiful advice, as groups are wont to do. After a time someone suggested that the question was not only how to get the patient back to work and to what kind of work, but that perhaps the question was to find out whether he really *liked* work, or preferred being at home with his managing but amiable wife. In short, what were the patient's aspirations and what kind of man was he? A long discussion followed.

At a follow-up report three months later, the doctor said that the seminar discussion had been helpful because the patient did not want to *leave* his work although he had stayed away for so long; nor did he feel angry with his employers. When the doctor listened again, the patient was able to say *what* he could do and what could be done and what he *wanted*. It seemed that he had not been able to be dominant at work, up to now, to "throw his weight about", but after the interview he had gone back to work and had felt quite well. He had been able to tell people to wait for him so that he could finish his job, instead of feeling rushed and bullied; he was in charge of the situation and did his work in his own way. The patient was able to assert himself more at home, too, and also with his doctor.

This patient had to say something and be understood before he himself knew, and could accept, one aspect of himself about which he had been only vaguely aware; he was then able to act upon it. The patient's conflicts and contradictions were not discussed but all that seemed to be necessary at that time was for him to find out, by talking, what kind of activity he was capable of and what he enjoyed. Some patients need more. They may seek psychoanalytic or other forms of treatment; or else trained general practitioners may be able to provide the "more".

Another patient, a women in her 50s, had to say and then to know, that she could be loved and loving. This was a patient who had visited her doctor for some years, principally with minor complaints like tension headaches. One day she came in complaining once more of headaches and said that she thought she had better leave her job because the noise in the factory was so great and this was what she thought caused her headaches; she added that she could not leave because her husband and she needed the money. The doctor knew that this was not quite true, and went a bit further with his enquiries into why she had to work. The patient then quite unexpectedly began to talk about her childhood. She had been brought up in an orphanage and remembered watching the parents and friends of other children when they came to visit them. She had spoken about this before — but never, as then, with emotion. The patient was never visited in the orphanage and was extremely surprised when anyone ever wanted her and astonished that her husband had offered to marry her, because she did not expect to be loved or wanted by anyone. She had never believed that her husband loved her, but at the interview, with the help of the doctor, she suddenly realised that she need not earn so much money: perhaps they did not need it. She still did not think that she was loved.

A few weeks later the patient visited the doctor again, this time with a sore throat. She told him that she was doing less work and that she had realised, on the way to the bus to see her doctor, that perhaps her husband did love her, and on telling the doctor this, to her surprise she burst into tears. Something apparently had happened in the previous interview to make her reconsider some of the things that she had assumed about herself, which had led her to realise also that perhaps she could be wanted and was lovable. But it was not until she verbalised this in the interview with the doctor on the second occasion that she burst into tears, and really felt cared for. Gradually, after this, her feelings about herself changed and she stayed at home more and she and her husband did more together. This, put as briefly as I have described it, sounds a bit simple and naive, but we have a long follow-up record to show that the changes were stable. It is important to know that the patient herself never connected the interviews with her doctor and the changes in her life following the interviews I have briefly described. However, the doctor seemed to be a key person in her life; a necessary link enabling her to change.

The doctors' aims in the two cases I have quoted seem very different, but the similarity between the two is that in both cases the patients verbalised a problem — which then led them to be active in a different kind of way. It is my view that it was this verbalisation in a particular kind of atmosphere, in a particular kind of setting at a time which suited them, which was needed.

Before proceeding, I must refer to the astonishing paucity of early writings on technique — particularly by Freud. This suggests that there were in him, as there are in most of us today, some feelings of reluctance in publishing this kind of material. He in fact was highly sceptical as to the value of "lessons in technique". He never ceased to insist that the proper mastery of the subject could only be acquired from clinical experience and not from books.

In spite of being well aware of this danger, I am writing this chapter, which I hope will be seen more as a signpost to treatment, and an introduction to the art of listening, than as a lesson on how to conduct it. I, too, still think that one can only learn to listen and to talk with patients by trying to do so, i.e. on the job, but I will add that one should, if possible, be able to discuss one's experience with some of one's colleagues, otherwise one may be unaware of what has taken place during the talk: it is important to have another person listen to oneself.

One of the difficulties of examining patients with emotional problems is that the doctor's own emotions have to be taken into account. They are very often involved and it is only natural, and certainly not unusual, for the doctor to feel angry or impatient, or sympathetic or protective, with the patient and sometimes these feelings cannot be controlled. If the doctor is aware of them, however, they are much less likely to interfere with the communication with his patient than if they are unconscious. They can even be helpful if understood.

As Ferenczi wrote (1919) apparently referring to a discussion he had with Freud:

> As the doctor . . . is always a human being and as such liable to moods, sympathies and antipathies as well as impulses — without such susceptibilities he would of course have no understanding for the patient's psychic conflicts — he has constantly to form a double task during the analysis; [we should say during any encounter with his patient where talking is important] on the one hand he must observe the patient, scrutinise what he relates, and construct his unconscious from his information and behaviour; on the other hand he must at the same time consistently control his own attitude towards the patient and when necessary, correct it; this is the mastery of the counter-transference."

This is asking a great deal of all of us, even for analysts who have plenty of time during their training to learn to use their feelings (counter-transference) in an appropriate way; still more for general practitioners in their surgeries; although from my experience it is not impossible. We still have very scant theories of personal relationships, and many about the structure of the mind. Freud himself had profound intuitive understanding of his patients and this gave him a therapeutic personal relationship with them. They got better partly because Freud understood them and they could understand some aspects of themselves which were preventing their development or their activities. Freud himself saw his cures, in the earlier years, as due to the removal of conflicts and anxiety due to the dammed-up tension of repressed instincts and the recovery of infantile memories related to primitive sexual fantasies. We tend nowadays to think that help is also given by the professional understanding a patient gets in the relationship with a trusted person, however brief it is.

Clinical experiences with therapeutic techniques are not necessarily reliable. Malan (1963, 1976 (1), 1976 (2)) and others have said that psychotherapy is one of the subjects least amenable to scientific study. Most writers have been unable to demonstrate from controlled studies that psychotherapy itself brings about any greater improvements than life experience alone, although it has been shown that dynamic psychotherapy can be more or less validated for psychosomatic conditions (Luborsky *et al.*, 1975). Malan, however, is hopeful about the outcome of studies and says that "all that is needed is . . . the objective handling by researchers of the subjective judgments gained by trained clinicians". His findings are very important and merit careful study by anyone wishing to brush talking treatments to one side.

SETTINGS IN WHICH TALKING CURES TAKE PLACE

Before proceeding to study in detail the settings in which talking treatments take place, I will give an example of one case which was studied in two different settings, to show how difficult it is to know the reason *why* the outcome was so different in the two occasions. Was it because of the settings in which they occurred; or because of the ways in which the doctors were able to listen; or the timing? We will see how difficult it is to answer these questions.

The case was first reported by a general practitioner in a training seminar. It was taped and transcribed and I can quote some of the discussion verbatim. The doctor started to describe his case and said:

One case I have got is a 35-year-old man, married, one child, who generally has an anxious personality. One day he jumped into the shallow end of a swimming pool and hit his head. After being X-rayed he suddenly said he couldn't feel the right half of his body, head, arms and legs. I think he finished up in various teaching hospitals. He had E.M.I. scans. He tends to be pushed to the psychiatrists who call him an anxiety depression. He has been put on various drugs; he's been reassured that there is no serious abnormality, yet he insists he can't feel the right side of his body, so you can prick him and he feels nothing. They say there is nothing wrong with him so he says, "Well why is it I can't feel the right half of my body?". When you ask him whether he has got problems and why he has got this terrible anxiety state he says, "Why is it when I am eating I can't feel the food on the right side of my cheek?" You say, "Well, that's all in the mind". "Well, why is it when I am on the lavatory I can't feel the right side of my cheek?" And this goes on forever and we are not just getting anywhere. He keeps saying he can't feel, and we keep saying it is in the mind. Various psychiatrists have suggested putting him on antidepressives but others are against it and he is awfully tense and he has got himself so that he just can't do anything or say anything but that he can't feel the right side of his body. And he says, "Why can't you give me some other tablets and make me better?"

Some of the doctors in the group asked about the patient's family life and the doctor said he had not found out anything; there had been masses of neurological examinations and the doctor said he just had to reassure him, that is all they could possibly do, but whatever they say, he just answers, "Why can't I feel the right side of my body?". The group tried to find out more about the patient but the doctor could only say how frustrating a case it was (and the group agreed). He had therefore passed him back to make another appointment with another teaching hospital.

It so happened that another general practitioner in the same group, who was working at the psychiatric department of this teaching hospital as part of his training course, saw the same patient. I will quote from the beginning of his report.

I have got a follow-up on last week's case — the chap with the hemi-anaesthesia. He came along full of the same problems. He's got quite a lot of guilt feeling. When he was 9 his sister died in a motorbike accident; she was 17 and she was admitted to hospital with multiple head injuries and he said at the time they had just had a row before she had gone out. "I hope she never comes back," he had said at the time, and of course she didn't come back. She died. Last September he and his wife had a row and she said, "Drop dead" and he went and banged his head in a swimming pool. His troubles all started from then and he reacts very strongly from the fact that his wife said "Drop dead" so he is going to die because of his sister.

The group asked the doctor how he got the patient to talk like this but he did not answer but continued, saying:

He is quite forthcoming. He has got a son of 6 and he resents the relationship between the mother and son. I think they are quite close together. He is a bit of an outsider. His wife works at the same school as the son goes to. They are there together all day. He is a bit resentful about that, but I have got to talk to him separately about that.

The discussion continued.

I quote the case rather fully because it is important to see the different way the patient used the two doctors and the different ways in which he talked. We cannot know whether this was because on one occasion he was in a general practitioner's surgery and in the other in a psychiatric department of a teaching hospital, or whether he was ready to talk on one occasion and not on the other. We must remember that he had been in the psychiatric department of many teaching hospitals before. From many years of experience with general practitioners we do know that patients can talk to their general practitioners in both ways demonstrated by these reports. The relevant factor may be that they perhaps can talk when the time is ripe *and* when the doctor offers to listen, i.e. when the setting in which he works makes it possible for him to tune in to his patients. I must state that the general practitioner who reported this case had very little time indeed in his surgery and was hampered by this factor, which some general practitioners might be able to overcome. If the doctor feels he has no time, the right kind of trusting atmosphere certainly cannot develop even if the patient is ready to talk.

We have a follow-up on this patient and it is interesting to note that, when our second doctor returned to the ward after the seminar meeting, the patient had abandoned his symptom and was playing ping-pong. One must ask why was he doing this; why at that particular time, and also why was he not able to do so on other occasions. His treatment continued, although there were few long interviews, and at the time of writing the patient is at home but visits his doctor regularly once a week in the out-patient clinic.

Let us now try to describe in general terms the kind of atmosphere that is needed for talking cures. How is the atmosphere created and what does it consist of? It is a setting in which the doctor can observe freely, not behave automatically, convey his observations so they mean something to the patient, not turn his back on unpleasant facts or confessions or asides. It would make it much easier for beginners if a kind of guide-book could be provided for doctors, with a plan of how to start the journey with the patient, pointing out the ways to look and where to go, and perhaps giving some hints about how to respond to various communications. Unfortunately, this is impossible, because no two patients are alike and no two doctor-patient relationships are the same. But if the right atmosphere is created, and the patient feels he can say what he wants and that he may be understood, he may feel far less alone and even feel that he is more related and similar to other people outside the surgery or consulting room than he previously felt. He may begin to feel that part of him corresponds with parts of other people, and ideas which he was only partly aware of, because of a feeling of shame or guilt or oddity, can be acknowledged by him, even though only in a half-understood way. In the case we have just discussed this seemed to happen and it enabled him to say he felt he was treated as an outsider by his wife and his son.

The setting in which the doctor sees the patient is not then made up entirely of the physical setting in which it takes place, or the training or lack of it in the doctor. It does not matter so much, perhaps, whether it is in a hospital ward, or the general practitioner's surgery, or in the psychiatric department of a hospital, but what does matter most is the doctor's personality, the way he behaves and thinks and the way he relates to and thinks about people. Words, it is true, bridge the gulf between the two people, the doctor and the patient, but more than words are exchanged between them; they are in a way emotionally involved with each other; in a special, professional way, both distant and intimate. I have already made it clear that I do not think that all patients want to be understood and listened to all of the time. It is sometimes difficult for doctors to know when a patient does *not* want to be understood or listened to, and it is important that he should take the timing of the patient's request for help into account. If doctors can leave patients alone when they want to be left alone on one occasion, it often seems to follow that patients will come back to their doctor when they do wish to talk and to be understood.

We recently had an example of this in a case mentioned by a woman doctor at a seminar.

The doctor reported that she was seeing a 12-year-old boy complaining of tummy aches. Various medicines had been tried but the boy still went on complaining and stayed away from school. The doctor had spoken to the school and they had said that the boy seemed to be in some trouble, but he was not performing too badly and they wished that he would come back and attend school and not be kept away by his tummy aches. The doctor felt that the boy was troubled and told the seminar that his mother had died a short time before and he was being looked after by an older stepsister. No one could talk to this boy about his mother's death or about his feelings for her, or about her long terminal illness, which the boy had witnessed in their home. The members of the group sympathised and felt too that it was impossible to talk to the boy about such a painful subject. They offered advice, suggesting various other remedies that should be tried for the tummy aches. Gradually, however, somebody ventured to say that perhaps the boy would like to talk, otherwise why did he come to his doctor? The doctor who was looking after him was delighted and said that, in fact, after a long silence at the last interview, the doctor had asked the patient what he was thinking about, and the patient had said, "I was wondering what question you were next going to ask me". The doctor said she would like to talk to the boy about his mother or to try to get him to talk about her. At a follow up interview later on, it seemed she had been able to do so and that the boy wanted to come back weekly.

This patient therefore did want to be listened to, but it was difficult for anybody to think that something as painful as one's mother's death could be spoken about, even in the trusting atmosphere which this particular doctor clearly provided.

A professional relationship exists usually only in the setting in which it takes place and it stops abruptly when the two people concerned leave it. Thus a kind of frame is put around the work and the patient need not leave the doctor feeling totally vulnerable because of what has passed between them.

Whatever the technique, the therapist's attitude to the patient will be as important as any verbal communication that takes place between them. This involves the therapist in having the courage to be himself (i.e. his professional self) and in being willing to accept his own peculiarities and weaknesses and strengths and limitations as a doctor, as well as those of his patients. He will certainly not be the same with every patient, because different people call for different responses, but he must certainly not "put on an act" with the patient and be, for instance, very friendly, very loving or very "professional", i.e. aloof. It is often only too easy for the doctor to present himself as a strong, dependable father figure, who may have some magic cure. This, however, is not very useful and it is easier for the patient if the doctor is relaxed and quiet and on the same level as his patients, not above him or beneath him, particularly so in difficult cases and when the patient feels that only a miracle can help him. It is very tempting for a doctor to think that his patient needs more love and for him to try to give it, but this is not his task; he furthermore cannot, for example, make up for early deprivations. What he can do, is to listen attentively to what is said and understand it in a professional capacity and, in particular, never forget that there is always something new to understand. He may have to wait, but it is often not the facts about the patient's past, or misunderstandings about his relation with, for instance, his parents which have to be understood, but odd trivialities which the doctor would never guess might be told him, so that he cannot prepare himself to hear them. It is very difficult indeed for the doctor to be attentive in this way, but if he does not feel in a hurry — even if he has only "six minutes" (Balint and Norell, 1973) — his attitude may enable the patient to say something quite quickly. We have found, in studying short interviews, that the capacity to waste, perhaps two out of six minutes of an interview, is well worth the time. If the doctor feels in a hurry and therefore rushes in with ideas, the whole of the six minutes will be wasted and not only the first two or three.

CLASSIFICATION OF TALKING CURES

Talking cures vary according to the training of the doctor and one way of classifying them is according to that training; or they can be classified according to the therapeutic goals. In the case I discussed (on p. 82) about the man who was seen by the two doctors, the training of the doctors was the same, as was their goal, which seemed to be only to remove the patient's symptoms: it was expanded later, as it often is.

We cannot discuss goals, of course, without discussing diagnosis, as our first task must always be to make a diagnosis — not one only consisting of labels — and on the basis of this diagnosis to decide on the goal. It quite often happens that the goal is to leave the patient alone with his symptom, or to see what happens for a time before deciding on what kind of therapy to try; it can be to keep in touch with the patient, or at other times to leave him alone and to let him get in touch with the doctor himself, if he wishes to do so. Some "talking" of course will have taken place between the doctor and the patient before any of this is decided. When I talk about diagnosis in this chapter I mean not only what is called a diagnosis in medicine, i.e. a traditional diagnosis — but what we have called, over the years, an over-all diagnosis, which can be described as an appraisal of the ways in which a patient sees himself, how he relates to and sees the people who are close to him, and how his illness or disturbance is shown in his life (Balint, 1968). This over-all diagnosis must also include a description of the patient's physical illness or disturbance, but not seen in isolation.

Many doctors and others — for instance, those who act as leaders of therapeutic groups — do so with apparently little specialised training in this field, and some of them learn "on the job". I think that training is needed, as in other branches of medicine. No one suggests that doctors should undertake any other kind of work without a thorough knowledge of the subject and the skills appropriate to the disturbance they are treating.

There are, however, many therapeutic groups in existence run by only partly-trained workers, who aim, for instance, to enhance the freedom of expression of the individual or the removal of some inhibition which is preventing him from being active. These are concepts similar to those which I have talked about earlier (*see* Loch and Dantigraber *op. cit.*) but the techniques used are different. They remind one of the early work by Alexander and French, who developed a therapy which aimed to provide "a corrective emotional experience" for the patient, in order to do away with the necessity of long-term psychoanalytic treatment (Alexander and French, 1946).

I must now briefly describe some differences in psychotherapeutic techniques in the different settings used by doctors where talking treatments are the main instruments used by them. I will not go into the general points which have already been made but will dwell upon the differences between one setting and another. I can only describe a few of the settings in which I myself have worked, or with which at least I am very familiar. I will start with the psychoanalytic setting.

The psychoanalytic setting

Classical psychoanalysis starts when a patient, after one or more preliminary consultations with the psychoanalyst, decides that he would like to, and is able to, spend years rather than months or weeks or days exploring the relationship between his unconscious mind and his relation to the world in which he lives. The work is based on the acceptance of the idea that there is an unconscious part of the mind which, although unconscious, influences the thoughts and behaviour of each one of us.

Analysts nowadays vary in their opinion about the frequency of sessions they offer their patients — most work about three to five times a week with each patient, and Freud himself sometimes saw his patients six times a week. Some analysts consider that they can do analytic work even when they see their patients infrequently. They presumably accept Freud's idea that anyone whose work includes an ability to use "transference" phenomena and is aware of the "resistances" can call his work psychoanalysis, thus leaving the frequency of interviews open (Freud, 1914).

It is difficult briefly to describe transference and resistance, I will refer to the definitions of Laplanche and Pontalis, which can be paraphrased thus: transference is a process of actualisation of unconscious wishes; it uses specific objects and operates in the framework of specific relationships established with these objects. Its context, *par excellence,* is in the analytic situation. Resistance is defined as "everything in the words and actions of the patient that obstructs his gaining access to the unconscious".

At the beginning of the work the analyst makes a diagnosis, i.e. tries to arrive at some idea of the patient's basic conflicts and of the way that these are interfering with his development and activity and feeling of contentment. The analyst must always be prepared to reassess his ideas and his diagnosis as the work proceeds. The normal technique is to ask the patient to say what comes into his mind, no matter how irrelevant or inconsequential this may seem. The analyst listens carefully, not only to the content of what the patient says, but even more to the association of ideas — how one idea follows another. It is by following the association of ideas, including those given in dreams, that the analyst can get into touch with the unconscious part of the patient's mind. The work is based on the idea that unconscious conflicts both within the patient, as well as with people in his environment, are largely responsible for his difficulties and for his suffering.

The psychotherapist's setting

Psychotherapy varies from simple advice and reassurance giving to very elaborate and well-studied methods of helping patients to change in their attitudes by talking to their doctor. I have had very limited personal experience of these methods, and will only describe one kind of psychotherapy which can be used in the setting of the hospital or in the doctor's consulting room.

Balint describes how he had been interested for many years in the possibilities of a therapy which would not last so long as the classical psychoanalysis (Balint *et al., see also* Malan, 1963). He saw that there might be disadvantages in this, but he thought that there were also advantages. He thought that if such work was to be undertaken, the results of the therapy must be comparable to those of an analytic treatment and must be stable in about the same degree. Fewer patients might be suitable for this sort of therapy, the chances of failure might be greater, and the work perhaps so difficult that it could only be undertaken by trained psychoanalysts. Balint decided that those trying to work in this way should concentrate on the interaction between the patient and his therapist and on the elaborate processes and techniques that developed as a result. It was felt that unless a focus could be found early in the work, this type of therapy was impossible. But it was important that if the focus proved to be wrong, i.e. if it was not continued during psychotherapy, it should not be adhered to and a longer form of treatment might prove to be necessary. A great deal of work has been done to validate these theories (*see* list of References, p. 92, under Balint, M., Balint, E., and Ornstein, P., 1972, *Focal Psychotherapy*). It is very difficult to make the kind of diagnosis required to arrive at a focus and the work can best be undertaken by psychotherapists and psychoanalysts working in a team or workshop.

General practitioner's setting

I have already reported some cases which have been treated by general practitioners either in their surgery or in hospital. I will therefore only enlarge on general practitioner treatments by describing work arising out of a study of ordinary short interviews during surgery hours. (For fuller discussion of the general practitioner's setting, *see* Balint and Norell, 1973.)

In this study, our aim was not to try to find short cuts in order to avoid longer psychotherapeutic interviews, but to measure, as precisely as possible, the therapeutic potential of the doctor-patient relationship in the general practitioner's everyday setting. In the work, which lasted more than five years with a group of seasoned general practitioners, we came to realise that, instead of solving exciting puzzles and problems, the doctor was expected to "tune in" to the patients' wavelength of communication, so that he could respond to them. The traditional aim of pinpointing the seeds of the trouble. or the suffering is not always appropriate. As an alternative, it was suggested that the aim of this kind of therapy should be to provide the patient with the opportunity to communicate whatever it is he wants, in a brief time. We found that this resulted in a brief, intense and close contact, which was then followed usually by less intense and less taxing meetings between the doctor and the patient. What comes up during the intense interview can be explored in subsequent interviews. The task of the doctor is to give a great deal of attention to what the patient is saying or is trying to say, or is trying to convey at that particular time, rather than in studying the underlying causes of his illness, though of course the latter may engage his attention on subsequent occasions.

This still seems to me to be the most suitable technique in general practice, but it is one in which experienced listening is more important perhaps than in any other setting. I am repeating what I said when I was talking in general about the nature of talking treatments. The aim in the general practitioner setting is, from time to time, to meet a patient's need in a short interchange without any guidelines and without any theoretical ideas present in the doctor's mind at the time of doing so. If he has theoretical concepts in his mind when he listens to his patient, it may block his ability to hear and he may not have the time to correct it during the short interview with the patient.

The setting of the general medical ward
A patient in hospital medical wards may also need to be listened to, and to talk. All the general observations I made earlier apply here too, but there is one striking difference, which is that no one doctor is in sole charge of the patient. In fact, each doctor is a member of a team, with a senior doctor at the head. Nurses, *aides*, consultants, registrars, housemen, are all working for a patient and it sometimes seems a matter of chance who the patient decides to talk to, or who decides to listen to the patient. This could quite easily be a nurse, and the nurse may not think it worthwhile reporting some of her observations to the doctor, or the doctor may not think it worth listening to some of the observations of the nurse. However, it does seem that such discussions between the team looking after a patient,

who is causing anxiety because he does not get well in the expected manner, can be rewarding. The variation here seems to be the communication between professional staff. In other settings it can be extremely important that the doctor should not tell anybody else what his patient has said; the need for *privacy* can be one of the most important needs that a patient has. He may feel that he has to be certain that what he says will be regarded as secret before he can trust his doctor at all.

The setting for marital therapy
It is not infrequent that patients approach their doctors with trivial problems which later turn out to be based on difficulties in the marriage. The doctor then has to decide whether to discuss the problem with the patient who comes to him, whether he should send for the spouse, whether he should see the two partners together, or whether he should refer them to another doctor. In some settings, for instance at the Institute of Marital Studies, two workers see the two partners, either together or separately, and some aspect of the marriage itself, rather than the problems of either one of the partners is taken as the focus for work. *In general practice* the partner who comes to the doctor first to complain should be seen as the patient and should be worked with before the spouse is sent for, even if the spouse is thought to be the sicker of the two. It has been our experience that unless some work can be done with the patient who comes first, then very little help can be given at all. It is also our experience that it is rare, if ever, that only one member of a family is to blame. However tempting it is to think that one person is the "guilty" party, it seldom turns out to be so at the end. It is common experience to note, for instance, that the wives of alcoholic husbands, or the husbands of alcoholic wives, are seldom without problems themselves. These do not arise out of, but dove-tail into, the spouse's alcoholism and it can be very helpful if, at the outset of the treatment, this is borne in mind. This is difficult work because the interactions that take place between marital partners are often hidden and complicated, and because of the difficulty in discovering these interactions the work cannot be undertaken in the normal "six minutes", not at any rate in the early stages of the work.

A case will illustrate the difficulties involved.

Recently a wife, who brought her baby with a cough, complained that her husband was angry with her because he said that she no longer looked after him properly. She was not interested in sleeping with him, as she had a baby. She said that her husband never left her alone, was very demanding and since her baby was born a year ago she did not like having him in bed with her, and often anyway she had to get up in the night and look after her baby when it cried and she then took the baby into bed to comfort it. The doctor wondered who needed comfort. There was a complicated interaction here between a woman who resented the demands her husband made, and preferred to respond to the demands of her baby; a husband who was jealous of the baby which comforted his wife, and who would have liked to have been able to care for both wife and baby. His greatest need was to feel he could look after someone rather than to be looked after, and hers was a need to manage alone. The wife had usurped his role and it was hard for the husband to bear it, or to realise he wished to care, and not be cared for. Once the couple understood this, it was easier for them to readjust. The couple were seen together after the second interview.

Other kinds of psychotherapy in various settings
Before concluding, I must state once more that I am well aware that there are very many kinds of psychotherapy. I have concentrated on a very few with which I am familiar, which will perhaps illustrate some of the general points I have tried to make earlier in this chapter. Most doctors give reassurance, and we have often asked the question whether the reassurance they give is for the patient or for themselves. If one examines the results of reassurance, we usually find that the patient gets addicted to it and asks for more and more. Simple reassurance may be what some patients want, but if it does not work it is no good repeating it, and it may be based on a faulty diagnosis.

Finally, when talking and listening to patients, much more goes on than the content of the talk itself: it is the way it is said, the order of the ideas that are talked about, the manner of the therapist and the relationship between therapist and patient which counts.

The object of this chapter is not so much, therefore, to confuse the doctor with advice about the dangers of this or that treatment, and the advantages of the other; what I want to do is to make it clear that, although there are variations in technique which can be described and arise out of the settings and goals and training of the doctor, *the same kind of two-way trusting atmosphere is needed in all of them,* and (so long as the doctor does not work in ways which he may have been taught but which he does not fully understand) only good can come of it.

REFERENCES AND FURTHER READING

Alexander, F. and French, T. M. (1946): *Psychoanalytic Therapy: Principles and Application,* Ronald Press, New York.

Balint, E. (1968): "Investigating the possibilities of patient-centred medicine", *Proceedings of the 7th A.P.A.P. Colloquium for Post*

Graduate Teaching of Psychiatry in New Orleans. American Psychiatric Association, Washington, D.C.

Balint, E. and Norell, J. S. (Eds.) (1973): *Six Minutes for the Patient,* Tavistock Publications, London.

Balint, M., Balint, E. and Ornstein, P. (1972): *Focal Psychotherapy, Example of Applied Psychoanalysis,* Mind and Medicine Monograph Series, Tavistock Publications, London.

Breuer, J. and Freud, S. (1955): *Studies on Hysteria* in Freud's *Complete Psychological Works,* Standard Edition, Vols. 2 and 14, Hogarth Press, London.

Ferenczi, S. (1919): *Zeitschrift für Psychoanalyse,* trans. in *Further Contribution to the Theory and Technique of Psychoanalysis,* Hogarth Press, London.

Freud, S. (1914): *Complete Psychological Works,* Standard Edition, Vol. 14, Hogarth Press, London.

Hampshire, A. S. (1972): *Freedom of the Mind,* Oxford University Press, London.

Laplanche, J. and Pontalis, J. B. (1973): *The Language of Psychoanalysis,* Hogarth Press, London.

Loch, W. and Dantigraber, J. (1976): *Changes in the Doctor and his Patient Brought About by Balint Groups,* Psychiatria Fennica, Helsinki.

Luborsky, L., Singer and Luborsky (1973): "Comparative Studies and Psychotherapies", *Archives of General Psychiatry,* 32, 995-1008.

Malan, D. H. (1963): *Study of Brief Psychotherapy,* Mind and Medicine Monograph series, Tavistock Publications, London, also published as a Social Science Paperback by Associated Book Publishers, London, 1975.

Malan, D. H. (1976 (1)): *The Validation of Dynamic Psychotherapy,* Plenum Press, New York and London.

Malan, D. H. (1976 (2)): *The Frontier of Brief Psychotherapy,* Plenum Press, New York and London.

Vel'vovskii, I. (1973): "The Health Service — If Your Nerves Play You up", *Pravda,* Moscow.

Useful Psychotropic Drugs

Dr. Robin Steel,
M.B., F.R.C.G.P., D.Obst., R.C.O.G., D.P.M.
General Practitioner, Worcester.

Useful Psychotropic Drugs

A doctor pours medicine (of which he knows little) into patients (of whom he knows less).

George Bernard Shaw.

INTRODUCTION

Treating patients with emotional problems by advising them to take chemical compounds is a multifaceted problem. Even to substitute the word "drugs" in the place of "chemical compounds" would raise the emotional tone of this opening remark, demonstrating how difficult it is to discuss this topic with absolute Olympian detachment. Yet to the busy specialist in clinic, consulting room or ward, or to the harassed family doctor seeing patients in surgery or their homes, it is a constant dilemma. The ideal Benthamite solution is to do the greatest possible good to the greatest number of patients, but it must also be added today with the least harm and cost, as well as in the shortest possible time. If there is a factor emerging from twentieth-century medicine, it is that demand is increasing with patients' expectations, while resources are limited either by personal purses, or, at one remove, by the taxpayers placing a ceiling on amounts, redistributed from the pockets of the mainly healthy, to provide health services as a whole, at lesser or no cost, to the sick when ill.

This chapter therefore discusses the problems and choices before the non-psychiatrist who is considering treating patients who have an emotional content in their illness with psychotropic drugs. Examples, such as the management of a hypertensive who develops phobic or stress symptoms, the gynaecological patient whose eyes water with tears when discussing a possible hysterectomy, the low-backache patients in orthopaedic clinics who wake early in the morning, as well as those with insomnia in the wards, are not rare, unknown phenomena to specialists and generalists. The treatment of migraine, colitis, asthma, non-ulcer dyspepsia and dysmenorrhoea may involve a decision in each case whether or not to prescribe or recommend a psychotropic drug. Holistic reappraisal of diseases regarded hitherto as mostly organic, such as rheumatoid arthritis, has revealed that psychological difficulties either co-exist with, or are caused by, the disease and, as such, need to be evaluated to see if they are susceptible to treatment alongside treatment for the organic component.

In an ideal world, the specialist should isolate precisely those presenting symptoms which are within his or her sphere of expertise. For those patients with symptoms outside this limited range the perfect specialist is expected in the ideal model to explain to the referring general practitioner that further reappraisal is required, either by the primary physician or by further referral to another agency. This is clearly impractical and although there may be tight knit little communities with such Utopian practices, I do not hear of them frequently, and I suspect closer on-the-spot observation might reveal a difference between the desirable ideals and the attained actual day-to-day practice. Many hospital clinics work on the "cascade" system and the longest attending patients are seen by the least experienced doctor, with little direction, who finds it prudent to allow a successor to review the patient in six months or a year, rather than discharge the patients back to the general practitioner. Those few pre-registration new brooms who attempt to discharge a high proportion of patients may unleash unexpected hostility to change. Similar hostility was evoked by the Balint group who attempted to discontinue patients' "repeat prescriptions" (Balint, 1970). Therefore, anyone in specialist, non-psychiatric practice, who says they never prescribe (or allow their juniors to prescribe) psychotropic drugs need read no further, although it is to be hoped they will carefully check, over the next month, that both amongst their patients, and in the family medicine chest, no evidence to the contrary could appear.

The general practitioner cannot escape from prescribing psychotropic drugs, unless his practice consists of extreme and devout Christian Scientists: some practitioners may proclaim they have, for example, nearly eliminated sleeping tablets in their practice, and fill us lesser mortals, who guiltily fear we may overprescribe, with gloom. Yet one G.P., whom I met at a conference and who claimed to have done so, mentioned he practised on a peninsula, and the nearest rival alternative doctor was seven miles away. Certain political states, behind iron and bamboo curtains, where personal car ownership is less common than in the West, may point out that restrictive state policy controlling this reduces certain difficulties, such as congestion and parking, ignoring limitations on personal freedom and mobility. It may be that single-minded, zealous practitioners have curtailed their prescriptions of hypnotics in a similar way to reduce problems connected with them, while ignoring the limitations. Since insomnia is not a notifiable disease, nor does it appear in morbidity statistics, it takes a more relaxed doctor to be more attuned to fulfilling the patients' desires and wishes than to currying favour with the D.H.S.S. by minimising prescriptions of hypnotics. It is always a matter of surprise that the N.H.S. *gauleiters,* who descend upon doctors spending more than so many standard deviations over the norm, do not also descend on those spending less than so many similar deviations *under* the norm to discuss whether their patients receive adequate modern, albeit expensive, therapy.

General practitioners are aware that their prescribing of certain psychotropic drugs, such as benzodiazepines, if plotted over the last fifteen years, produces a graph curve like that of a modern aeroplane taking off and only just levelling off, and the graphs of antidepressants are similar. Total hypnotic prescribing remains static and fairly constant, with barbiturates losing to safer, modern, but more expensive hypnotics. These trends are illustrated in the November 1971 supplement of the *R.C.G.P. Journal,* "The Prescribing of Psychotropic Drugs in General Practice" by Professor Peter Parish (Parish, 1971). However, more recent figures are hard to find to see if, with experience, a steady state has been achieved. Even "Trends in General Practice", published with the authority of the Royal College of General Practitioners in late 1977 in an impressive chapter on prescribing, only gives totals of prescriptions up to 1974, with breakdowns up to 1970, and no reference after 1975 (Royal College of General Practitioners, 1977). To those accustomed to searching for statistics this comes with little surprise, neither does the time-lag between collecting data, through official sources, via official publications, and appearance in review chapters such as this. What is happening to prescribing trends for psychotropic drugs in the present year may not be evident officially for five years, and if it shows a plateau it may not be so newsworthy as some new pharmacological growing point.

General practitioners have been presented as gullible dupes of the mass media, who react to the latest tranquilliser on impulse, from advertisers' blotting paper or film strip, and who force unwanted prescriptions upon patients who do not need them. Whilst overprescribing is a real problem, especially to the Treasury paying an open-ended cheque for N.H.S. scripts, or to house physicians washing out drug overdoses, I believe these attacks are over-simplistic. The Office of Health Economics 1977 *Second Compendium of Health Statistics* reveals that in 1967 pharmaceutical services cost the N.H.S. 10.6 per cent of its budget, falling to 8.4 per cent in 1975, and I fancy those in administration in a few years, when the statistics become available, may find administrative costs have risen extravagantly, while drug costs fall proportionately. General practice, which used to claim 9.5 per cent of the N.H.S. budget in 1951, has *pari passu* fallen by nearly a third to 6.1 per cent in 1975. With the houseman or sister, washing out stomachs full of Valium or Librium, in mind, it is pertinent to ask whether an overdose of paracetamol, bought over the counter and quickly attacking the liver, would be in some ways preferable. It is my contention that British general practice, with its independent contractor status, is far more sensitive to the patient *qua* consumer than other larger units of the N.H.S. The increase in the use of psychotropic drugs has been paralleled by increased alcohol consumption, and by the discharge of patients from secure asylums to the community, who may or may not care but who know that the one person to phone on a Saturday evening is the general practitioner.

General practitioners can be mildly paranoid when denounced by specialists in medical or non-medical fields for not knowing enough of their pet topic, yet I fancy a study of changing attitudes over the years towards abortion might reveal practitioners altering their approach more as a response to public-patient pressure than to official policy of Big Brother or professorial edicts. That practitioners can resist combined blandishments from lay and *avant garde* medical groups, is, I believe, instanced by the present slowness of adoption of hormone replacement therapy by the average general practitioner. Bearing in mind these reasons, perhaps the general practitioner can usefully reappraise his or her psychotropic prescribing, away from the heat and pressure of the consultation, by considering in the study some aspects of this problem.

This review of useful psychotropic drugs for generalist, or family doctor, deals with the problems under the following headings:

1. Differing Facets of Psychotropic Drug Prescribing Problems.
2. Updating.
3. Approaches Towards Prescribing Psychotropic Drugs.
4. Psychotropic Drug Treatment by the Non-psychiatrist.
5. Treatment by the Psychiatrist.
6. Super Treatment.
7. Conclusion.

DIFFERING FACETS OF PSYCHOTROPIC DRUG PRESCRIBING PROBLEMS

I will lift up mine eyes into the pills which everyone takes from the humble aspirin to the king-sized, multi-coloured, three decker, that which puts you to sleep, wakes you up, stimulates you, and soothes you, all at once.

Malcolm Muggeridge, 1962.

It is said that if the average engineer had as little information when asked to build a bridge as a doctor has of his patient or of other relevant variables, the bridge would never be built. Nowhere is this more apparent than with psychotropic drugs. Some of these variable factors are considered later with regard to the intricacies of decision, but the problems extend beyond the consultation. The academic in the ivory tower sees the statistics and comments upon the lack of precision of control without appreciating the problems of completing out-patients or morning surgery, knowing that an urgent problem on the ward or a home visit, exists. Yet if we turn to academics and ask them to measure depression or anxiety, reliably and consistently, few will confidently predict their ability to do so. Those few who do, if placed together in a conference, will probably attack each other in internecine combat, rather than produce a simple method of value, comparable to the haemoglobin or sedimentation rate, which is of use clinically. Rating scales that are used by trained observers such as the Hamilton Scales, or the more scientific Present State Examination of the Maudsley questionnaires (Wing *et al.*, 1974), given to patients (so that they are not contaminated by bias masquerading as clinical expertise) have been developed, of which the Beck (for depression) is popular and the later General Health Questionnaire (again from the Maudsley) appears more scientifically based (Goldberg, 1972). In many earlier examples, the original scale was developed in a population differing culturally, racially, and socially, from the population at risk under present surveys. It behoves all investigators who use such instruments to go back to the original book or paper, to see the criteria used to collect the original patients on whom the scale was based. If quoted research was dealing with those patients depressed enough to warrant E.C.T. as an alternative to phenelzine, imipramine or placebo, as in the 1965 M.R.C. trial, there may be less problem in agreeing the diagnosis than, for example, in the more profuse minor depressions that would never warrant E.C.T., and yet are so disabling.

Even if scientific psychological measurement is difficult, little extra useful assistance is available from laboratory tests, such as blood levels of metabolites, C.S.F. amines, E.E.G.s, twenty-four hour urine analysis, etc. all of which have been assiduously studied, with every available body chemical that is accessible being plumbed and measured. Our knowledge of the normal control of mood and emotion is as incomplete as the early explorers' knowledge of African geography, when all they had discovered was the coastline and the rivers. The future will undoubtedly reveal much, but this is of little consolation in dealing with today's patients. Today's ignorance may in future look as quaint as past debate over the source of the Nile.

It is ironic to realise that powerful therapeutic weapons, such as the anti-depressants, tranquillisers, lithium and hypnotics, have been developed upon an empirical basis far outstripping our knowledge of the underlying pathological processes. It is as if research in this field of mental illness could be compared to giving doctors iron,

B_{12}, folic acid, vitamin C, and other haematinics, and asking them to work out the indications for each by asking patients questions and gazing at the colour of the conjunctiva. To those who like to glance at yesteryears' journals and books, the problem of deciding whether cholera was due to a miasma, or if consumption was ever present in those cured of it, long before bacteriology or radiology were day-to-day tools, may not be dissimilar to our present perplexities. Our views on the genesis of today's psychiatric ailments may seem in the "brave new world" as ludicrous as the Victorian explanation that *paterfamilias* contracted tabes dorsalis by standing with his back to the household roaring fire. Ignorant of disease, but supplied with alternative remedies, can scientists not assist hard pressed clinicians? Mapother wrote in his 1936 Bradshaw lecture, albeit of psychotherapy:

> There is practically no evidence in existence as to the efficacy of psychotherapy which is guarded against fallacy in such a way as would entitle it to serious consideration in a court of law. Among those "cured" by any novel remedy are those who have never had the disease, those who still have it, those who have never had the treatment, and those who would have recovered equally well without it. All these classes are generously represented among those cured by psychotherapy.

The same could be said of drug treatment. Even in the most severe breakdown, schizophrenia, recent research has shown that America and Russia differ from the rest of the world in the criteria of diagnosis, making multinational trials or the extrapolation of results from one nation to another difficult. A new therapy for leukaemia, or aggressive hepatitis, may more easily be translated world-wide, than a new treatment for deviant psychological behaviour.

Another facet is the layman's perception of increasing psychotropic-drug prescribing. To those ageing unhappily, "Happy Pills" are a sign of decadent youth and evidence of professional pandering, yet, sadly, the ageing psyche probably heals itself less effectively than the youthful, in a manner comparable to similar less effective constitutional response to somatic insults. To the man from the Treasury posted to the Department of Health empire, it must seem the height of economic lunacy to read that anorectic drugs cost the N.H.S. several million pounds a year, for which a sizeable hospital could be built, and especially when Holy Writ states they are of no proven value: "Appetite suppressant drugs have little place in the management of the obese patient", says the National Formulary.

Even within the political spectrum, opinions diverge on psychotropic drugs, as on other issues. One view sees them as a modern alternative to opium for the masses, subduing the ground-swell of the have-nots, whilst at the same time, enriching pharmaceutical capitalist multinational companies. These drug companies make their ill-gotten gains by battening upon the sick and frail, bribing doctors with free meals for them and their wives, to collusively swell profits, whilst hiding legally behind defensive positions when tragedies, such as that of thalidomide, become apparent.

The opposite extreme point of view lays stress on the suffering relieved by modern treatments, asking how many remedies which save lives in Britain today were produced by the D.H.S.S. or a State drug industry? The advocates of this view ask if the second and third generations after revolutions are prepared to accept minimal standards or sacrifices, or if later pressure of consumerisms will want more personal medicine, leading to situations as in anecdotes of increasing private practice in Russia and its satellites. The sociologist sees the intricate patterns that cause one person to consult a medical practitioner, whereas another ignores the complaint and a third seeks solace elsewhere. The Health Safety Officer organises campaigns to hand-in unwanted medicines and is aghast at the hoards that are hauled in and wonders what lies in the cupboards of less public-spirited non-participants who continue to hoard rather than hand-in. Yet waste in society is regrettably replacing parsimonious attitudes as drug consumption increases, parallel to alcohol consumption.

With all these factors the public debate continues over psychotropic drugs. Should all motorists stop driving if they take a tranquilliser or sleeping tablet? Should prison medical officers prescribe psychotropic drugs for prisoners who react badly to containment, or is this an easy way out of the difficulties of reality? Would much of literature or music or art produced by persons of above average sensitivity have been produced if they had not suffered emotional distress? These problems abound so much that the average doctor, if he became too involved, might be a less effective doctor. In his Bradshaw lecture of 1957, "Between guesswork and certainty in psychiatry", Aubrey Lewis recalled the philosopher Cratylus who, as told by Aristotle, decided never to say anything but that which was certainly true, and so ceased to talk at all, limiting himself to wagging his finger (Lewis, 1958). Those modern doctors disheartened over this may take comfort from the past, from Aubrey's *Brief life of William Butler* (Penguin Books), a physician who lived for eighty-five years from 1533 to 1618.

Butler lived at Clare Hall, Cambridge, but "never tooked the Degree of Doctor", though he was the greatest physician of his time. He did attend a parson of Newmarket who hearing he was to preach before King James "who had a reputation of a great scholar" —

... the Clergyman studied so excessively that he could not sleep, so somebody gave him some opium, which had made him sleep his last, had not Doctor Butler used this following remedy. He was sent for by the Parson's wife. When he came and saw the Parson, and asked what they had donne, he told her that she was in danger to be hanged for killing her husband, and so in great choler left her. It was at that time when the Cowes came into the Backside to be milkt. He turnes back and asked whose Cowes those were. She sayd, her husband's. Sayd he, will you give one of those Cowes to fetch your husband back to life again? That she would, with all her heart. He then causes one presently to be killed and opened, and the parson to be taken out of his Bed and putt into the Cowes warme belly, which after some time brought him to life, or else he had infalliby dyed.

This historical perspective has two messages. It reminds us that the use and the abuse of psychotropic drugs is not wholly recent: whilst a physician has always to take some immediate resourceful action.

UPDATING

The principal goal of education is to create men capable of doing new things, not simply repeating what other generations have done.

Jean Piaget

It may seem imprudent, if not impudent, to introduce at length this topic in a review of psychotropic drugs, yet the half-life of medical technical information is decreasing. Pluck a journal from the shelves of five or ten years ago and the reader will find revolutionary treatment that came to nought, or minor snags such as the headaches with monamine oxidase inhibitors (M.O.I.s) that led to matters of great interest, and practical therapeutic importance. A medical school dean used to tell his graduates that one half of what they had painfully learned in their studies would be out of date within ten years, but no one knew which half. As a doctor, aged 45 at the time of writing, I find myself uncomfortably poised, Janus-like, between qualification at 25 and possible retirement at 65. In the fifties, at University College Hospital, London, the earliest hypotensives were being given by injection, like soluble insulin, with oral diuretics and hypoglycaemic agents still undiscovered around the corner. The impact on society and medicine of antibiotics, oral contraception, hypotensive drugs, has altered the face of prescribing habits and hopefully anti-tumour agents will extend from control of the blood proliferative disorders, to such scourges as cancer.

Yet if a cohort of students were stopped on graduation day and interviewed by searching sociologists on how they had been instructed to keep up-to-date over the next forty years, I fancy uncomfortable answers would emerge. Nor, I suspect, would a random survey of their teachers be wholly comforting. An International Congress in Pisa, for example, may make a gastronomic impact or one of camaraderie, but detached analysis may reveal from the set contributions that little was learned of value that would not shortly be in the literature. It is said, cynically, consultants learn most generally from a succession of registrars and housemen, except within their own small area of expertise. The Postgraduate Centre has performed the same function for general practice, for those who visit it, and when an enlightened organiser arranges programmes based on learners' needs, rather than on bravura displays of rare, fascinating, but statistically irrelevant illnesses. Yet what of the practitioners who do not attend their local centre, or the specialist who attends increasingly specialised conferences, learning more and more about less and less? Traditionally, the answer is that general reading covers this, but I suspect if we all kept a notebook of what we read for one month, it would reveal that we read what interests us, of which we have already above average knowledge. What we should be reading is in our area of deficiency.

I was immensely encouraged to learn that in the States (for a fee, of course) you can complete an M.C.Q. at home over a range of subjects, and be told that, for example, your knowledge of ophthalmology and orthopaedics is below par, whereas you need not read any learned articles with colour pictures of psychosexual problems for several years. Just as medicine is moving from the era of more reliable appraisal before action, so in postgraduate education we need to diagnose the defects before prescribing the remedy. We discovered in a local vocational training course for trainees in general practice, by giving a simple half year M.C.Q., that all trainees were very weak in factual knowledge of practice organisation. Teachers had assumed, working all day in the milieu, that trainees would have imbibed knowledge by osmosis without formal instruction. Once the diagnosis had been made, it was no problem to remedy a defect we had not realised existed. It is more important that we know where we lack knowledge in common day-to-day problems and seek actively to improve them, than to spend our hours in stage-one drowsiness, in a darkened lecture theatre, being impressed with hi-fi scientific technology of a disease that occurs once a decade in the hospital district.

Increasingly, groups of doctors, in the communities they serve, are meeting to answer day-to-day problems. How frequently should blood pressure be checked in a patient treated for hypertension and how often should the patient have a repeat prescription? How often should the diabetic have the retina examined? How often should a swab or smear be taken with vaginal discharge; is a script given, with a half-promise of examination when less rushed, if the discharge does not clear up, sufficient? The same questions can be asked of antibiotics given with minimal examination or, nearer the theme of this chapter, we can ask how often has a houseman written up a few sleeping-tablets for bed twelve, without knowing why the occupant is not sleeping?

Traditionally, postgraduate education suggests the answer is to be found in the conference or the archetypal lecture of forty minutes with five minutes of questions. I suggest many of these are pleasant and comfortable, but pretty irrelevant. Our reading is disordered and many journals we get because we belong to the B.M.A., or this, or that, Royal College. My accountant queried the fact that I spent an annual sum of three figures on new books, but agreed this above average sum might be justified as necessary to the tax inspector, as providing resources for chapters such as this. Benjamin Jowett, the famed Sage of Balliol, in another age, once was quoted as saying "an educated man should aim to spend a tenth of his income on books".

If lack of insight into intellectual deficits is the first major problem in personal updating, the second is the explosion of knowledge. Dr. Blakemore, in the 1976 Reith lectures "Mechanics of the Mind", postulated that man could extinguish himself by over-accumulating facts (Blakemore, 1976). The earlier doom-sayers prophesied a Malthusian excess of demand for limited natural resources: later gloomy prophets felt that pollution, possibly by radioactivity or hydrocarbons from aerosols, may lead to the end of civilisation as we know it. Dr. Blakemore postulates that in this age of photocopiers, computers, and data banks, we accumulate information faster than we can destroy it. Mercifully the brain can forget: whereas we can remember yesterday's dinner and, with difficulty, last week's, last year's is not remembered unless exceptional. It has been estimated, for example, that a conscientious reader, who sat down to read one month's publications of the world's literature in the English language on liver diseases alone could spend a lifetime reading only this. As I write this section, for example, I receive an advertisement for a handbook [sic] of studies of depression, the contents of which are of the highest relevance and fascination, but which has 440 pages and costs 68.95 dollars.

The third problem of updating is our childlike desire for steadystate knowledge. We learn early that two and two are four, and research is not likely to alter that. As we progress through school, especially in evolving subjects, such as the sciences, from time to time we have rare and occasional glimpses that our teachers and textbooks have old-fashioned knowledge that has been fossilised and is not up-to-date. At Medical School, increasingly, we became aware that scientific controversy exists. Professor X anticoagulates all coronary artery diseases, even those just with angina, whereas the eminent Dr. Y will not give his patients rat poison, and clever young Dr. Z is giving his patients aspirin. It is only as time expires after qualification, or if a young student has a premature interest in medical history, that it is realised yesterday's heterodoxy is today's orthodoxy, and yesterday's orthodoxy is now a quaint anachronism. Did we really keep coronary patients on absolute bedrest for three weeks? Did we always try to force young girls to have babies and suffer the trauma of seeing them adopted? Whoever treated diverticultis with a low-residue diet? We need to think of knowledge as fluid and constantly changing. The history of graphic representation of events has evolved from the cave drawing, to the oil painting, to the photograph, to instant video-visual playback in colour, and possibly eventually with three dimensions and smells. Donald Schon in the 1970 Reith lectures, discusses in "Beyond the Stable State" public and private learning in a changing society (Schon, 1970). He quotes from Tolstoy's *War and Peace* the understanding of real life uncertainty:

> For people accustomed to think that plans of campaign and battles are made by generals — as any one of us sitting over a map in his study may imagine how he would have arranged things in this or that battle — the questions present themselves: Why did Kutuzov during the retreat not do this or that? Why did he not take a position before reaching Fili? Why did he not retire at once by the Kalunga Road, abandoning Moscow? And so on. People accustomed to think in that way forget, or do not know, the inevitable conditions which always limit the activities of the Commander-in-Chief. The activity of a Commander-in-Chief does not at all resemble the activity we imagine to ourselves when we sit at ease in our study examining some campaign on the map, with a certain number of troops on this and that side in a certain known locality, and begin our plans from some given moment. A Commander-in-Chief is never dealing with the beginning of any event — the position from which we always contemplate it. The Commander-in-Chief is always in the midst of a series of shifting events and so he never can at any moment consider the whole import of an event that is occurring. Moment by moment the event is imperceptibly shaping itself, and at every moment of this continuous, uninterrupted shaping of events the Commander-in-Chief is in the midst of a most complex day of intrigues, worries, contingencies, authorities, projects, counsels, threats and deceptions, and is continually obliged to reply to innumerable questions addressed to him, which constantly conflict with one another.

The following three facts are essential in updating personal professional knowledge.

1. A knowledge of one's own personal deficiencies is essential, if painful, and a necessary pre-requisite of planning any learning as opposed to bumbling or browsing through a few comfortable, passive, postgraduate exercises with a "satisfied feeling that duty has been done".

2. The difficulties of selection are immense and a sensible compromise has to be reached.

3. Knowledge is in a fluid state and maintenance work has to be planned accordingly.

Many years ago, when I was soliciting donations for our first small Worcester postgraduate lecture theatre, a doctor senior to me, asked what all the fuss was about as "I thought what I learned at St. Swithins was meant to last me for life". It is an indictment of the medical profession's attitude to postgraduate learning (which I fear it shares with the legal profession) that it is still, as far as keeping up-to-date is concerned, locked into the *olde worlde* attitudes of the previous centuries. Yet academics at university, working a much lesser week than clinicians, have sabbatical study, every seven years. Ph.Ds. in industry are alleged to need to return to the basic laboratories every few years, or retire into non-scientific executive posts, and many hard-headed industries retire their brain workers at 55 or 60, on the grounds they are past their peak. High Court Judges and general practitioners, many of whom work into their seventies, seem to have escaped from the procrustian retirement age of 65. If the D.H.S.S. was passionately interested in the quality of their consultants or general practitioners, perhaps they would fund, with adequate locums and on full pay with allowances, study leave, comparable with the practice of industry, or some non-medical university posts.

APPROACHES TOWARDS PRESCRIBING PSYCHOTROPIC DRUGS

A desire to take medicine is the great feature that separates man from other animals: nickel-in-the-slot, press-the-button, therapeutics are no good because you cannot have a remedy for every malady: One of the first duties of a physician is to educate the masses not to take the medicine.

Aphorisms of William Osler (1849-1919)

The doctor
It has been my melancholy experience, both in previous practice as a psychiatrist lecturing to primary physicians, or a general practitioner talking to his peers, that notebooks appear and audience arousal occurs when the nitty-gritty of drug prescribing is discussed. Preach as I may that treatment consists of a balance between psychological methods and social manipulation together with the appropriate physical and drug treatments, it is the latter than interests the audience. The reason for this is self-evident, when I consulted a recent audit of a two-week period in my own practice, when I gave 1,501 items to 611 patients, of which items 184 (12.2 per cent) were tranquillisers, 121 (8.1 per cent) antidepressants, and 129 (8.6 per cent) hypnotics. Antibiotics were only 123 (8.2 per cent), simple analgesics 114 (7.6 per cent), gastrointestinal drugs 119 (7.9 per cent), topical steriods 54 (3.4 per cent), whereas I only once prescribed a cough suppressant, and never an expectorant (not all prescriptions are listed here). Also from the same figures the ratio between the first prescription and a renewal, either by consultation, or by our repeat system, was for tranquillisers 1 to 3.2, for antidepressants 1 to 3.9, for hypnotics 1 to 0.52 (i.e. of 129 scripts for hypnotics 85 were the first for that illness and only 44 were repeats for those patients seen again or given by remote control to messengers), whereas topical steroids were evenly balanced between new scripts and repeats. It is of interest that over the period the 611 patients were seen, only 475 were given a prescription, but 122 patients received repeat prescrip-

tions without being seen. With our repeat copy system, each doctor writes out his own repeat from evidence he has initiated treatment. Faced with such prescribing pressures (and I know of no audit of a hospital doctor's pattern) we need much periodic information. In the April 1982 issue of *MIMS* (a monthly index of medical specialties, issued free to all general practitioners and certain hospital doctors and pharmacists), the volume has a section (3) of twenty-nine pages dealing with drugs acting on the central nervous system. Section 3B on hypnotics lists twenty-five preparations, 3C on sedatives and tranquillisers forty-eight, and 3C on antidepressants forty-one.

There is evidence that an average doctor uses not more than one or two hundred preparations with any degree of regularity, i.e. more than once or twice only. Leaving aside special specific remedies for rare diseases, patients being treated under specialist advice, addicts to their bottle of medicine, tonic, or nostrum, prescribed by a doctor long departed from practice, if not this world, our repertoire is limited. If we, as prescribers, are psychiatrists rarely using non-psychiatric drugs, we can use our repertoire to cover a wide range of psychotropic alternatives. If we are general physicians with especial interest in leukaemia, Wilson's disease, or brucellosis, we can use part of our repertoire to give these diseases several alternatives. However, the more general the interest and the busier the workload, the more we descend to rule of thumb. Nor does an interest in psychotherapy decrease psychotropic prescribing. Balint *et al.*, who wrote *Treatment or Diagnosis: A study of repeat prescriptions,* revealed they were writing 27 per cent of their scripts for C.N.S. drugs (Balint *et al.*, 1970), as opposed to the British norm of 25 per cent.

We like to imagine that we balance all factors with deliberation before prescribing, but I fear this hope may not always be realised. When once I was personally involved with market research interviews about which oral contraceptive a particular practitioner chose, it was difficult to isolate factors influencing choice; brand image, chance, local consultant's advice, happy advertising, a patient's commendations, partners' experience, cost, bad experience in a single side-effect: all seemed to be jumbled together. Watching this topic evolve it does not appear that experts are unanimous so sometimes it may be there is little to choose. Choice is sometimes influenced by prejudice or personally idiosyncratic factors. Publicity in a popular radio talk, such as on the Jimmy Young show, can be counterproductive in persuading some doctors to try a new drug.

The patient
There is an old Yorkshire saying, "There's nowt so queer as folks". Even if the medical practitioner in his infinite wisdom has strong, well-validated views of what he will prescribe in certain circumstances, the active co-operation of patients is needed, much to the

chagrin of those with a depersonalised scientific approach who some-times give the impression that medicine would be an interesting intellectual occupation were it not for the tiresome patients. A very old Worcestershire lady patient, whom I inherited when starting practice, always used to take one glyceryl trinitrate tablet every morning and suck Digoxin when she fancied she had angina, and my efforts to alter her habits only damned me in her eyes as inexperi-enced, as I certainly was. Other patients have returned enraged, adamant that Largactil or Valium really suit them and my generic substitution of chlorpromazine or diazepam is of no value, which I find difficult to accept on the grounds of failure to put it to the test alone, as some have only read the name on the bottle before protest-ing, and have not consumed any of the contents.

Even with excellent psychotropic drugs and an enlightened doctor, consultation patterns influence prescribing. Some patients consult over minor matters, even as to which colour their front door should be painted, contrasting with the lady who phoned me in the early hours after the birth of her second child asking for phone advice how to deliver the placenta because, as she was fully dilated during the night-time, she did not want to disturb her midwife or doctor. It is understandable that a psychotic who thinks he is Napoleon does not consult, but such is the fear of insanity and the stigma of emotional illnesses that some patients, especially reliable extrovert men, will suffer weeks of insomnia or unpleasant symptoms before consulting, often with some pretext even then. One executive with an excellent war record developed palpitations, following his wife's and widowed mother's illnesses, accepting with reluctance tranquil-lisers "only because you say so, doctor", but subsequently being almost lyrical as to the relief and well-being they gave him.

The family attitude to medicine, whether the patients are con-vergers or divergers, whether the pharmacist puts in a good word or the woman next door approves, are all factors which affect accept-ance. Coloured tablets are better than white as Schapira showed (1970), and all who visit patients' houses must have been mortified to have found caches of untaken tablets, even collected while seeing the doctor regularly. I always ask patients what they are taking before prescribing and am surprised how much can be learned. Glyceryl trinitrate was given four times a day rather than when required, until Dr. William Murrell listened to a patient recorded as "Mr. A. B." at Westminster Hospital in the 1870s, who noted that the tablet relieved the pain as this occurred far better than taking the tablets regularly, and Dr. Murrell reported to the medical press that this patient's observation was well-founded, deservedly enhancing his professional reputation on this occasion. Similarly, taking antidepres-sants mostly at night, has become established through similar information from patients, as has the fact that the minimal doses to start with are often most useful in psychogeriatrics.

The patient's constitution may influence the desired results. Acetylators may metabolise some monomine oxidase inhibitors faster than non-acetylators and blood levels of nortriptyline reveal great variations and we have little idea of brain levels in man. A patient taking phenobarbitone may have accelerated liver metabolism, whereas an alcoholic with a diseased liver may have below-average drug clearance. It has been suggested that too high a blood nortriptyline level may be counterproductive. Absorption, metabolism, hepatic and renal clearance all can perplex the clinician who may have overlooked non-compliance.

Dr. Porter, a general practioner in Surrey, marked active agent and placebo with riboflavin in a trial of imipramine in general practice and found that some patients who were even bringing empty containers for further medication could not have fluorescence demonstrated in the urine, indicating that they had not taken the medication (Porter, 1970). Even in an elite psychiatric hospital some patients given chlorpromazine by trained nurses were revealed by urine analysis to be non-takers, as was illustrated in the film *One Flew over the Cuckoo's Nest.*

The drug

Arthur Bloomfield (1888-1962) once said, "Every hospital should have a plaque 'There are some patients we cannot help: there are none we cannot harm' ". Some factors concerning the interaction of the patient and the drug have been considered, but as a medical profession we often overlook the debt we owe to pharmacists, pharmacologists, and manufacturing chemists. Although I am frequently critical of occasional misguided promotions, regaining research costs by high prices, or "me too" drugs, evolved by molecular roulette in place of new concepts, I consider we are fortunate in the high English pharmaceutical standards set and achieved. From the general practitioner's view point, a highly efficient service is at his disposal, so that nearly any item in *MIMS*, however esoteric, can be produced within a day or so, and relied upon. When defects in industries such as car manufacturing are considered, or the prosecutions of bakers for foreign bodies in bread are recollected, the low level of complaints in all branches of pharmacy is as remarkable as "the dog that did not bark in the night".

Drug representatives, or detail men, are frequently criticised, but they can be a mine of information if approached correctly, they can answer or get answered queries, and, most importantly, can take back messages to H.Q. from the front-line troops. Those doctors who never see representatives, or only listen uncritically to sales patter, are not only losing a valuable source of information and influence, but shutting off feedback.

The evaluation of new psychotropic drugs, especially those for the commoner and less often referred emotional ailments, can only be assessed in general practice, but using the same scientific methodology with appropriate modification. Dr. David Wheatley has pioneered this work of general practitioner co-operative drug research and his book *Psychopharmacology in family practice* explains both the methods and hazards, whilst illustrating some results (Wheatley, 1973). The threat of drug toxicity hangs like the sword of Damocles over the head of the patient and the conscience of the prescriber. Some toxic effects are known and are a calculated risk, but others, in spite of all precautions, declare themselves like the practolol reactions. It has been estimated that 2,000 patients, under the closest scrutiny, will have sampled a drug before the Committee on Safety of Drugs will release it, and, although for further surveillance specially coloured prescription pads, or mailing questionnaries to patients have both been proposed, it is clearly necessary for all prescribers to have enhanced suspicion, and to remember to post off yellow information cards. These yellow cards should be familiar to all those who practice in the N.H.S. of the U.K., but for others it should be explained that they are reply-paid cards, regularly distributed to all doctors, encouraging reporting to a control agency of all adverse actions. In return, the doctors receive a horrifying printout of death and disaster attributable to the drug these have reported.

PSYCHOTROPIC DRUG TREATMENT BY THE NON-PSYCHIATRIST

The choice of drug either to relieve anxiety or promote sleep is therefore either a matter of fashion or convention.

National Formulary

It will have become evident that I am no pharmacologist, but a hard-pressed front-line physician, who judges it frequently necessary to prescribe psychotropic drugs. General practice has an infinite variety and the concept of orthodoxy is anathema. "There are nine and sixty ways of compiling tribal lays and-each-and-everyone-of-them is right", wrote Kipling. What I shall attempt to do in this section is to summarise my present attitude and approach in the four fields of (1) hypnotics, (2) anxiolytic drugs, (3) anti-depressants and (4) treatment of psychosis. I have not included, for example, the antibiotic treatment of G.P.I., anti-convulsants, nor the vain attempts to slow the ravages of arteriosclerosis.

Although some patients may seek omnipotent physicians, I have either developed insight into my poor memory or developed sufficient maturity to consult reference books, even during consultations or at the bedside. In my drawer and in my bag I keep the *National Formulary* and *MIMS* as an infantryman carries his pack and rifle. In the practice's library, less than ten seconds away from any consulting room, we have the lastest edition of Goodman and Gilman's *Pharmacological Basis of Therapeutics*, painlessly updating it by hiring annually from Lewis's Lending Library, so that the cost (£11 in 1982) is not a deterrent to replacement. In extremis, as a third line of defence, I consult (either in the postgraduate library, or more conveniently, at my local pharmacist) the incomparable Martindale (*The Extra Pharmacopoeia*), whose encyclopaedic twenty-seventh edition (which cost £30 in 1982) has 43,000 entries, 26 per cent more than the previous edition. It passes relentlessly from adrenalin via alcohol ending with water and has twenty-three close-packed pages on antidepressants and fifty-four on tranquillisers.

Having reached the state where I may consider a trial of psychotropic drugs worthwhile in a consultation, I attempt to assess briefly if the patient agrees with me and check from past notes any previous prescription. Clearly, if the patient has been helped in the past and the problem is similar, the same drug, even though not in my repertoire, is the first choice. If one of my favourites has been tried and discontinued, then either an alternative or extra sales-talk is needed. All other factors being equal, I prefer to use a few drugs frequently, than use many for minimal indications. Trethowan, in a personal view, postulates he can practice psychiatry with only five psychotropic drugs, but I would find it difficult to manage for long even with seven.

Hypnotics

Thomas Dekker wrote: "For sleep is the golden chain that ties health and our bodies together. Beggars in their beds take as much pleasure as kings. Can we therefore surfeit on this delicate Ambrosia," but Hippocrates' aphorism, "Sleep and wakefulness when both immoderate constitute disease", is still true 2,000 years later. Babies sleep sixteen hours a day, at 10 years this falls to ten hours, again falling to six hours at pension age. Forty per cent of children have a sleep problem, peaking at 2 to 4 years old.

Turning to adults, Hodgkin in *Towards Early Diagnosis*, suggests ten to eighteen consultations per year per 1,000 N.H.S. patients were for insomnia (Hodgkin, 1963). Shepherd took a random sample of nearly 2,500 patients from fourteen practices in South London in 1962: 15 per cent of men and 25 per cent of woman said "yes" to "Do you have great difficulty in falling asleep or staying asleep?". This rose from 9 per cent in young men to 23 per cent in male pensioners, and 13 per cent in young women to over 25 per cent in female pensioners (Shepherd *et al.*, 1966). In *Medicine Takers, Prescribers, and Hoarders*, (1972) Dunnell described a sociological survey from the Institute of Social Studies in Medical Care. They surveyed, with great sampling accuracy, 969 households in England and Wales, and 71 per cent responded. They tried to interview the 598 general practitioners of these households, but I regret only 56 per cent replied. One in five houses have tranquillisers or sleeping tablets hidden away. Over two weeks, those surveyed kept special health diaries in which 16 per cent of adults and 4 per cent of children admitted sleeplessness. Again of the 16 per cent of adults there were 20 per cent of women to 12 per cent of men, but I wonder if the fact that the difference between men and women was meaningful, since the percentage of non-sleeping children is more relevant than differences in the central nervous system between the sexes. Even more relevant to this is that a quarter of scripts were repeats. Eight of one hundred adults were taking drugs acting on the C.N.S. prescribed by remote-control repeats, having last seen the doctor over a year previously. The final nugget from this book for the medical reader was that 1,412 patients and 307 doctors were asked should a doctor be consulted if "they had difficulty sleeping for about a week": 53 per cent patients said they would see a doctor, but 17 per cent would do something themselves. Only 58 per cent of doctors felt this was a problem suitable for consultation. A similar question asked to patients five years before had produced a figure of only 45 per cent of patients that would consult for a week's insomnia in 1967 compared to 53 per cent in 1972 — this 8 per cent increase in demand in five years seems perhaps to support the pressure we allege we all feel, although denied by some of the statisticians of general practice, who say we "are working less hard and complaining more".

Malted milk drinks (e.g. Horlicks), hot milk itself, decreasing noise, increasing warmth, and even sex, all aid sleep, as does allaying anxiety and explaining that with age we need less sleep. Bennet reported in the *Lancet* that a single-handed Atlantic sailor woke briefly every half-hour of his thirty-eight day crossing with no gross ill effects (Bennet, 1973). Alcohol as an aid to sleep is expensive and crude and can produce early wakening, as well as the traditional hangover; it is, in my view, for physiological not pharmacological use. I stick to the old and tried rule-of-thumb to use benzodiazepines for initial insomnia, and tricyclic antidepressants for early wakening, but when in doubt, the former.

From an audit of my prescribing in May 1973, I found I prescribed 683 items at night of which 420 were true hypnotics (including benzodiazepines). The difference was chiefly due to 228 scripts for promethazine — chiefly for children or adults with a cough — which, although a relative of chlorpromazine, usually is classified as an antihistamine. Its safety and its absence of side effects makes this an undervalued drug, and having observed my own three small children, I felt that a good night's sleep for the mother of a catarrhal child is very worthwhile. Of the 420 true hypnotics, 177 (42.2 per cent) were for tricyclics (chiefly amitryptyline, trimipramine, and nortriptyline), 126 (30.0 per cent) for phenothiazines (121 for prochlorperazine), 100 (23.8 per cent) for benzodiazepine (nitrazepam 77 and diazepam 18 and 5 others), 15 barbiturates (3.6 per cent), chloral 2 (0.5 per cent), and 17 others. The D.H.S.S. will, if given an undertaking that it is for personal research, return each year a random month's prescriptions some months later, fully priced. Following this, I realised in 1973 that a year's nitrazepam cost £7.02, whereas diazepam cost £1.95, and a year's trimipramine cost £8.58 and amitriptyline was £27.20 as elixir, but £6.90 as tablets, whereas imipramine was £4.03 a year. After this, my current practice is to try diazepam with initial insomnia, but imipramine for early wakening (using 10 mg tablets for those starting over sixty). Sleep laboratories' research such as that of Oswald, is revealing more of different sleep types and the importance of REM (Rapid Eye Movement) sleep, when profound different metabolic changes occur. Dr. Felicity Edwards of the Employment Medical Advisory Service, speaking at the Royal College of Physicians "Health Risks at Work" symposium, quoted Nicholson, the expert on aviation medicine, as showing that, in 1976, diazepam 10 mg at night had no imparing effect on laboratory tests of work next day, which was not the case with nitrazepam or flurazepam. Research has also shown hospital wards may be as noisy as a London street, so sound control and ear muffs may be worth a trial as an alternative to hypnotics. Even in enlightened hospitals waking at around 4.00 a.m. can occur and it was also interesting to read Jill Tweedie write in the *Guardian* of October 20th 1976 "Now on valium I still wake at four in the morning, but I lie contentedly staring at the ceiling . . .".

A recent introduction is temazepam (Enhypnos, Normison) given in doses of 10-30 mg at night in soft gelatine capsules. The benzodiazepines mentioned earlier, when taking into account their active metabolites, have half-lives that may exceed twenty-four hours (and even forty-eight hours). Temazepam has a genuinely short half-life and should theoretically give less hangover.

Hypnotics are relatively safe and helpful, if used skilfully, as an adjunct to dealing with a sleep problem. The real art is to tell patients that they are for short term use and that once the circumstance for stress which causes insomnia has passed, the patient must be willing to wean herself or himself off the drug even at the risk of an occasional night with broken sleep. The regular repeat prescriptions for insomnia initiated by the doctor should be regarded as a rare occurrence. It is inevitable that many patients will be seen who have for years been on sleeping tablets and the ability to wean *these* patients off their drugs depends on the ruthlessness of the doctor and the sophistication of the patient in trying to find alternative sources of supply.

Anxiolytics

"Do I look pale? . . . I'm very brave generally . . . only today I happen to have a headache," so said Tweedledum in Lewis Carroll's *Alice Through the Looking Glass.* Discussion of anxiety and its treatment with drugs has a major problem of nomenclature, in that the physiological and pathological states of anxiety have the same name both to patients and professionals. There is no differentiation, linguistically, between protective anxiety and morbid anxiety, as there is between, for example, the words "sound" and "noise". For the same reasons, some doctors often unconsciously decry patients' morbid anxiety, possibly because these doctors fear lest their own defence mechanisms may contain personal fears. It is as if a patient with a fractured finger is advised by a doctor who, too, had a hurt (but only bruised) finger, which responded to rubbing it better, that increasing the degree of rubbing should cure the fracture.

The plethora of treatment for anxiety over the ages shows that suggestion, authority, placebo response, the passage of time, and the removal of stress are all powerful factors. The twentieth-century equivalents include psychotherapy, biofeedback and behaviour therapy amongst the alternatives to anxiolytic drugs. From alcohol to bromides to barbiturates to modern drugs, time and ingenuity have produced more specific drugs and, more importantly, less dangerous drugs. Their value was recognised by this table, extracted from data in the Office of Health Economics *Compendium of Health Statistics* (1977), showing number (in millions) and costs of N.H.S. prescriptions (in millions of pounds) for England and Wales.

	Barbiturates	Other Hypnotics	Tranquillisers
1964	16.1 (£1.9m.)	2.6 (£0.3m.)	9.0 (£3.9m.)
1966	16.8 (£2.0m.)	3.5 (£0.8m.)	12.5 (£5.9m.)
1968	15.3 (£1.9m.)	5.8 (£1.8m.)	16.0 (£8.2m.)
1970	12.2 (£1.7m.)	6.6 (£2.5m.)	16.0 (£9.2m.)
1972	10.5 (£1.8m.)	8.4 (£3.4m.)	19.5 (£11.5m.)
1974	8.6 (£2.4m.)	9.5 (£4.7m.)	21.5 (£9.6m.)

It is of interest to consider what further development is needed for a "perfect" tranquilliser. Even the rigorous *Drug and Therapeutic Bulletin* (which should be compulsory reading for anyone who prescribes) admits in the October 1977 issue the relative safety of benzodiazepines, except for a few unstable patients who become tolerant and need to be rapidly identified, as they increase the dose, which they probably would in the use of alcohol, cannabis, or placebo.

Aldous Huxley in 1932 wrote *Brave New World* predicting the future, describing in the year 184 A.F. (After Freud or After Ford as they recorded time) "soma" the new psychotropic drug which was produced by 1,800 chemists. This was to combine the advantages of Christianity and alcohol with none of their defects. It was a super-tranquilliser euphoriant and publicised with guilt-relieving jingles, such as "A gramme in time saves nine", "A gramme is better than a damn", but the central figure of Huxley's book was a primitive man who would rather be unhappy than have a false-living, chemical happiness. He finally chose rather than having drug-induced comfort to claim the right to be unhappy and freedom to protest. To re-read the book today is an uncomfortable and salutary experience.

Again, for the treatment of anxiety, I use diazepam as my first choice, substituting oxazepam or chlordiazepoxide if the patients had tried diazepam, or had heard ill of it from a neighbour or workmate. Probably the major disadvantage of diazepam is its wide range of uses and the fact that, as with most drugs, it is easier and far less time-consuming to prescribe it, than to sit down and talk to the patient.

Some benzodiazepines with a shorter half-life have been marketed for the treatment of anxiety (e.g. lorazepam). The conventional drugs are 1 : 4 benzodiazepines. Now clobazam (Frisium) which is a 1 : 5 benzodiazepine, is available. In spite of a fairly long half-life (eighteen hours) this was found to be less sedative than diazepam but equally tranquillising both in the laboratory and in a G.P. trial.

Controversy still abounds over the relative problem of long term consumption of anxiolytics. Many general practitioners such as Dr. M.R. Salkind feel that some 10% of patients are in chronic danger of being submerged by morbid anxiety and can be saved by the life-belt of anxiolytics. On the other hand the Institute of Psychiatry has found that some patients who have been on lengthy, heavy doses of benzodiazepines have visual hallucinations when withdrawn, and have required in-patient treatment to wean them off the drugs. The 64 thousand dollar question is whether after withdrawal there are long-term effects even months after they are off the drugs, or whether the residual effects are due to the psychiatric illness that caused them to be put on the medication originally. Stopping any psychotropic drug suddenly, without weaning, and monitoring of withdrawal effects may be an indictment of the method of withdrawal rather than the drug. It might equally be said because of the disastrous effects of dismounting from a motor car doing 70 m.p.h. on a motorway that such travel is dangerous.

Other drugs that I use in the treatment of anxiety I prescribe less frequently. In the section on hypnotics, the phenothazine drug pro-chlorperazine (Stemetil) was mentioned. In the chronic tense patient, with migraine or tension headache, two 5 mg tablets at night, or half a 25 mg tablet, can be more helpful than diazepam alone. Children who complain of bellyache or have the periodic syndrome, especially if they have a family history of migraine, can also be helped by pro-chlorperazine. The other somatic symptoms of anxiety, especially those of palpitations or sweating, can respond to propanolol (once thyrotoxicosis has been excluded). It is as well to explain to the patient with cardiac neurosis that the same tablets are used to treat a "nervous heart", as well as organic heart complaints, or *further* anxiety may occur after a chat at the chemists. Dixarit (clonidine) is a boon to many menopausal women with or without diazepam, especially as it does not have the embolic or withdrawal bleeding hazards of hormones. It is also one of the drugs where I prefer the proprietary name to avoid confusion with the two strengths of clonidine. The antipsychotic drugs have been used for severe anxiety but they are more toxic; they are used if diazepam or one of its family fails and, even then, in the lowest dose. If sedation is required, chlorpromazine 10 mg can be added, or substituted, whilst Stelazine 1 mg (which I find easier to remember than trifluoperazine) is alleged to be less sedative. The place for barbiturates is in the museum, although excellent and cheap for many patients in their day.

Antidepressant drugs

Burton (1577-1640) in *The Anatomy of Melancholy* wrote, "If there be a Hell upon Earth, it is to be found in a Melancholy Man's Heart". If anxiolytics are over-prescribed and might with value be curbed, then antidepressants are probably under-prescribed. The present range produce no rapid response to symptoms, and therefore are not so instantly popular. Furthermore, most have side-effects, including dryness of the mouth, drowsiness, or make special demands at a time of emotional distress, such as having to remember to avoid certain foods. Furthermore, even with the most successful drug therapy, there is a lag of some ten to fourteen days before an effective therapeutic response and during this time suicide may occur. Two Oxford psychiatrists, Keith Hanton and Eileen Blackstock (1977) interviewed 130 patients referred for depression, mostly having taken a drug overdose. In 122 cases the general practitioner was interviewed and it was found that 63 per cent of patients had seen their general practitioner within a month and 36 per cent within the last week (Hawton and Blackstock, 1977). Shepherd (1966), surveying a sample of several thousand from fifty London practices, found 7 per cent of men and 13 per cent of women said they felt unhappy and depressed, with 2 per cent of men and 6 per cent of women "wishing they were dead and away from it all" (Shepherd). Barraclough (1977) and Sainsbury, in a series of articles, have found that many successful suicides had seen their doctor recently and many other deceased depressives had an open verdict given, as suicide is still a stigmatised cause of death. Although the national suicide rate is falling, a fact that has been attributed both to North Sea non-toxic gas and to the help of the Samaritans, every general practitioner has, on average, a "successful" suicide every three years. It is a pity that the Royal College of Psychiatrists do not have a confidential enquiry into suicide, on the lines of the enquiry into maternal deaths, so well organised by the Royal College of Obstetricians and Gynaecologists. Watts, in his outstanding book *Twenty Years Observation of Depressive Disorder in a Community* (1966), calculates that an average practice would need two or three depressives a year to be referred to a psychiatrist, the G.P. would see and treat some forty that presented, and as many as 450 may be there to be detected. The last figure is corroborated in surveys conducted in other practices with the General Health Questionnaire.

The evidence is substantial that a real mortality risk and considerable morbidity risk attend the treatment, or rather lack of treatment, of depression. Tearfulness, illnesses such as glandular fever, flu, or hepatitis, early-morning wakening, fatigue, the T.A.A.T. ("tired at all times") syndrome and the request, "Can I have a tonic?" can all start the hunt for depression. The old, the lonely, the alcoholic, the physically ill, and those who have made a previous suicide attempt, should make the prescriber extra vigilant against suicidal attempts, as should patients who say gloomily all symptoms are due to their own fault, however superficially plausible.

My current management, when I feel a depressive illness to be present, is to ask five questions.

(a) What organic illness may masquerade as, co-exist with or have precipitated this? Especially with the first depression in the elderly it is worth doing thyroid function tests and an E.S.R.

(b) What social faults play a part or what psychological stresses exist?

(c) Is there a risk of suicide?

(d) Is there concomitant anxiety? If so may it be worth treating the anxiety in the first instance, evaluating at a second consultation the depressive remnant.

(e) What antidepressant regime will suit this patient best?

Antidepressants can be divided into tricyclics, mononamine oxidase inhibitors (M.A.O.I.s) and others. Tricyclics are of most value in the older patient with physical organic type symptoms of depression, such as weight loss, retardation, early-morning wakening and gloom. I now start with imipramine, giving as much as possible at night and varying the dose with symptom-relief and side-effects. In general practice one can give, say, two 25 mg tablets at night (less to elderly patients), and then review after five days to check tolerance and encourage perseverence during the phase of side-effects. The occasional one in a hundred of severe depressions may need the dose pushing rapidly up to a 25 mg tablet three times a day, and from three to six at night, but to do this to ninety-nine mild depressions seen in practice, will guarantee discontinuation of therapy or loss of confidence in the doctor.

I warn patients of the dry mouth, blurred vision, and constipation, and also that it takes two weeks before the depression can be expected to lift. I also warn that if the patient is better after a few weeks and they stop medication on their own initiative it will be several weeks before relapse can be excluded. Most of the tricyclics work similarly, acting, it is thought, to prevent the re-uptake of amines in the nerve terminals of the C.N.S. It is claimed that some act quicker and some have less side-effects. Although it may incur the wrath of those marketing one or other branded products, it is in my opinion more important to spend intellectual energy seeking out depression in its occult form and gaining the patient's co-operation, rather than to differentiate between individual tricyclics or rivals.

It is salutory to consider that imipramine was first synthesised in 1889 and was originally being tried out as a phenothiazine alternative when Kuhn astutely, in the mid-fifties, noted its antidepressant action. It comes as a surprise to me that I calculate I have been using it since 1958, being involved then, at a lowly level, in one of the first British-double blind trials. However, having tried out several newer preparations, hoping for less toxic or quicker actions, I find myself back with imipramine. To the minor side-effects must be added its cardiac effect, as it can lower blood pressure and alter rhythms (the last effect being dangerous in overdose or with myocardial damage).

The M.A.O.I.s were also discovered earlier as antidepressants by serendipity. Iproniazid was being studied as an alternative to isoniazid in tuberculosis, but the cheerfulness and euphoria it generated was disproportionate to its chemotherapeutic effect. As a group of drugs they are controversial and have two major defects.

Firstly, they are not so effective with the severe depression where E.C.T. is being considered, so that those doctors chiefly seeing in-patients, or non-private out-patients, do not see the small group who benefit most from M.A.O.I.s. In my experience, the atypical depressive of Sargent (1948), or phobic-anxiety-depersonalization

syndrome of Roth (1959), respond best. These patients are obsessional, timid, and only confess to symptoms of depression, phobias, or
unreality with reluctance; if they see a psychiatrist it may be
privately. Many truly housebound housewives fall into this category,
and these patients hide from state psychiatrists. Depression with
phobias should always mean that M.A.O.I.s are considered.

The second disadvantage discovered was that foods rich in tyra-
mine, especially cheese or yeast extracts, can precipitate a hypertensive crisis, with death from a cerebrovascular accident, or render
anaesthetics and other drugs hazardous. It is just the sort of patient
who benefits most who is terrified to receive the warning card that
must be given if they are to avoid forbidden foods. In Britain this
card is available from the Association of British Pharmaceutical Industries (A.B.P.I.) or any manufacturer making M.A.O.I.s. My drug of
choice is phenelzine (Nardil), starting at 15 mg t.d.s. and again
warning of the latent period when side-effects outweigh benefits.
Others include iproniazid (Marsilid) or tranylcypromine (Parnate).
The latter, which has a more stimulant effect, is also available with
Stelazine as Parstelin. All can produce hypotension and ankle swel-
ling. If no response is evident in a month, or earlier, or if depression
worsens, tricyclics should be tried, but after an interval of washout.
E.C.T., if severity warrants it, is still worth while in spite of the back-
lash against it. The newer antidepressants in my hands have been
disappointing. The tetracyclic compounds, such as mianserin (Bovi-
don, Norval) or maprotiline (Ludiomil), in trials do almost as well
as tricyclics, but although they lack the cholinergic problems of
tricyclics my patients complain of greater drowsiness. Mianserin is
being used increasingly if concomitant heart disease exists or if cholinergic symptoms from older and cheaper tricyclics cause distress.
Tryptophan, although good in theory and occasionally helpful, is
not regularly useful. Viloxazine (Vivalan) is unrelated to other
psychotropic drugs, does not give the usual tricyclic side-effects, but
produces nausea in some patients. Many others are advocated by
their champions, but in a fluctuating disease diagnosed only clinically,
and where placebo responses are high, it would be surprising if the
best placebo was not a drug that an enthusiastic physician believed
in and sold as really effective. Depression has been the subject of an
exhaustive and authoritative monograph (Paykel and Coppen, 1979)
in which the opinion is expressed that E.C.T. is warranted for severe
depression, tricyclics are the drugs of choice for moderate depression,
and M.A.O.I.s are worth trying in milder depression with phobias.
Yet there is still a need for a quicker less toxic remedy for depression
as has been written 300 years ago of depression:

It is also called the Scourge of Physicians because they who have it are continually asking
new medicine, and presently wearied therewith and daily complain to the Physician
and often change them.

The Practice of Physic — Riveri (1661)

DRUG TREATMENT OF PSYCHOSIS

Canst thou not minister to a mind diseas'd,
Pluck from the memory a rooted sorrow,
Raze out the written troubles of the brain,
And with some sweet oblivious antidote
Cleanse the stuff'd bosom of that perilous stuff
Which weighs upon the heart?

Macbeth V. iii. 41-4

It is difficult today for a young doctor to realise the plight of schizophrenics and other patients condemned to lengthy stays in large asylums when the editor and I were learning undergraduate psychiatry. My first psychiatric ward sister, a fount of wisdom, nearing retirement as I started as S.H.O. in psychiatry in 1957, gave, as her considered opinion, that "the new Largactil was not here to stay and they will never beat paraldehyde or morphia combined with hyoscine". Again, first developed for its antihistamine effect, chlorpromazine (Largactil) has revolutionised psychiatry, emptying wards so well that some cynics fear the pendulum has swung too far, filling prisons, lodging houses, river banks, and doorways, with patients discharged after intermittent therapy and a community that cares little more than in Poor Law days. Following the introduction of chlorpromazine, as soon as its value became apparent, many anologues appeared. The occasional jaundice or blood disorder produced by chlorpromazine meant that it was particularly hazardous to those sensitive to it, while if the dosage was pushed up, uncomfortable extrapyramidal effects were noted. I have personally appreciated its wide drug therapeutic range, having slept for two days after receiving only 25 mg intramuscularly, whilst I have seen an over-active patient with G.P.I. roaming the wards "searching for his elephant", on 400 mg q.i.d. taken as a syrup (to ensure compliance). For the acute psychotic, whether for manic schizophrenia, or organic delirium in acute illness, chlorpromazine or one of its analogues should be in the repertoire of all physicians and practitioners. It is more important to know the actions of a drug range of one of them well and confidently, than to have one-tenth of the experience with ten different drugs.

Schizophrenia has also been reviewed recently (Crow, 1979). Long-term treatment with drugs seems justified by preventing relapses, and a time lag in producing rises in prolactin in blood levels only deepens the mystery over the elusive cause — presumed to be a biochemical defect — leading especially to increased dopamine receptors. The fact that several drugs have equal antipsychotic effect with varying extrapyramidal side-effects is hypothesised to be due to the latter action being at *corpus striatum* whilst the researchers dispute whether the A.10 area, medial to the *substantia nigra* and involving the nucleus *accumbens*, may or may not be the critical area of metabolic fault in schizophrenia. None of the present remedies seem likely to exclude others in this field so far, but the tempo of original work makes possible the provision of a specifically tailored new product.

The more potent preparations have a higher risk of extrapyramidal effects which can be counterbalanced by anti-parkinsonian drugs, but these effects are disturbing to the patient who may well stop all medication unless closely supervised. As with antidepressants (and unlike the anxiolytic drugs) the side-effects of phenothiazines (which include chlorpromazine) are more apparent to the patient than the benefits, so that non-compliance is common for both these reasons and because of the features of the illness for which it is prescribed.

Chlorpromazine, of course, is of great value in organic illnesses or anaesthesia, and other phenothiazines have been used in non-psychotic illnesses. Prochlorperazine in migraine and tension headache has already been discussed and some severe tension states may benefit from a trial of Stelazine, or your favourite alternative phenothiazine, in low doses, with or without diazepam, if the latter alone has failed and environmental factors have been re-explored. Chlomipramine (Anafranil) is particularly well worth a trial in tense, obsessional ruminators, even without overt depression.

With certain exceptions, if drug treatment fails, it is more likely it is not the incorrect drug that is at fault, but it is that it is not being taken, or the dose is wrong, or that extraneous stresses exist. A similar drug in an alternative disguise can be more profitable if presented in a more attractive light, rather than ringing the changes on the same first choice.

Injections of phenothiazines in depot preparations overcome the disadvantage of compliance and are discussed in a later chapter as treatments not likely to be initiated by a general practitioner or non-specialist.

TREATMENT BY PSYCHIATRIST

Psychiatry is Neurology wthout Physical signs. A psychiatrist is often the first doctor to take a full history.

Neurologist Extraordinary — Henry Miller

Indications for referral depend on many variables: the experience, motivation and time available to the primary physician, his *rapport* with, and the tolerance of, the patients (with influence of families and friends) as well as the referral facilities available. Clearly, if the patient is not prospering and the family doctor feels it is likely that a second opinion may help, it is essential that this should be arranged. However, if the general practitioner equips himself or herself with appropriate skills, knowledge and attitudes, then most patients with anxiety should be able to be helped in general practice. A high proportion can only be supported, rather than cured, because of intractable personal, marital, or housing problems, and are not likely to be helped more by a psychiatrist. Some may be made worse or find that if they need life insurance, or a full medical for employment in future, the referral can raise queries. A second reason for referral is request by the patient or relative. The prudent, mature general practitioner, aware of the patient's rights under the N.H.S. terms of service, will rarely allow himself or herself to be manoeuvred into a position where a second opinion is refused outright, although by the time some appointments come through the patient may have improved with treatment, or the crisis be passed, so the appointment can be cancelled. A third and more valid reason for referral is that the psychiatrist has at his or her disposal weapons not available to the practitioner. These include possibly more time, a fresh approach with a new start from a mystical specialist who deals with the mind, the chance of in-patient treatment, referral to a psychologist for assessment or treatment, behaviour therapy, as well as physical treatments, such as E.C.T., or differing forms of psychotherapy. To these may be added treatment with medication such as lithium, where the rarity of its initiation and complexity of control make it usual that specialists, rather than G.P.s, start patients on such regimes, although once stabilised, the patient may return to attend only the G.P., being discharged from psychiatric follow-up. Finally it must be admitted there are some patients whose clamours and demands precipitate their referral, in which case the letter should read "take this patient off my back", although in these days, when patients or their lawyers in certain conditions can obtain photocopies of all their N.H.S. notes, including referral letters and the family doctor's N.H.S. Record Envelope contents, it is rarely expressed so bluntly. With time and experience the average practitioner realises that such referrals produce but temporary respite, the patient returning, harpy-like, reinforced by titbits as to what the consultant, the nurse, or non-English speaking S.H.O. said, often at variance with correspondence. For this patient it is not referral that is needed, but a Balint seminar group for the practitioner to explore, in a skilfully-led peer group, why such patients react in the way they do.

When I was the only psychiatrist in South Arabia for two years, patients and unit medical officers had no local alternative psychiatric second opinion. It was then possible to realise that the more sophisticated the primary physician, the less useful advice the psychiatrist could give, except by evoking therapies not available to the referring doctor, such as admission or invaliding. The reasons for psychiatric referral are few in personality disorders. The reasons for referral in selected neuroses are where the effort of special treatment is worth while, and in alcoholics who need drying out, or who will co-operate in treatment. For depression, referral is often necessary if there is a suicidal risk, or if response is incomplete. Most psychoses, such as mania or schizophrenia, need to be referred, unless they are transient, whilst for organic brain states referral depends on the speed of physical response, the tolerance of home or hospital ward, and whether psychotic or physical symptoms are being controlled.

What then are the special drug regimes that the psychiatrist can order that I would not initiate? It may be a new drug with all its blandishments to be used speedily "while it still works" before it disappears into limbo. A glance through the old notes of some patients attending psychiatric clinics for years reveals the whims of psychotropic fashions, with vague memories of Oblivon, Miltown and Drinamyl, and as Aubrey Lewis wrote: "the medley of tranquillising drugs may pass into the like chiaroscuro of approval and rejection." For examples of current regimes initiated by psychiatrists that I see helping my patients are: depot injections of neuroleptic drugs, lithium, Antabuse, and haloperidol.

Depot injections of neuroleptic drugs

These have produced a tool for managing schizophrenics of a dimension similar to the first introduction of phenothiazines. First, as these patients are undergoing treatment by injection, they cannot be forgotten, and this places the onus on the specialist in co-operation with community nursing to follow up such patients till well established, when they can return to the care of the primary health team alone. Furthermore, by injection much of the filtration by the liver is prevented, so more active drug enters the systemic circulation. Modecate (fluphenazine decanoate) is the local favourite, usually being given every three or four weeks, whereas Moditen (fluphenazine enanthate) is given usually every two or three weeks, and Depixol (flupenthixol decanoate) is alleged to be less depressing.

Unless the patient is a very dulled schizophrenic with the temperament of a stoic, the extrapyramidal side-effects may need Kemadrin, Disipal, Cogentin, or some similar agent for drug-induced parkinsonian effect. Of great importance to the practitioner is to realise that depression can re-occur not infrequently and needs active extra treatment with regular imipramine and possibly also diazepam for rapid relief of agitation in a crisis. Once the schizophrenic is stabilised on injection, if the practice has a nurse and, most essential, a system to recall defaulters, many of these patients can attend their local surgery or health centre. A major problem is for how long to continue injections. So far, no convincing long-term survey has worked out length of treatment for oral phenothiazines or the newer, injectable forms. Certain studies where placebo injections have been substituted, unknown to the patient, have revealed that a proportion of patients relapse, becoming psychotic again. Having had to deal with the excitement of relapses in early days when courses of injections were shorter, I consider that in view of the enhanced quality of life for the schizophrenic (unless some toxic reaction emerges generally or individually) treatment should be long-term. However, this conservative long-term approach may be modified if the newly-reported tardive dyskinesia accounts appear to be substantiated. From a few centres, patients on heavy long-term phenothiazine were seen to develop neurological extrapyramidal signs which persist long after the drug is stopped. Only time and observation in other centres will decide the significance of this.

Lithium

Lithium was used to treat gout over a hundred years ago, and fell into disrepute because of unexplained fatalities. For the patient who has had more than one attack of mania or where mania alternates with depression, it is invaluable and fairly popular, even with patients. The debate is, whether it is worth using in recurrent depression without mania. It probably depends on the frequency of the swings, how easy it is to combat depression, whether E.C.T. is needed or not, the value of long-term imipramine, and facilities available locally. It is a treatment not lightly to be undertaken, as toxicity can develop leading to death, with neurological effects at blood levels over 1.0 mmol/L, more serious damage up to 2.5, leading to a coma and death between levels of 4 and 5 mmol/L. The therapeutic range varies with laboratories and is often aimed to keep between 0.8 and 1.2, the figures 1.0 mmol/L being a convenient target. It is suggested that patients carry cards similar to M.A.O.I. warnings and need to watch salt intake and diet. Recently a case of intoxication induced by sauna and dieting was reported. If weight gain or concomitant cardiac failure occurs, diuretic treatment means more frequent blood tests.

Antabuse

This can be of value in helping alcoholics deal with their problem, but probably occupies a place only peripheral to the other methods of: group therapy, attending Alcoholics Anonymous (A.A.), dealing with underlying anxiety and depression and sorting out life stresses. A.A. are not in favour of Antabuse, but seem to tolerate it locally. It is tempting fate to give it to ambulant patients who have not been first dried out, rehabilitated and given a test dose, hoping the experience of a bad reaction to drinking on the drug will be severe enough to make Antabuse act as a deterrent. It is most useful in those living with a partner so they can take the tablet when observed and in the morning when motivation is highest but temptation least. Taken this way, it can make sure that a drink is not taken after the office or factory, or just a little gin before lunch and tea to "buck up" the spirits of the isolated wife of the over-busy husband, whose family has grown up. Analysis of relapses of those taking Antabuse often reveals that binges are premeditated and not so spontaneous as superficially appears, since the Antabuse has been stopped a day or two previously. A further refinement developed in Europe since 1955, is to implant ten or more tablets subcutaneously, but a recent Canadian series, although claiming 60 per cent abstinence at six months, confirmed my personal conviction that the alcohol experience, either due to low disulfiram blood levels or habituation, is unpleasant rather than devastating. A patient of mine, whom I saw with delirium tremens, having celebrated his forty-second birthday, told me he attended his first A.A. meeting after his twenty-first birthday. This patient has his implant supplemented by daily oral calcium carbimide (Abstem). A disulfiram injection with some basic research involving blood levels could be a most promising development in a field where the problems are increasing. Chlormethiazole (Heminevrin) is a useful alternative to diazepam or chlorpromazine in withdrawal states, but should only be used in short courses, as many alcoholics develop an ominous liking for it and a few use it to complement alcohol.

Haloperidol
Haloperidol is an excellent example of a drug which an average general practitioner would initiate so infrequently that good experience in its use would neither be gained nor sustained. For the one hundred and twenty general practitioners in the Worcester area, there are three consultant psychiatrists, therefore the opportunities for specialists to use potent but tricky drugs must be some forty-fold over the generalist. The chances of precipitating extrapyramidal reactions are great, although I have seen it used by a consultant psychiatrist in a patient's home with great skill and effect intravenously, with Kemadrin to follow, to tranquillise miraculously a most disturbed schizophrenic.

SUPER TREATMENT

People rather admire what is new (although they do not know whether it is proper or not) rather than what they are accustomed to (although they know already to be proper); and what is strange, they prefer to the obvious . . . . It is a good remedy sometimes to use nothing.

Hippocrates (400 B.C.)

Household surveys reveal statistically that most deviations into ill-health are self-limiting and settle with time, subjects such as "catarrh" giving rise to alternative topics of conversation other than the English weather. A relative or a neighbour may be the first source of advice and nurses, factory first-aiders, local healers, doctors' receptionists, and pharmacists all filter a proportion of ailments before the sometimes mildly paranoid family doctor (who fancies he sees *all* trivial illnesses) is first consulted. Some surveys have suggested general practitioners view three out of four consultations as trivial, but ask two out of three patients to come back, thus producing a category of trivial illness so serious a doctor cannot treat it at one consultation! Nine out of ten episodes of illnesses that seek medical attention are dealt with by the doctor or primary health care team. Of referrals, many are for technical reasons rather than that the primary doctor does not know what to do, e.g. repair of a hernia, or removal of a lump in the breast. With the increasing technology of medicine, sophisticated therapy must become commonplace. Will Pickles, the founding President of the Royal College of General Practitioners who practised in the Yorkshire Dales, would obtain second opinions from local colleagues and operations would either be done in the patients' homes or at a large town or city, like Leeds, often at a teaching centre.

One of the major benefits of the health service has been that specialists have been distributed nearer to where they are needed, in places of higher morbidity rather than nearer to the lure of private practice. Before the Second World War, a Worcester sick child, to see a paediatrician, would have to visit Birmingham or even London, whereas the first 1948 N.H.S. paediatrician, on recent retirement, has been replaced by two paediatricians. At the same time technology has simplified the cure of many illnesses: for instance, my grandfather died of a cerebral abscess following an ear infection, in spite of the best of medical attention in consultations with a youthful doctor establishing his reputation before becoming famous as Lord Cohen; I spent months in hospital with bilateral mastoidectomy, yet my son with nine attacks of otitis media in one winter rarely missed school; my brother's tonsils were removed, not quite on the kitchen table but in our guest bedroom at home, deemed to be safer than operation in hospital, yet of the one hundred and nine mothers I examined ante-natally last year, only two exerted their right, which I offered, to have their babies at home. Before the war our local asylum (which once employed Elgar as a professional musician as part of the therapeutic milieu) had a special unit built for operations to remove teeth, tonsils, and other focal sepsis. After the war, a unit was pioneered to abreact patients with L.S.D. Visiting surgeons performed leucotomies before the pendulum swung against this and insulin therapy (while even E.C.T., which has proven scientific validity, is currently under attack in the press and on television as barbarous and abused, being banned in certain parts of the world).

If one is fortunate with above average local psychiatric facilities, supported by psychiatrists and community nurses, what psychiatric treatments of value exist today that are not available locally? In the organic field of medicine patients are referred to centres for super treatments, for instance a patient of mine from the Worcester area is now at Oxford having his subarachnoid assessed for surgery; at St. Mary's Hospital, London, a young boy with hypertension and coarctation was restored to fitness and to being normo-tensive after a most involved operation; a keen golfer is playing again after the specialist fitting of a new aortic valve, having previously suffered nocturnal left ventricular failure; and a child with a Wilms's tumour is having chemotherapy under a trial protocol in Birmingham: in all these cases local investigations isolated the problems that require special treatments at regional units or centres of excellence. In psychiatry, although opinions are sought outside the local district they are more for "leaving no stone unturned", or for prestige, rather than for super treatment. Perhaps a girl with anorexia nervosa may go to an adolescent unit, or an exhibitionist (thus a law-breaker) attend a psychologist specialising in forensic problems. In my own experience of local treatment I can cite the case of an American (on a year's exchange programme), who had had twelve years' psychotherapy for depression (with supportive drugs) and requested psychoanalysis; the nearest Freudian analyst fifty miles away and another in London did not fit into the American private practice model to which he would return, so he settled for a year of my prescriptions for drugs (with supportive G.P. psychotherapy), presenting to me, on his return to the States, a volume of the Freud/Jung letters inscribed "For considerate and considerable help this year".

There are certainly psychotropic treatments being evolved experimentally, not yet available as routine. Involved cocktails of tricyclics, monamine oxidase inhibitors, tryptophan and lithium for depression, depot injections of fluspirilene (Redeptin) for those tense beings who cannot control their own tranquillisers, intravenous antidepressants as an intensive alternative, without any memory disturbance, to E.C.T., or the latest antipsychotic that acts better, quicker, safer and more expensively. There are existing treatments which seem to have gone out of vogue without good reason, such as Pentothal or Dexedrine intravenous abreaction useful for a block in psychotherapy, perhaps because psychiatrists using drugs favour minimal psychotherapy, and psychotherapists hope to use psychological techniques, not drug-assisted techniques. Psychiatry, technically, is going through a phase of regrouping and consolidating. Existing therapies are being re-evaluated in depth, whilst retreating from the omnipotence of a decade ago when any deviant or society reject was curable by psychiatry and no discussion of soccer hooliganism, nor shoplifting, was complete without euphoriant claims of success. It is difficult to think of examples of super treatments of proven value, available under the National Health Service, that take a significant proportion of my patients out of Worcester for psychiatric treatments that compare with those examples described in organic medicine. That there are experimental units, pioneers with bees in their bonnets, registrars with papers to write and reputations to make, alternatives to psychiatry and also the lunatic fringe, is undoubted, but the useful treatment that could be recommended to a relative or personal friends seems fortunately, although perhaps complacently, to be available locally with local psychiatric colleagues well-tuned to community needs.

CONCLUSIONS

> Guérir quelquefois, soulager souvent, consoler toujours.
> (To cure sometimes, to relieve often, to comfort always.)

Psychotropic medication draws such extreme points of view, from practically putting antidepressants in the drinking water, to almost-religious denunciation of the total concept of drug treatment, that to attempt to strike a balance may appear trite or impossible. It is easy to dismiss the floods of tranquillisers as being issued by the lowest medical therapeutic reflex involving a black ball-point pen and a white prescription pad but not the intervening grey cells. It would be nice if in primary care we could live up to our ideals of scientific prescribing, but in the issue of psychotropic drugs, as with antibiotics or skin applications, it far too often has to be a probability decision. It may be better to accept this and analyse how probability decisions can be improved. After all a skill such as car-driving employs many small instant decisions based upon incomplete factual knowledge, and also using probability decisions based on previous experience, rather than rigorous problem solving techniques using the hypothetic deductive technique. Professor Marshall Marinker, asked how he prescribed psychotropic drugs, responded by saying those patients who made him tense got diazepam, whilst if he felt sad with them he prescribed antidepressants, and those who drove him mad needed chlorpromazine.

If a proportion of patients on health surveys suffer from chronic insomnia it is possible they may be helped by long-term hypnotics, just as myopics are helped by glasses, some deaf by hearing aids, without being labelled addicted to long-term support that does not cure. When one hears "psychotropic drug policy" discussed as a political or social problem it is helpful to consider a comparison of the discussions in the same plane on "the problem of the motor car". Both drugs and cars have been boons in the personal life of millions, widening the range of their lives and relieving hardship and inconvenience. They both are only widely available in modern affluent societies, and increasingly a higher proportion of under-privileged "have nots" become the "haves"; both cars and drugs are surrounded by licences, restrictions, tests of safety and limitations of use; both are costly, although true costs, especially of development and supportive facilities, are often concealed; both are potentially dangerous, especially when rules are broken, leading to personal and family tragedy, and financial burden on the community and hospital facilities. In both cases of cars and drugs those who denounce the existing system often are in a minority position where they do not need that which they attack, or if they did, could rationalise their use in special circumstances, or see the problem from a very atypical angle, rarely face to face with the individual user with an immediate need. I think both psychotropic drugs and the personal car are here to stay, unless society alters radically. It is our job to improve, simplify, cheapen, and rationalise what we can afford in cost and efficiency, whilst realising that patterns of demand and attitude are greatly influenced by national planning, public debate and democratic choice. Seen in this way some of the emotive overtones of discussing psychotropic drugs can be viewed in perspective. For the doctor in the busy out-patient department waiting for nurse to show in the next patient, or a practitioner pressing the buzzer to signal he is ready for the next, the problem is real, immediate, and not solved by philosophical debate, sociological pleading, or bankruptcy of the N.H.S. The balance has to be struck, risks taken and decisions reached with psychotropic medication as with all medicine and its practice.

> The essential unit of medical practice is the occasion when in the intimacy of the consulting room, or sick room, a person who is ill, or believes himself to be ill, seeks the advice of a doctor whom he trusts. This is a consultation, and all else in the practice of medicine derives from it.
>
> Sir James Spence, *The Journal of the Royal College of General Practitioners*, April 1977, p.197.

REFERENCES

Balint, M., Hunt, John, Joyce, R., Marinker, M. and Woodcock, J. (1970): *Treatment or Diagnosis — A Study of Repeat Prescriptions in General Practice,* Tavistock Publications, London.

Barraclough, B. N. *et al.* (1977): "The effect of inquests on relatives of suicides", *Brit. J. Psychiat.,* 131, 400-4.

Bennet, G. (1973): "Medical and psychological problems in 1972 transatlantic yacht race", *Lancet*, ii, 7832.

Blakemore, C. (1976): "Mechanics of the mind", *Reith Lectures*, B.B.C., London.

Crow, T. J. (1979): in *Recent Advances in Clinical Psychiatry (3)*, ed. Kenneth Granville-Groseman, Churchill Livingstone.

Dunwell, Karen and Cartwright, Ann (1972): *Medicine Takers, Prescribers and Hoarders*, Routledge and Kegan Paul, London.

Goldberg, D. (1972): *The Detection of Psychiatric Illness by Questionnaire* — Maudsley Institute Monograph No. 21, Oxford University Press, London.

Hodgkin, K. (1963): *Towards Earlier Diagnosis*, Livingstone, Edinburgh and London.

Hawton, K. and Blackstone, E. (1977): "Deliberate self poisoning: Implications for psychotropic drug prescribing in general practice", *J. Royal Coll. of General Prac.*, 27, 560-3.

Lewis, A. (1958): "Between guesswork and certainty in psychiatry", *Lancet,* i, 227.

Mapother, E. (1936): "The integration of neurology and psychiatry", *Bradshaw Lecture*, Royal College of Physicians, London.

Office of Health Economics (1977): *Compendium of Health Statistics*, 2nd edition, Office of Health Economics, London.

Parish, Peter (1971): "The prescribing of psychotropic drugs in general practice", *J. Royal Coll. of General Prac.*, Supp. 4.

Paykel, E. S. and Coppen, A. (eds.) (1979): *Psychopharmacology of Affective Disorders*, Oxford University Press, Oxford.

Porter, A. M. W. (1970): "Depressive illness in general practice: A demographic study and controlled trial of Imipramine", *Brit. Med. J.*, ii, 446-9.

Roth, M. (1959): "The phobic anxiety-depersonalisation syndrome", *Proc. Roy. Soc. Med.*, 52, 587-595.

Royal College of General Practitioners (1977): *Trends in General Practice: A Collection of Essays by Members of the Royal College of General Practitioners*, British Medical Journal, London.

Sainsbury, P. (1968): in *Recent Developments: Affective Disorders*, ed. A. Copper and A. Walk, R.M.P.A., Heddley Brothers, Kent.

Salkind, M. R., Hanks, G. W. and Silverstone, J. T. (1979): "Evaluation of the effects of clobazam, a 1, 5 benzodiazepine, on mood and psychomotor performance in clinically anxious patients in general practice", *British Journal of Clinical Pharmacology*, 7, supplement 1, 113-118.

Sargent, W. and Slater, B. (1948): *Physical Methods of Treatment in Psychiatry*, 2nd edn., Livingstone, Edinburgh.

Schapira, K., McClelland, H. A., Griffith, N. R. and Newell, D. J. (1970): "Study of the effects of tablet colour in the treatment of anxiety states", *Brit. Med. J.*, ii, 446-9.

Schon, D. (1970): "Beyond the stable state", *Reith Lectures*, B.B.C., London.

Shepherd, M. Cooper, B., Brown, A. and Kalton, G. (1966): *Psychiatric Illness in General Practice*, Oxford University Press, London.

Watts, C. A. H. (1966): *Depressive Disorders in the Community*, John Wright, Bristol.

Wheatley, D. (1973). *Psychopharmacology in Family Practice*, Heinemann, London.

Wing, J. K., Cooper, J. E. and Sartorius, N. (1974): *The Measurement and Classification of Psychiatric Symptoms*, Cambridge University Press, Cambridge.

FURTHER READING

From the very nature of the subject any review of psychotropic drugs begins going out of date like a decay curve of radioactivity. For information on a new drug the pharmaceutical companies often embarrass with a plethora of information, but by its very source, selected for its positive nature. To counter balance this, critical reviews, especially those such as *Drugs and Therapeutic Bulletin* need to be consulted. The perplexing field of the newer antidepressants is reviewed in Vol. 1. No. 2. January 1978, *Journal of Pharmacotherapy* by P. K. Bridges and T. R. E. Barnes.

Trends in General Practice (*see* Royal College of General Practitioners reference above). Chapter 8 reviews prescribing, whilst "The Future General Practitioner" (learning and teaching) *B.M.J.* 1972 delineates general practice especially from an educational point of view. Chapter 8 "General practice — the team approach and social services" in *Comprehensive Psychiatric Care* (1976), edited by A. A. Baker (published by Blackwell Scientific), discusses management with psychotropic drugs as one method of containing the psychiatric workload.

The National Formulary and *MIMS* (which appears monthly) are freely available to practitioners and Martindale should be available at the Postgraduate Library.

The Diagnosis and Management of Sexual Inadequacy

Dr. Alan J. Cooper,

M.D., F.R.C.Psych., D.P.M., Dip.Pharm.Med.

Associate Professor of Psychiatry, University of Western Ontario and Director of Psychiatry, Sarnia General Hospital, Sarnia, Canada.

The Diagnosis and Management of Sexual Inadequacy

INTRODUCTION

The aims of this chapter are to:

(a) define the main types of sexual inadequacy encountered in contemporary practice;

(b) outline the essential steps in taking a history and arriving at a diagnostic formulation;

(c) detail a short-term mainly practically-oriented treatment approach; and

(d) offer a guide to prognosis.

The therapy described has evolved out of personal research findings (Cooper, 1967) together with relevant borrowing from some other contemporary workers, notably Masters and Johnson (1970). Give or take an "ingredient" it is very similar to many other behavioural models in current use which are now generally accepted as being the treatments of choice for sexual inadequacy (e.g. Bancroft, 1975; Ansari, 1976; Kaplan, 1974; Lobitz and LoPiccolo, 1972).

The method which is suitable for an N.H.S. setting can be applied with or without minor modifications by any reasonably intelligent person, able to communicate adequately, in the vernacular if necessary, who has no sexual "hang-ups" and has a confident, empathic manner — in short any competent general practitioner or other health professional interested in the field.

Traditionally, in the recent past most sexual problems have been managed by psychiatrists using various types of individual psychotherapy. Ranging from classical psychoanalysis on the one hand, to simple reassurance and sexual education on the other, the majority of these methods, to satisfy their own theoretical requirements or simply out of custom, have tended to exclude the sexual partner. It is perhaps ironic that it was left to the innovative research of Masters and Johnson, respectively a gynaecologist and a social worker, to make crystal clear that there can be no such thing as an "uninvolved partner" in sexual inadequacy and that therapy, to be optimal, must involve the active co-operation and participation of both (Masters and Johnson, 1970). Furthermore, without minimising the importance of a good relationship, Masters and Johnson pointed out that the bulk of problems could be successfully treated by short-term, mainly practical measures, with very little psychotherapeutic content — a view in sharp contrast to psychiatric thought and practice at the time. Although some psychiatrists believe that Masters and Johnson place undue emphasis on the "behavioural" at the expense of the "psychological", most present-day counsellors take something from them for building into their own systems.

The writer conceptualises sexual inadequacy, however precipitated, as being variable failure in various physiological responses, i.e. erection, ejaculation, lubrication in the female etc. A logical treatment approach, therefore, aims to establish or re-establish these mechanisms by mainly practical means. Analogously (and it may seem too obvious to state) learning to swim at some stage involves getting into the water, however much prior discussion (e.g. psychotherapy) is enjoined. This is not a denial of the importance of psychodynamics, but a plea for perspective. In a rapid-treatment programme the optimal role of the discussion lies in creating, as far as possible, a climate favourable to the proper implementation of a suitable practical regimen. Clearly in some circumstances this is easier than in others. For instance, in the case of a young, sexually naïve male, with a normal drive, impotent because of inhibitory anxiety, who has a good marital relationship and is motivated for treatment, psychotherapy should mainly be concerned with providing relevant factual information on the physiology, anatomy and psychology of sexual arousal, stimulative techniques, reassurance and support: to boost confidence, successes are praised and failures analysed. Such superficial counselling requires no great sophistication, nor a detailed knowledge of psychodynamics; it needs mainly intuition and common sense, which can be refined with experience.

On the other hand, if the impotence is symptomatic of grave personality and relationship problems, then *a priori* these will need to be resolved sufficiently by psychotherapy to enable an appropriate physiological programme to be instituted. In such complicated cases a greater knowledge of dynamics is required, which usually puts it outside the scope of the non-psychiatrically-trained.

The therapist's skill lies in assessing the many possible often interwoven causal factors, making a valid diagnostic formulation, and thereafter in blending psychological and physiological elements into a suitable treatment plan for the individual case.

EVALUATION OF THE SEXUALLY INADEQUATE COUPLE

Sexual inadequacy *never* affects individuals, only couples. This is a maxim which should never be forgotten and it is probably unwise to attempt treatment without the active co-operation of both partners. Repeated failure of one or other to attend either the initial interview or subsequent sessions, however excused, should make the therapist ask himself whether the couple are sufficiently motivated. As a general rule it is inadvisable to continue with persistent defaulters, since the basic therapy requirements can rarely be met.

Ideally, the first interview involves seeing the couple separately for about ten minutes each and then together for forty-five minutes. There is no place for the embarrassed evasion of threatening topics and even if "keep off" signs are posted, the therapist must be diplomatically singleminded in securing accounts of sufficient detail to enable an accurate diagnosis to be formulated. In the majority of "simple" cases this can be made within one hour. More "complicated" issues, involving personality and relationship difficulties, may take longer to unravel. If these latter prove daunting, the therapist may choose to refer the couple for the more specialised attention of an appropriate psychotherapist. However, in the writer's experience this is a comparatively rare eventuality.

A history-taking scheme for use in sexual inadequacy is set out in the appendix to this chapter. With experience, it soon becomes apparent which items are especially relevant in the individual case and the protocol can be pruned accordingly. Additionally a physical examination should be conducted in every case and, when indicated, appropriate laboratory tests performed (but *see* p. 179).

CAUSES OF SEXUAL INADEQUACY

It is convenient to consider the many possible causes of sexual inadequacy in four arbitrary categories as follows:

(*a*) organic;
(*b*) psychosocial;
(*c*) constitutional;
(*d*) biological.

They are not mutually exclusive; in the individual case one or more factors from each category may co-exist and overlap or interact to a lesser or greater degree. The main ones are set out in Table 1.

An illustrative example is the impotence of diabetes mellitus. Although initially this may have a predominantly organic aetiology, the majority of patients develop performance anxiety which exacerbates and/or perpetuates the erectional failure, even if the diabetes is adequately controlled. The best treatment plan must, therefore, combine appropriately medical and psychosomatic elements.

TABLE 1. CLASSIFICATION OF MAIN CAUSES
OF SEXUAL INADEQUACY

Organic (see Table 2)	Psychosocial	Constitutional (Mainly genetic)	Biological
Any debilitating physical illness, such as diabetes and side-effects of drugs, e.g.: antidepressants sedatives hypotensives tranquillisers anticholinergics alcohol, etc.	Anxiety Personality and relationship problems Hostility Disgust Inhibition Sexual inversion Sexual ignorance Faulty stimulative techniques Depression Sexual boredom	Probably determines the strength of sex drive. Low sex drive may limit sexual learning during adolescence and early adulthood and thus compromise adult proficiency, apparently much more important in the male.	Pregnancy and post-partum Ageing Climacteric problems Menstrual cycle

Organic conditions

Possible organic causes of sexual inadequacy which have been culled from the literature are elaborated in Table 2. In perspective these are rare, probably not contributing significantly to more than 5 per cent of cases. The two most important are diabetes and the side-effects of drugs; although it should be remembered that *any* moderately serious physical illness can inhibit libido and performance at the time.

It may helpful to take the example of diabetes and look at its features in contributing to inadequacy. The association between impotence and diabetes which was first made in 1798, has become well recognised only during the past two decades. It has been estimated that up to 60 per cent of all diabetic men will develop impotence of varying degrees at some stage of their sexual lives (Cooper, 1972). Clinically the impotence of diabetes takes three main developmental forms:

(a) usually the condition manifests after diabetes has been (biochemically) established for several years;

(b) impotence may be the first or an early sign of diabetes, present before the diagnosis is firmly established;

(c) any diabetic whose illness gets out of control may become impotent temporarily.

The underlying cause of impotence in diabetes remains as yet unknown. Nevertheless, it has been postulated that at least three mechanisms may be responsible, which may coexist and overlap:

(a) it may be a type of diabetic neuropathy;

(b) it may be due to arteriosclerotic changes in the penile blood vessels which impair the pooling of blood, thereby reducing erectile capacity; and

(c) it may be due to generalised "metabolic abnormality".

The position in female diabetics is somewhat different. Although, in general, they are probably less sexually responsive than non-diabetic women, they appear to be relatively immune from the severe impairment which may be seen in men. This may be due to the fact that psychological and emotional considerations are proportionately more important in determining a sexual response in women; for men physical influences are pre-eminent.

TABLE 2. ORGANIC DISORDERS AND PHYSICAL CAUSES
ASSOCIATED WITH SEXUAL INADEQUACY[1]

Organic disorders	Other physical causes
Cardiorespiratory	*Anatomical*
Myocardial infarction	Castration
Emphysema	Congenital deformities
Angina	Testicular fibrosis
	Hydrocoele
Endocrine	Intact hymen
	Episiotomy scar
Acromegaly	Perineal prostatectomy
Addison's disease	Vasectomy
Adrenal neoplasms	Hysterectomy
Chromophobe adenoma	Sympathectomy
Diabetes	
Feminising interstitial cell	
Testicular tumours	*Interference with sensitivity reactions*
Infantilism	Condoms
Ingestion of female hormones	Pessaries
(e.g. oestrogens)	Douches
Antiandrogens, e.g. cyproterone	
acetate	
Myoedema	
Obesity	
Thyrotoxicosis	

NOTE: 1. With the exception of diabetes and the side-effects of certain drugs, all are extremely rare and in many cases debatable.

TABLE 2. contd. ORGANIC DISORDERS AND PHYSICAL CAUSES
ASSOCIATED WITH SEXUAL INADEQUACY[1]

Organic disorders	Other physical causes
Genito-urinary	*Side-effects of the following drugs*
Prostatitis	(*see* note 2. below)
Phimosis	Alcohol
Priapism	Amphetamines
Urethritis	Amitriptyline
Cystitis	Atropine
Fibroids	Benperidol
Laceration of broad ligament	Bethanidine
Peyronie's disease	Chlorodiazepoxide
Endometriosis	Chlorpromazine
	Guanethidine
Infections	Methantheline bromide
Candida albicans	Reserpine
Trichomonas	Thioridazine
Genital tuberculosis	Pesticides
Gonorrhoea	
Mumps	
Endometritis	
Neurological	
Amyotrophic lateral sclerosis	
Transection of the cord	
Multiple sclerosis	
Parkinsonism	
Peripheral neuritis	
Tabes dorsalis	
Temporal lobe lesions	
Vascular	
Haemorrhoids	
Thrombosis of aortic bifurcation	

NOTE: 2. At the time of writing over forty commonly prescribed drugs are alleged to be capable of causing or contributing to sexual inadequacy.

Side-effects of drugs

Many drugs are stated to have adverse effects upon sexual response (*see* Table 2). In a few instances these are well documented and can be predicted from pharmacological knowledge; in others, however, the evidence is vague and inconclusive. Perhaps nowhere is this uncertainty greater than in the case of contraceptive hormones. In some women there may be an enhancement of libido, possibly because they feel secure against an unwanted pregnancy, whilst in others, concern about reported side-effects (especially depression, anorgasmia and thrombosis) which are represented as being inevitable, or at least highly likely, take their toll in increased sexual morbidity. In fact there is no real evidence for an effect on orgasm either way but, of course, individuals may experience increased or decreased libido coincidentally. The area has been well surveyed by Weissman and Slaby (1973).

All hypnotics, narcotics and tranquillisers, being cerebral depressants, may impair libido and sexual response if large enough doses are used. However, paradoxical effects are sometimes observed, depending on dose and the emotional state of the user at the time (Cooper, 1978). Although, in general, the situation is confusing and arguable, there are a few classes of drugs which most authorities agree, specifically depress sexuality in a sizeable minority. Thus, hypotensive agents such as guanethidine and bethanidine which block adrenergic impulses in the peripheral sympathetic nerves may delay or arrest ejaculation in up to 41 per cent of users (Bulpitt and Dollery, 1973). Although there are no precise figures, medicines with powerful anticholinergic properties, such as tricyclic antidepressants and major tranquillisers, including thioridazine and chlorpromazine, may cause impotence as well as delaying and inhibiting ejaculation, depending upon dosage. Indeed thioridazine has been used with some success as a specific treatment for premature ejaculation (Mellgren, 1967). It has also been claimed that such drugs, by inducing relaxation, might attenuate the function of the pubic muscles sufficiently to impair a female's capacity to respond to orgasm; this returns to normal on stopping the medication (Renshaw and Ellenberg, 1978). It is mandatory, therefore, to enquire about drug habits in all cases and to make an assessment of any probable aetiological significance.

In practice, because of the underlying medical condition, it may not always be wise to discontinue a drug. However, if it is suspected that it might be playing a major role in the sexual inadequacy, then the matter should be discussed with the patient, and, whenever possible, the prescriber, to explore the feasibility of reducing the dose. Clearly, the patient's motivation for improved sexual function as well as the severity of the medical condition being treated must influence the final decision. In many instances, however, it has been possible to reduce the dose of a hypotensive sufficiently to improve sexual response without jeopardising the patient's medical status. On the other hand, in malignant hypertension, such a course may be fraught with danger and unacceptable. Each situation demands careful review and must be treated on merit.

Psychosocial factors

Despite the paucity of adequate studies (but *see* El-Senoussi *et al.*, 1959; Fisher, 1973), the majority of experienced clinicians dogmatically assert a central role for various psychosocial factors in up to 90 per cent of all cases of sexual inadequacy. However, it should be pointed out that these are just some of a group of many and diverse possibilities and they should only be adduced positively and in perspective, never by default. Psychological causes should never be presumed: if operating they should be elicitable in all cases during a searching examination even if subtle or disguised.

The following are the commonest psychosocial causes of sexual inadequacy which may be unearthed during a searching diagnostic interview.

Anxiety

Although its central aetiological significance is well recognised it is incumbent upon the therapist to judge the relevance of anxiety in the individual case. This is best done by asking the patient to introspect and describe his feelings during attempted coitus or other forms of love-play. The somatic and psychological manifestations of anxiety can then be appraised. For instance, in a case of severe vaginismus or premature ejaculation the presence of tachycardia, sweating, dry mouth, together with a subjective experience of dread, may be overwhelming and there is no room for argument. On the other hand, in many cases anxiety may be playing only a minimal role and scrupulous questioning may be required to make an accurate assessment of its causal contribution. Even if not the original cause, anxiety is a common bed-fellow of sexual inadequacy, and invariably exacerbates it. The range of anxieties expressed during a clinical interview are protean and reflect specific concerns of the sufferer. Illustratively Table 3 shows some common male worries experienced during actual or imagined coitus (Cooper, 1969 (1)). Fear of failure itself, i.e. of not living up to the current media sexual stereotype of a sexual superman, capable of sustaining an erection for hours on end and performing repeated acts of coitus, is far and away the most frequent.

Apart from the differences inherent in her procreative role, the female is subject to the same sort of fears as the male. It is perhaps only necessary, therefore, to highlight some differences. In women various worries about the penis are common. Very often they feel threatened by its size and, believing it might be damaging in some way, may develop variable levels of avoidance anxiety, in some cases of phobic proportions (i.e. severe vaginismus). Probably it is a sign of the times that an increasing number of women, especially the more emancipated, who have "hang-ups" about the traditional dominant sexual role of the male are anxious (although more often angry) about letting themselves go, i.e. of being exploited and forced to respond against their will; this may preclude a full response.

TABLE 3. SPECIFIC ANXIETIES MOST FREQUENTLY ASSOCIATED WITH COITAL ATTEMPTS IN A GROUP OF POTENCY DISORDER MALES

Specific anxiety reported	Number of times mentioned	% (n = 46)
Fear of failure	26	56.3
Fear of being seen by wife as sexually inferior	20	43.5
Fear of ridicule (from wife)	19	40.0
Fear of pregnancy	11	24.0
Anxiety over size of genitals	7	15.2
Fear of physical disease	7	15.2
Pervasive anxiety (no specific cause)	5	11.0
Fear of detection (i.e. of being caught by a third party)	3	6.7

NOTE: Table 3 refers to manifest anxieties experienced by the patient during coital attempts. Only anxieties specifically and spontaneously (sometimes with a minimum of prompting) mentioned by the patient, were included. No attempt was made either to "interpret" the statements, or to unearth fears that may have been "unconscious". The majority of the patients complained of three or more specific anxieties.

Although fascinating psychopathologically, since it provides insight into personality structure and neurotic predisposition, the expressed "content" of the coital anxiety is less relevant in a treatment context than the associated pathophysiology. In both the male and the female the basic neural (physiological) control of the sexual response is the same and consists of spinal reflexes and autonomic and somatic components, subject to facilitation and inhibition by higher nervous centres. In the spinal cord there are two main centres involved. The first has its outflow through the second and third sacral roots (S2 and S3) via the *nervi erigentes* to the genitalia. This is parasympathetic and concerned with the vasocongestive mechanisms underlying sexual arousal in both sexes, i.e. erection, lubrication, etc. The second centre is sympathetic, via the first and second lumbar roots (L1 and L2) which subserves the orgasmic phase of the sexual response. Anxiety or other disruptive emotional states by increasing sympathetic or decreasing parasympathetic tone may cause erectional or ejaculative problems in the male and orgasmic difficulties in the female. In the author's experience these are normally best tackled directly at the physiological rather than the psychological level.

Personality and relationship factors
For both men and women, sexuality is much more than being able to conclude satisfactorily the physical act of coitus, although that of course is important. It is a significant segment of personality, encompassing among other things body image, sexual confidence and attitudes, gender identity, and many facets of behavioural interaction with the opposite sex, overt as well as subtle.

Ambivalence or apprehension of a sexual commitment, with all the implications, may be one aspect of generalised inadequacy which may disadvantage the individual in many life spheres. Such people, but especially men, for whom potency is the epitome of masculinity, are oversensitive to criticism, fear physical sexual failure above all and dare not risk initiating a relationship with a member of the opposite sex. Instead, they often opt for a life of loneliness.

The diagnosis of personality abnormality may cause problems to the non-psychiatrically-trained. It relates to a definite and durable disturbance in an individual's pattern of relationships with others, chiefly excessive dependency, immaturity, withdrawal, egocentricity, or hostility. The author has previously recognised three broad personality-type abnormalities which may predispose an individual to sexual inadequacy (Cooper, 1967) and these are given below.

(a) Hysterical personality abnormality. These individuals show to an excessive degree several of the following traits: desire to obtain attention, superficial relationships, self-centredness, tendency to exaggerate symptoms or complaints, manipulative behaviour, dramatic behaviour, emotional lability or immaturity, insincerity, impulsiveness.

(b) Psychopathic personality. These conform to several of the following descriptions to an excessive degree: asocial; impulsive; feels little or no guilt; unable to form lasting affectionate relationships; unreliable; lacks a sense of responsibility; shows a pronounced ability to rationalise behaviour; lacks consideration for accepted moral standards; unable to form mature judgments; unable to profit from past experience; aggressive.

There is some overlap between the hysterical and psychopathic type of personality.

(c) Obsessional personality abnormality. These may fit the following descriptions: rigid, organised, meticulous, with controlled emotions, over-conscientious, tending to ruminate, cautious.

Clinically, the more disturbed the personality the greater the difficulty in resolving any co-existing sexual problem. Such cases, which are probably outside the scope of the non-specialist, require prolonged psychotherapy to change attitudes before any practical approach is feasible.

Hostility
In all its nuances, hostility or aggression is probably the most pernicious of human expressions. It is a common enough finding in sexual
inadequacy and may be causal or consequential; however, even if the
latter, its presence must be expected to worsen the original problem.
The aetiological significance of hostility is best assessed by exploring
the relationship of the partners during the joint interview. Additionally, this allows the therapist to get a good idea as to the likely level
of co-operation between them in any therapeutic plan.

Sexual hostility which may be part and parcel of a generally affec-
tionless or acrimonious marriage may take several forms, but most
commonly is expressed as an explicit (or implicit) belittlement of
the other's sexual prowess. In some instances this may be a direct
adverse comparison with another lover past or present, in others an
oblique or snide reference. Sometimes verbal castigation may be
absent but in behavioural terms the message is clear enough. Gutheil
aptly refers to this scenario as "The War Between the Sexes": in
his opinion it commonly underlies various manifestations of sexual
inadequacy (Gutheil, 1959).

When the relationship seems to be irreparably damaged, the interview often provides a suitable forum for one or other to declare
their intention of parting or at least of negotiating a sexual truce,
which normally means abstinence or a much reduced frequency —
much to the chagrin of the still interested partner; at this juncture,
some couples agree to live together but to go their own ways. Yet
other couples, who may have already decided that the partnership is
over, attend for several interviews before the pronouncement is made.
If after a few sessions it is apparent that the situation is more intractable than it seemed, then it is wise to refer the couple to a psychiatrist or marriage guidance counsellor.

Positive emotional feelings especially of security and belonging
seem to be proportionately more important in therapy for women
than for men who usually are more interested in the intensity and
variety of direct bodily erotic stimulation. However, this is not invariably so and a small minority of females can be "physical" in a way
unmatched by any man (Kinsey *et al.*, 1953).

Disgust
In both sexes the presence and causal significance of disgust may be
gauged by exploring attitudes towards menstruation, sex play (including masturbation), own and partner's genitalia, and particularly
sexual smells and secretions such as sweat, saliva and "slime" —
semen and vaginal mucus.

Disgust is frequently associated with an obsessional type of personality and may be one facet of over-concern with orderliness and

cleanliness and the polar opposite, fear of dirt or of becoming contaminated. Although not impossible to treat, sexual disgust is certainly a more difficult proposition than coital anxiety.

Sexual inhibition

At some stage during a diagnostic interview an assessment of sexual inhibition is mandatory. This may proceed somewhat as follows.

> *Therapist:* "Is there any type of sexual activity or experimentation that you think you would like to do but just can't?"
> *Patient:* "Yes. I have often wished to have sex from the rear, with her lying on her stomach, but something always seems to stop me. I simply knot up inside and try as I might I can't even discuss it with her. I suppose I'm afraid of being thought 'kinky'."

Inhibition is often associated with a rich fantasy life in which the patient enjoys those very same activities which he cannot perform in real life. Sexual inhibition may be, but is not always, found in "emotionally constipated" individuals who, although experiencing feelings inwardly, often are unable to express them (Mackay, 1977). These are to be distinguished from the affectively flat who, it is conjectured, are just biologically incapable of experiencing any type of intense emotion.

The elegant prose of Walker and Strauss (1948) is descriptive.

> There is a disposition on the part of some married couples to feel that while certain methods of love making are right and proper others are illegitimate and degrading . . . . It is chiefly because the British pay great respect to convention that their method of love making rarely departs from a certain accepted model. Love has not always been so conventional. In the *Khama Sutra* we read of at least seven different ways of kissing; eight varieties of touch, eight playful bites, four methods of stroking the body with the hands and eight sounds which may be emitted whilst doing so. For the India of *Khama Sutra,* sexual congress was looked upon not merely as a conjugal duty, the necessary preliminary to the obtaining of children, but as an activity from which both partners could view pleasure and eroticism as among the riches which life could provide them. In writing his great work of love, the author was in no way pandering to the sensuousness of youth. On the contrary, there is every reason to believe that when he penned it he was himself living the life of a religious recluse in Benares. In undertaking this work at such a time, he must of necessity have felt that in sexual love there was no element that need be in enmity with, or in any way contradict, the highest spiritual aspirations of mankind.

In the more mundane surroundings of clinical practice, the commonest thorny areas relate to oral sex, extended manual stimulation, the use of certain aids like vibrators, creams and lotions, etc., and variations in coital positions. Many men and women who would probably delight in such refinements, find it impossible even to broach the subject fearing that they will be rebuffed as perverted. Consequently the couple, in (not-so-blissful) ignorance of each other's innermost desires, may have been operating under suboptimal conditions for years.

Sexual inhibition, which varies enormously from person to person, is probably laid down during adolescence in response to two variable, opposing forces. On the one hand there is the biological imperative of sex drive itself, whilst on the other there are a multiplicity of social pressures which in Western culture traditionally serve to discourage sexual activity until marriage. This positive/negative reinforcement equation is crucial. In its simplest form it states: the greater the physical and emotional rewards from any particular form of sexual activity, the greater the likelihood of this being repeated and ultimately established as permanent. If, on the other hand, negative consequences such as feelings of guilt, fear of detection, fear of pregnancy are overwhelming, then it is unlikely that an adequate pleasure-response pattern will develop and the seeds of dysfunction might have been sown. It should be stressed that this is neither a plea for permissiveness nor a condemnation of the status quo; it is simply a statement of probable fact which is supported by a great deal of anthropological, sociological and clinical data (Mead, 1939; Ford and Beach, 1952; Burgess and Wallin, 1953; Kinsey *et al.*, 1953; Cooper, 1969 (2)).

It is an interesting observation that learning to respond sexually during adolescence, from masturbation or coitus, seems of much greater developmental importance in the male than the female, for whom the apt term "sleeping beauty" has been coined (Friedman, 1962). Women seem better able to compensate for such a hiatus if and when they are exposed to sexual opportunities later (Kinsey *et al.*, 1953).

Sexual ignorance
Despite a vast increase in health education both in the schools and via the popular media such as television and magazines, which has done much to break down supersitition and myth, depressingly ignorance remains an all too common finding in many of the sexually inadequate.

The commonest misconception in both sexes relates to masturbation which not only may be viewed as innately wrong, but also capable of causing physical and emotional disorders. Arising out of a preoccupation with moral turpitude, and no doubt believing that it was in the public interest, misinformation has been promulgated even by highly respected organisations considered by many to be bastions of society. For instance, the U.S. *Boy Scout Manual* of 1954 exhorts the youth to "avoid wasting the vital fluid" (i.e. masturbation). Dire consequences were promised to transgressors. In similar vein, some people continue to believe that excessive sexual intercourse, even if desired, is weakening and should, therefore, be avoided.

Other areas for clinical concern may include the similarities and differences between male and female sexual anatomy, physiology and psychology. Incredibly, many sexually-inadequate men have no idea what the clitoris is, where it is, or how it responds to stimulation. Perhaps even more surprising is, that some women do not know either.

A common phallic fallacy, which may threaten some men, is that "size wins the prize" and those who perhaps are only of average dimensions believe they must be at a performance disadvantage when compared with the more "fortunately" endowed. In fact, the size of the penis has been shown to be comparatively unimportant in determining either male potency or female satisfaction. The latter is much more dependent on good technique and, of course, emotional commitment, preferably within a stable relationship.

Faulty or inadequate stimulative techniques may play an important causal role in many types of sexual inadequacy. For example, a proportion of premature ejaculators have practised coitus interruptus as a birth control measure over many years. By its very nature, this prevents the male from acclimatising to "the feel of the vagina" which simply becomes a thing to be got out of as quickly as possible. Within a comparatively short time span this pattern may become habitual, persisting even if replaced by safer and aesthetically superior contraceptives later. Some premature ejaculators have a prior history of "forced" self-masturbation dating back to adolescence. Usually they will have been told, or it may have been implied by parents, a clergyman or a teacher, that masturbation was wrong and sinful, even harmful to health. Consequently, when engaged in it, often under furtive circumstances, the youth would try to get it over as quickly as possible. Sometimes at home, and especially at school or other semi-public place speed might have been the difference between the ignominy of being caught literally "with his pants down", or merely appearing with creased clothes, a red face and breathing rather hard. Once learned, such a brisk response tends to generalise to other situations, such as partner-masturbation and especially coitus. Yet other sufferers have a story of early prostitute exposure, when it was made clear that the quicker the emission the better. Not only this, but the type of relentless demanding stimulation likely to be meted out adds physical to verbal imperative. Since greed may be best satisfied by speed, prostitutes have the strongest commercial motives for plying a brisk trade. It would only take a few similar experiences, subsequently, to consolidate the initial ejaculative pattern as the usual.

Even in the security of a caring relationship, ignorance about stimulative techniques may be equally damaging. For instance, many chaste and inexperienced couples believing that the object is to reach climax as quickly as possible go at it like a "bull at a gate". Since they know no better, there is no attempt to prolong the experience by skilful and intermittent stimulation. Both may suffer, the male with prematurity, the female with dyspareunia, anorgasmia, pelvic congestion and frustration. Unfamiliarity with contraceptive techniques, or an unwise choice, by interrupting continuous smooth stimulation, may have similar unhappy consequences. If the author has learned anything in sexual medicine, it is never to take anything for granted. However well-turned-out and articulate a couple appear, it is judicious to examine comprehensively their knowledge. Ignorance, together with faulty stimulative techniques, probably accounts for more sexual morbidity than any other single cause; the aetiological role of these two factors must, therefore, be defined precisely if optimal treatment is to be designed.

Sexual orientation
As a matter of routine the patient's attitude towards, and any experience of, homosexuality, fetishism, transvestism, etc., should be explored, even if seemingly irrelevant or greeted with hostility. Surprisingly, perhaps, some individuals come straight out with the fact that they are "gay"; others are much more guarded and skilful probing over several sessions may be required to establish their true diathesis. It is a salutory reminder that up to 20 per cent of male homosexuals and 8 per cent of females have been or are married; they may be quite competent with a same-sex partner, but inadequate with their spouses.

The commonest forms of sex variants which may be associated with heterosexual impairment are:

(*a*) homosexuality, both male and female; and
(*b*) autoeroticism: that is a preference for masturbation and other forms of self-stimulation. Autoeroticism may be one facet of an excessively narcissistic or egocentric personality; however, some individuals are simply afraid of the opposite sex and resort to self-stimulation as a "second best" outlet.

Sexual orientation may have a decisive bearing on the outcome of treatment. Thus, a committed homosexual will rarely be genuinely interested in embarking on a treatment plan, if this involves being made more heterosexual; in any event, this is rarely possible (Bancroft, 1969). Married homosexuals who present such a request often do so out of deference to a spouse, or in an attempt to preserve the marriage; they should be referred to a suitable psychiatrist for evaluation.

Depression
In both males and females some reduction in libido and coital satisfaction may be the initial symptom of a mild or atypical depression. Thus, the "fed up" housewife is especially susceptible to ups and

downs in libido and this may portend the development of more typical symptomatology which clinches a depressive aetiology. In the
more severe retarded cases, libido fluctuates less. Indeed, in both
sexes, it may be totally suppressed and sexual activity nil until the
illness remits.

From the standpoint of practical therapeutics, a first-time sexual
complaint, without an obvious cause, should alert the practitioner
to the possibility of an underlying depression and a diligent search
made for confirmatory symptoms such as general fatigue, an increase
in irritability, mild hypochondriasis etc. Until the patient recovers
from his illness improvement in sexual function is at best unlikely.
Even then it should be remembered that successful treatment with
appropriate medication or E.C.T. does not in itself guarantee an
uneventful return to former levels of sexual proficiency. Interruption
of regular outlets, especially if prolonged, may complicate the picture
-- Dr. Alex Comfort says, "if you don't use it you lose it". Therefore,
as soon as libido has recovered sufficiently it may be judicious to
prescribe a modified sensate-focus programme in all cases as a safeguard.

Constitutional factors
"Constitution" in the shape of an unusually low sex drive may be
an important cause of sexual inadequacy as well as limiting a therapeutic response.

Sexual strength is not as straightforward a concept as might be
imagined: indeed there is a good deal of controversy. Kirkendall's suggestions fit the facts better than most. He subdivides strength into
three components: "sexual performance" (what one actually does),
"capacity" (what one can do) and "drive" (how strongly one desires
or strives to do) (Kirkendall, 1967). According to Kirkendall sexual
capacity is determined by the ability of the nervous and muscular
systems to respond to stimuli with orgasm and to recuperate to the
point where it can be experienced again. This ability, which is governed mainly by genetic factors, varies greatly from person to person
and it probably represents the actual physiological difference between individuals.

Performance, although limited at its upper extreme by capacity,
fluctuates according to physical and psychological circumstances at
the time. Performance is not an accurate measure of capacity because
few, if any, persons conform to full capacity. Kirkendall's concept
of performance is roughly equivalent to Kinsey's statistic of "strength
of sex drive". Kinsey simply charted the actual frequencies of sexual
outlets to orgasm, from all sources (i.e. self and partner masturbation,
coitus etc.) for various age groups. He found that sex drive was normally distributed (like intelligence) and for males varied inversely

with age, reaching a peak in the late teens and declining thereafter. It was remarkably constant throughout life — high responders tending to reach puberty earlier and retain their potency longer than low responders. Like Kirkendall, Kinsey also believed that there was a very strong underlying genetic influence.

Drive, according to Kirkendall, is the strength of the intensity with which the individual wishes to perform. This seems to be largely a psychologically conditioned component, varying enormously from individual to individual as a personality trait. However, it is feasible that the functional availability of sex hormones both during intra-uterine life, as well as later, plays a significant role. During a clinical interview, it is possible to get an idea as to the strength of the sex drive by enquiring about the frequency of sexual outlets to orgasm both from coitus and, where it applies, masturbation.

Like "inhibition", which might curtail learning during adolescence, "sexual apathy" may also compromise future proficiency. This is not innate: it needs to be acquired and consolidated by appropriate pleasurable exposures during adolescence and early adulthood. A low sex drive seems to disadvantage males proportionately more than females and, in the writer's opinion, those who neither masturbate nor engage in heterosexual outlets during adolescence, rarely develop completely satisfactory adult sexual response patterns (but *see* p. 166). Sexual drive in the female seems somewhat different. Although it may be influenced by the same general factors as in the male it does not necessarily peak during the late teens: neither does it decline in parallel fashion. Physiologically speaking, women generally seem better able to contend with the vicissitudes of time. Ordinarily later developers, they seem to retain their responsiveness or at least their potential longer than most men.

It is clinically important to distinguish between the "inhibited" patient with a definite sex drive, even if this is below average, who is prevented from performing to capacity by constraining attitudes and the individual who is "just not interested". Despite some opinions to the contrary, the latter do exist and rarely do well in treatment. In sexual terms it's just not possible to "make a silk purse out of a sow's ear" and a treatment goal should be realistically modest.

Some psychiatrists, and especially psychoanalysts, affirm that a proportion of abstinent individuals have sublimated their sexual drives into other channels, usually of an aesthetic nature. Frequently, the concept is illustrated by reference to certain narrow religious sects who practice celibacy and harsh austerities. Untroubled by prurient desires, apparently sublimated, they sail serenely through life. However, Kinsey's compelling statistics (Kinsey *et al.,* 1948) augmented by clinical experience suggest otherwise. Thus many celibates, of one religious persuasion or another, driven by strong libidinal needs which they cannot suppress, resort to self-masturbation or other forms of release. Some, unable to come to terms with their urges, become guilt-ridden and suffer other emotional upsets. In the author's opinion, sexual drive cannot be altered or displaced to any great extent without resulting in psychological upheaval of one sort or another.

As well as limiting the strength of sexual drive, constitutional factors may decisively influence the speed of response and thus be causally important in a complaint of premature ejaculation. There is no counterpart condition in the female. Schapiro was among the first to recognise the significance of heredity in prematurity (of ejaculation), which he divided into three overlapping aetiological types (Schapiro, 1943). An oversimplified profile of a "Type A" sufferer which Schapiro believed was largely genetically determined is as follows: he experiences normal or enhanced sexual desire in the coital situation; erections may develop on the slightest stimulation, but they may be lost just as easily; on psychological tests, he scores as anxious and neurotic; frequently he complains of somatic manifestations of anxiety such as sweating, palpitations, dry mouth, etc. In lay terms, he is often referred to as "highly strung". Often such patients have suffered from prematurity constantly since the early days of adolescence. Brisk even during self-stimulation, they are twice as quick in coitus with their partner. The condition possesses some of the characteristics of an exaggerated reflex, perhaps based on innate instability or lability of the autonomic nervous system. In learning terms, it is possible that high levels of anxiety, evoked during coitus, minimise habituation and play a large part in consolidating the ejaculatory disorder. Although superficially this type of prematurity might be viewed as a manifestation of high sexual drive closer scrutiny indicates otherwise. Thus, very few sufferers are able to proceed to a second coitus and in those that can, there is a much prolonged refractory phase. If, in addition, the opinion of the female partner is considered there can be no room for argument. Often frustrated because of his precipitancy, her rueful complaints label him for what he is — sexually inept.

Biological factors

Patterns of sexual response, particularly in the female, may be subject to biological variation at certain times. The underlying causes are not known with certainty but it is probably a combination of endocrine and psychological factors (Cooper, 1969 (2); Masters and Johnson, 1966). For instance, libido may fluctuate according to the time of the month. Unfortunately, there is no general rule and some women report a temporary increase and some a decrease in libido; in yet others this remains relatively constant. During pregnancy, changes in responsiveness tend to be more predictable. According to Masters and Johnson the majority of pregnant women are less libidinal in the first than in subsequent trimesters, the second generally being the period of maximum interest and responsiveness (Masters and Johnson, 1966). During the postpartum period, in a minority of women sexuality may wax and wane haphazardly for months. For most, however, libido returns to former levels within eight to twelve weeks, unless progress is complicated by psychological factors such as depression, anxiety and especially persisting feelings of sexual unattractiveness.

The effects of the menopause have probably been overstated, but up to 20 per cent of women do complain of mild symptoms which are more of a nuisance than anything else. The overwhelming majority pass through this time of life without any problems whatsoever. The single most significant hormonal change at the menopause is a marked reduction of oestrogen: this has widespread effects on various target organs and may influence sexual functioning adversely. Thus, a few women who have never previously been uncomfortable during sexual activity complain of pain on and after intercourse, vaginal burning, pelvic aching, and dysuria. These symptoms are probably due to marked thinning of the vaginal mucosa, which becomes less distensible, and an absence of lubrication. Pelvic pain, due to uterine (orgasmic) contractions, may be severe in a small minority of cases. Although these symptoms can cause great distress, in perspective they trouble comparatively few and in virtually all they can be ameliorated by appropriate hormonal replacement and supportive counselling.

That the change of life represents the end of a woman's sexuality is a myth. Education, communication and research spell out a different message, which needs to be repeated at every opportunity. In truth there is no reason why any woman should not continue to enjoy her sex life during and following the menopause, and neither her libido nor her orgasmic capacity will be necessarily reduced. It is true, however, that some women who were previously ambivalent or neurotic about their sexuality and coitus may develop an acute dislike or repugnance during the change. These feelings may be strengthened by an attitude still prevalent, that sex during and after the menopause is "unnatural" and undignified. The increasing number of sexually active septuagenarians belies this myth, which should ultimately be dispelled.

The clinical significance of this is for the therapist to be aware that such fluctuations in libido and responsiveness do occur in women, in a way not seen in men, and may require no more than simple reassurance and the passage of time to revert to normal.

Ageing

Age *per se* is not necessarily a significant factor in sexual inadequacy; however, it may certainly limit the response to therapy and this should always be borne in mind.

Research has demonstrated that for elderly males the availability of an affectionate and sexually empathic partner is the greatest influence in preserving potency into longevity. The late Professor Kinsey, a biologist, concluded that much of the impotence seen in old men was a type of "psychological fatigue" (sexual boredom), consequent upon many years of sexual experience (Kinsey *et al.*, 1948, 1953). He supported his thesis by citing cases of elderly men impotent with their wives, but sexually competent with other, usually younger, women. This he ascribed to a resurgence of sexual interest sparked by the new partner. However, it should be cautioned that although some older impotents may indeed improve with a new, younger female, or more exciting stimulation from their old partner, this is often comparatively short lived. Habituation is rapid and responsiveness and performance slowly wane to former levels usually within a few months.

Although perhaps the deleterious influence of advancing years on potency has been overstated there is no doubt that ageing has progressive effects on all physiological systems, including the sexual, which may ultimately defeat every treatment modality. Curiously, libido is often retained beyond physiological capacity. That the spirit is willing but the flesh is weak, is an adage only too familiar to many old and not-so-old men who, unable to reconcile themselves to this biological inevitability, continue to strive, hopelessly, after former glories. Age seems to be less detrimental to the female who, perhaps because of her receptive role, may be able to engage in coitus until death. If a male cannot get erect then he cannot perform, however much he might wish to.

DIAGNOSTIC FORMULATION

After a measured assessment of all relevant aetiological factors the next step is to make a diagnostic formulation which is a prerequisite of treatment. This should consist of a clinical label, i.e. impotence, vaginismus, etc., together with a brief summary of the presumed aetiology. An illustrative formulation might be as follows.

Clinical label

Mr. Smith, aged 44, is suffering from secondary impotence.

Summary of presumed causes:

1. Biological/constitutional

Mr. Smith has shown progressive decline during the past five years of his sexual interests and potency. Early morning and spontaneous erections are less frequent than formerly; he is less interested in coitus and requires greater stimulation to become fully aroused.

2. Psychosocial

Mr. Smith is under a great deal of "general" pressure. He has just been promoted to sales manager and is overworking. He is particularly concerned about his "targets", which he thinks are unattainable; he is having too many late nights and has been drinking excessively. Mr. Smith's initial failure occurred when, at the insistence of his wife, he made a half-hearted attempt which was unsuccessful. Subsequently he developed considerable performance anxiety; anticipating failure he often tries too hard, and his expectation is fulfilled. Latterly he has been avoiding coitus whenever he can, pleading a headache or being too tired. Ashamed of his failure, he has been unable to discuss it with his wife; she has been wondering if there is somebody else. Communication has dried up and their relationship is at an all-time low.

Such a thumb nail sketch of Mr. Smith's problem points to several different areas which require attention in a treatment plan.

Important treatment principles

Once a diagnostic formulation has been made a treatment contract can be negotiated with the couple, i.e. agreeing on treatment priorities, defining roles and aims; the likely number of sessions etc. It is made clear that regular home assignments form an essential part of the programme. Therapy is tailor-made according to key features in each case, but incorporates various permutations of the following principles.

1. Training in relaxation techniques

Both in the male and the female, satisfactory coital performance depends upon the maintenance of "dynamic" equilibrium between the sympathetic and parasympathetic components of the autonomic nervous system. Physiologically speaking, penile erection and vaginal lubrication are predominantly parasympathetic responses, ejaculation being a sympathetic one. Unpleasant emotional states such as anxiety, anger and hostility may be associated with an increase in sympathetic activity, or a decrease in parasympathetic, or both, which may inhibit or disrupt arousal or performance, resulting in either failure of erection or a disorder of ejaculation in the male, and varying grades of orgasmic dysfunction or vaginismus in the female.

Relaxation aims to reduce sympathetic influences reciprocally by increasing parasympathetic activity. This may be accomplished by instructing the patient in the art of deep abdominal breathing and the simultaneous use of appropriate visual imagery as a means of inducing calmness. The format is very similar to standard antenatal relaxation exercises taught to pregnant women to ease childbirth. Therefore individuals suffering from sexual dysfunction of any type are advised to take time out whenever they can, at work, on a bus, or preferably in the more conducive surroundings of their homes to practice self-relaxation, even for a few minutes. Mastery of this art makes it much easier to implement the other more specific components of therapy.

Relaxation is of most value in those in whom very high levels of anxiety are in evidence. However, it is probably true that the majority of people with sexual problems suffer from some degree of secondary tension, which at the very least exacerbates their condition; therefore a modicum of relaxation training is recommended in all.

2. Provision of optimum sexual stimulation from the partner
Optimum sexual stimulation is that combination of psychological and physical stimuli which allows any individual to respond to full erotic capacity ("sensate focus activity", Masters and Johnson 1970). No two people are alike sexually and what excites one may repel another. It is, therefore, imperative during the diagnostic interview to get explicit and detailed information on the sexual likes (and dislikes) of the couple; only then is it possible to examine as to whether the likes can be provided by the partner and the dislikes eliminated. It is a melancholy fact that many sexually dysfunctional couples have been operating under poor conditions for years. Commonly, this is due to severe inhibition which not only limits their sexual repertoire but also precludes two-way communication.

The therapist's main task at this point is to act as a catalyst and encourage the couple to vocalise their sexual preferences and to discuss with them how far these might be incorporated into the treatment plan. A fairly typical schedule in the case of, say, an impotent male, might be as follows. (The same general principles would apply for virtually any type of sexual inadequacy.)

From the outset it is made clear that coitus is prohibited until such time as the couple mutually agree that they feel sufficiently confident to make an attempt. The great fear of all impotent males is of being compelled to penetrate, knowing full well that failure is probable. The fact of "letting them off the hook" for many represents a relief beyond measure. Perhaps for the first time in many months they can forget about performance anxiety and let things develop naturally.

The couples are instructed to engage in mutual bodily pleasuring and simply to explore and test out their erotic potential and to confirm their likes and dislikes. It is stressed there is nothing to prove; they should simply let themselves go without there being any predetermined end point. The aim is to feel both relaxed and yet at the same time to focus on the sensual pleasure of body caresses. No attempt should be made to "force" sexual arousal, i.e. erection. This is a physiological impossibility. It occurs naturally, if an individual is relaxed, comfortable and receiving good quality stimulation from a caring partner.

If anxiety is marked, hierarchical desensitisation may be employed: when fully relaxed, various grades of stimulation, discussed and agreed previously between the couple and the therapist are introduced; "least threatening" first and "most threatening" last. Such a hierarchy might be as follows:

(a) simply lying in intimate bodily proximity, without any additional stimulation;

(b) relaxed "non-sexual" stroking of neck, arms and shoulders, calves, thighs etc. As the male becomes able to accept such approaches without feeling anxious, it is in order to proceed to more demanding and more obvious erotic measures. In the majority of cases such sensate focus activity elevates sexual tension and leads naturally to direct genital stimulation, which may soon become imperative. The watchword is "gradual". The male is instructed to tell his partner his precise needs and if it be conducive to optimal stimulation to guide her hands to his sensitive areas. Once more there is no question of forcing a response. He should simply lie back and wallow in sensual pleasure.

(c) When strong and durable erections become commonplace, the tease technique should be incorporated into the proceedings. This involves allowing an erection to wax and wane by modulating stimulation accordingly; thereby countering the fear that as soon as erection occurs it will be lost unless used promptly. If successful, this manoeuvre gives an added boost to the male's self-confidence.

(d) Sexual arousal might be further enhanced by the judicious use of fantasy and other provocative stimuli such as appropriate "sexy" photographs, erotic literature and music, perfumes and moisturising lotions. However, these issues should be broached late and cautiously and only with a full understanding of the involved personalities, since many couples may see them as idiosyncratic or "kinky". The revelation and discussion of erotic fantasies may be especially delicate, the more so if these concern sexual partners other than the spouse, or particularly uninhibited sexual practices. If the therapist suspects such matters are likely to be beyond the couple's emotional resources, then they should not be introduced. It is infinitely preferable to hasten slowly than to risk losing the patient.

These "home assignments" form the central core of the programme and the therapist must do his best to commit the couple to follow instructions explicitly. In practice, at each clinical session a behavioural goal (i.e. in sensate focus terms) is set. At the next session progress is reviewed and if appropriate the next (more difficult) goal is agreed. As confidence develops, with a co-operative couple, it is normally possible to consider a coital attempt within five sessions. In the impotent male, for a number of reasons, this is best made in the female superior position.

During sensate focus activities it is mandatory for the male to stimulate his partner reciprocally. A sexually satisfied female is a motivated female. Masters and Johnson's phrase "to give to get" is short but completely descriptive.

3. Sexual education

Relevant sexual information should be given as required to rectify false beliefs or fill any gaps in knowledge, resulting from inadequate or defective education during adolescence. A common stumbling block is the conviction that certain sexual practices are innately abnormal and, therefore, taboo. Some people even today believe that masturbation and oral sex can result in mental or physical illness. It should be stressed to both partners that any variety of stimulation which is mutually pleasurable and emotionally acceptable is perfectly normal and can be indulged in without fear of guilt. However, it is equally important to make clear that being unable to engage in the same activities as other couples, such as oral sex, does not make them abnormal or prudish or mean they are missing out. Although they should be encouraged to experiment and be more adventuresome in their love-making a couple should not be pushed into stimulative techniques beyond their emotional tolerance. If they find that any particular activity is particularly anxiety evoking they should revert to a more familiar one until confident to proceed further.

Many sexually ignorant individuals can benefit from "middle of the road" literature such as the book, *The Joy of Sex* (Comfort, 1975), and the article, "Anatomy of the Female Orgasm" (Cooper, 1974(a)). Appropriate films on sexual anatomy, physiology and stimulative techniques also may be a boon to selected couples. Two very different but equally good productions with which the writer is familiar are: Martin Cole's *Sexual Intercourse,* and *Sexuality and Communication* made available by Organon Laboratories. The former is concerned more or less exclusively with stimulative and coital techniques, whilst the latter concentrates delightfully on sexual relationships and communication. However the optimal use of such aids in sexual therapy remains to be determined and will perhaps be more important in the future (but *see* Gillan and Gillan, 1976).

4. Superficial psychotherapy

Providing there is a reasonable relationship between the partners, psychotherapy consists in the main of reassurance, explanation and in developing and maintaining motivation to proceed and persevere with the practical measures. Commendation in line with improvement is also important: any behavioural goal failures are discussed and analysed and appropriate counter measures prescribed. No serious attempt should be made to change personality and intense transference situations are discouraged. If there are major interpersonal difficulties between the couple, it is wiser to refer them to a psychiatrist.

5. Drugs

Apart from the occasional use of antidepressants already referred to, anxiety-reducing agents may have a legitimate role for patients who develop high levels of tension during coitus or other love play; if absent or minimal, then it is probably a disservice to prescribe these cerebral depressants. Instead of helping, such preparations may actually worsen things by dampening down libido and limiting physiological arousal.

The best candidate for the use of small doses of a minor tranquilliser is the highly-strung patient. These are relatively easy to spot. Characteristically during a clinical interview they look uneasy or agitated, they fidget, have difficulty with talking because of a dry mouth, exhibit a fine tremor, or show palm-sweating and other tell-tale signs of sympathetic overactivity. In such cases it may be helpful to prescribe small doses of benzodiazepines such as diazepam 5 to 10 mg, to be taken thirty minutes or so before a coital attempt. The object is to promote muscular and concomitant mental relaxation without loss of libido. To achieve this some trial and error experimentation may be necessary, and the patient is instructed to calibrate the dose accordingly.

Anxiety-reducing drugs are seldom used alone. They are generally employed simultaneously with a practical training programme, appropriate to the sexual dysfunction being treated, e.g. sensate-focus in the case of impotence or orgasmic inadequacy, the squeeze technique for premature ejaculation, progressive dilatation in vaginismus, etc. Occasionally intravenous sodium amytal, as a relaxing agent, might form part of a visual-imaginary desensitisation programme for certain highly anxious patients (Cooper, 1964; Friedman, 1968). However, this procedure, which demands considerable skill, requires specialised training, and it is outside the armamentarium of most medical practitioners.

6. Sexual aids

At present sexual aids are very much a growth industry and "sex" shops and mail order firms have mushroomed to market what seems a bewildering array of rings, splints, love-balls, vibrators and so on. In the author's opinion, much of what is purveyed, generally with a money-back guarantee, is at best ineffective and at worst hazardous. Furthermore, since very few of the devices have been tested medically, there is no validity for the invariably enthusiastic claims made for them by the distributors. If they are to be treated seriously, sexual aids should be viewed in precisely the same way as drugs: unless both safety and efficacy can be demonstrated under "blind" conditions, where the patient is unaware of the nature and expected effect of the aid, they should not be sold.

Despite these cautionary remarks, there is some evidence that penile rings and vibrators might be beneficial in certain limited circumstances (Cooper, 1974(b); Haslam, 1976). Such devices should not, therefore, be condemned out of hand, but rather be viewed with healthy scepticism, as possible adjuncts in a few cases.

7. The squeeze technique for premature ejaculation

This technique (Semans, 1956) is described fully on p. 172.

8. Progressive vaginal dilatation for vaginismus

A discussion of this technique can be found on p. 182.

Treatment is a dynamic process and as it evolves, in the light of new information derived from increasing knowledge of the couple or of amelioration or exacerbation of symptoms, it should be constantly reappraised and, if indicated, changes in emphasis made. Inertia or reluctance in one or both partners can be countered by threatening termination, or by suggesting that if no further progress is made they will have to seriously consider the alternatives open to them including separation or a "sexless" relationship. In such cases the therapist should make it clear that the responsibility for such action lies with them.

As a general rule, ten to fifteen fortnightly sessions should be the longest treatment contract. Improvement when it occurs is usually apparent within two or three sessions and is maximal after about eight to ten. Protracted therapeutic effort much beyond this time is rarely worthwhile (Cooper, 1967; Bancroft and Coles, 1976).

Summary of treatment steps

(a) In the first session each partner is seen separately for history taking, then jointly for about fifteen minutes. Intercourse is banned, and precise and detailed instructions are given on "sensate focus" home assignments. Any factual gaps in relevant sexual knowledge are filled. If there are reasons to believe the couple might "forget" or "misunderstand" what is required of them, especially regarding specific stimulative techniques, the information should be provided in writing.

(b) At subsequent meetings the couple are always seen together. The sessions are devoted to discussing the extent to which previously agreed behavioural goals have been attained. Relevant sexual attitudes are explored and attempts made to modify these whenever appropriate.

(c) Channels of communication are promoted between the couple who are encouraged to express themselves both verbally and emotionally.

(d) New behavioural goals are set in a hierarchical fashion until by mutual agreement coitus is attempted.

(e) Once successful, variations in technique are introduced to enhance enjoyment and consolidate the sexual gains.

(f) If, after the agreed number of sessions, there is no improvement in the sexual problem the situation is reviewed and treatment is either terminated by mutual agreement, or different, mainly relationship, goals are negotiated. Occasionally, if the relationship is beyond repair separation or divorce may become a legitimate issue for discussion.

COMMON SEXUAL PROBLEMS ENCOUNTERED IN PRACTICE

Table 4 below sets out the commonest problems encountered in practice and indicates the relative emphasis of the individual treatment principles used. Although arbitrary and an approximate guide only, it confirms the pre-eminence of a behavioural component in uncomplicated difficulties, which present overtly as failures of physiological responses.

Psychotherapy, although used generally, is proportionately more important and necessarily more analytical in complicated cases and where there is no "sexual" complaint as such, the patient presenting with a substitute symptom, such as pelvic pain. Psychotherapy is also more important when the quality of the relationship between the partners is so bad that a direct behavioural approach is not possible without radical changes in attitude. These latter categories, which are generally tougher treatment propositions, additionally require a much longer therapeutic commitment than the average practitioner can afford, even if he possesses the requisite knowledge and expertise. The most important conditions will now be described individually.

TABLE 4. COMMON SEXUAL PROBLEMS
WITH THE RELATIVE EMPHASIS OF TREATMENT PRINCIPLES

Diagnosis	Relaxation training	Provision of optimal sexual stimulation (sensate focus)	Psycho-therapy	Drugs	Sex aids	Squeeze technique	Progressive vaginal dilation
Impotence	+	+++	++	+	+		
Reduction in/ dissatisfaction with/ absence of female orgasmic response (i.e. "frigidity")	+	+++	++	+	+		
Premature ejaculation	++		+	+		+++	
Ejaculative incompetence		+++	+				
Male/female sexual dissonance		+++	+++	+			
Vaginismus	+++	+++	++	+			+++
Male/female dyspareunia	++	+++	+++	+			
Male/female pelvic pain	++	+++	+++				
Sexual problems in the elderly		+++	++	++	++		
Sexual problems associated with: diabetes, myocardial infarction, physical disability, etc.	++	+++	++	++	+		

Level of emphasis: Least: +   Moderate: ++   Greatest: +++

Impotence

Impotence is the inability to develop or sustain an erection sufficient to allow orgasm and ejaculation to be satisfactorily concluded during coitus. It may be partial, or complete, temporary or permanent, primary or secondary. Primary implies that the male has never been competent in coitus, whilst secondary, which is by far the commonest, denotes at least one prior success.

Traditionally, impotence has been classified according to presumed aetiology, by developmental history, or by typology. In the author's view this is somewhat arbitrary and has little or no use in practice. Thus, with the arguable exception of the "primary — secondary" distinction, which is relevant prognostically, features such as level of performance anxiety and aspects of the partner relationship are of much greater significance in determining both the form of treatment and the likely outcome.

The following illustrative cases of primary and secondary impotence are fairly typical.

A case of secondary impotence

Dr. G., aged 56, attended his diagnostic interview alone. This was despite previously agreeing on the phone that he would bring his wife. He complained of increasing difficulty in developing and sustaining erections over the previous seven months. Sometimes he had been able to manage coitus satisfactorily; but latterly more often not. He was becoming obsessed with the thought that he was "failing his wife" and that he would never regain his former potency.

At the interview Dr. G., highly intelligent and articulate, impressed one as being a somewhat neurotic man with an obsessional type of personality. Over the years he had suffered intermittently from a multiplicity of neurotic symptoms from which he had undoubtedly derived a considerable secondary gain in the shape of various significant psychological concessions from his wife and children.

The initial failure seemed related to the fact that he had instigated sexual overtures when neither he nor his spouse had really desired coitus. In fact, she had been downright unenthusiastic. However, since he had already started he decided (intellectually) to see it through. Unfortunately, his wife's indifference coupled with his own ambivalence were sufficient to preclude a full response and penetration proved impossible. Determined to succeed however he tried to force an erection by "willpower". Nothing happened and becoming more anxious with every minute he tried to "shovel" his penis in manually. At this point what erection he had completely disappeared and the débâcle was over. Subsequent attempts had been marred by the same fear of failure, with limited or no precoital stimulation from his spouse, and more often than not coitus had been impossible or unsatisfactory.

The diagnostic formulation was that of a middle-aged man with secondary impotence. Although there was some evidence of biological sexual decline, the main cause seemed to be high levels of performance anxiety, in a setting of inadequate precoital stimulation from his spouse.

At the next meeting, when they were seen together, it became clear that the couple were as different as "chalk from cheese". Mrs. G. came over as an extremely dour woman who contributed very little to the proceedings. Although she agreed that her husband did have erectional difficulties, she felt that he was overstating his problem and that he enjoyed worry. Despite some very obvious areas of conflict, their interpersonal relationship appeared strong enough to make a predominently behavioural approach immediately possible. Mrs. G., albeit reluctantly, agreed to co-operate fully in any treatment plan.

Treatment and progress. During the second half of the second session Dr. G. was given some instructions in the methodology of muscular and mental relaxation as a means of reducing his extremely high levels of coital anxiety (*see* p. 155). It was made crystal clear that he had nothing to prove and intercouse was prohibited. If erections occurred during these preliminary sensate focus exchanges, they were to be seen as a bonus. The agreed goal was simply to give pleasure to each other with non-genital caressing.

During the third session two weeks later the couple admitted that they had gone beyond their brief: erections had developed readily and mutual masturbation had occurred. During the remainder of this session, the next behavioural goal was set: that of manual genital stimulation, incorporating the tease technique to allow waxing and waning of his erection, but coitus was still forbidden. An attempt was also made to rouse Mrs. G. out of her sexual passivity. It was explained that if she was able to let herself go a little more, even if she had to force it initially, then her own pleasure would be increased.

Two weeks later during the fourth session, the couple confirmed that durable erections were now the rule and both felt that they would like to proceed to coitus, which was now set as the next behavioural goal. It was to be accomplished in the female superior position following the usual extensive mutual precoital sexual play. It was stressed that on no account was insertion to be attempted unless he was powerfully erect and in a high state of erotic arousal. Once accomplished, Dr. G. was advised to introduce pelvic thrusting at a depth and rate paralleling his sexual tension.

At the fifth session the couple confirmed a 100 per cent success rate (coitus twice a week) in the female superior position. Mrs. G. admitted to being less inhibited than formerly although, as she put it, she found it "difficult for a parson's daughter to let her hair down". During this session specific advice was given relating to different coital positions, in particular the lateral which allows maximal unrestrained movement of both partners, as well as adding variety, which is a good thing in itself. This position, because of anatomical considerations, is maximally conducive to good female response.

The next session, which was to be the last, was cancelled by Dr. G. over the telephone. Coitus had occurred satisfactorily three times a week and both felt perfectly satisfied. Dr. G. still complained somewhat about his wife's relative passivity, but he admitted that things had improved. Six months later coitus had stabilised at once or twice a week which was agreeable to both partners. Although Mrs. G. felt her husband still tended to introspect unduly about his performance, she had accepted that it was just "part of his personality" and would probably never change.

Case of primary impotence
Mr. D., was a short, plump and somewhat aggressive man. He attended a diagnostic interview in the company of his wife; she contributed very little to the proceedings. The stated complaint was that of primary impotence since their marriage ten years ago; however, it soon became obvious that their main reason for seeking a consultation was because they both wished for a child.

Mr. D. seemed to have reached puberty extremely late at 14 or even 15. He denied ever practising manual masturbation, which he believed was both sinful and abnormal, although under pressure he did admit to occasional ejaculations induced by rubbing his penis against the bedclothes. He did this out of curiosity only and practised it only intermittently over the years. There was no other type of sexual outlet.

He courted his wife for two years before they married. There was little or no petting during this time and although he recalled occasional erections these were generally only partial and temporary. Both he and his wife described themselves as "religious and highly moral" people who did not believe in premarital sexual activity. They decided to "save themselves" until later; difficulties were not anticipated, both believed (naïvely) that coitus would just happen naturally.

Their first attempt on the honeymoon was a disaster. Abysmally ignorant about anatomy and stimulative techniques, neither was able to assist the other in becoming roused. Mr. G.'s erection had been poorly formed and penetration impossible. Subsequent attempts to consummate their marriage had also failed, seemingly due to a combination of low libido, sexual ignorance and performance anxiety. Over the years, his already low libido had waned further and at the time of referral he was almost totally apathetic; his last attempt at coitus was made six months previously, on the insistence of his wife, who desperately wanted to be pregnant.

Treatment and progress. In an extended first session, almost forty-five minutes were devoted to appropriate sexual education, including details of stimulative techniques. Coitus was banned and the usual sensate focus goals were scheduled in a strict hierarchical fashion to allay performance anxiety and encourage arousal. After twelve home assignments, durable erections were occurring on about 80 per cent of occasions, and it was agreed that a coital attempt was in order. Surprisingly, they were successful the first time, although ejaculation did not occur. Six months later they had settled down to an intercourse pattern of about once a week. Although not always completely successful, both were delighted with their progress and felt that they would get even better with time.

Comment. The author was extremely surprised that Mr. D. overcame his impotence so readily, since there seemed so few favourable prognostic pointers. The decisive factors appeared to be a high level of motivation and the relationship between the couple, both of whom out of affection were able to commit themselves unreservedly to the treatment suggestions. It seems unlikely that Mr. D. will ever be highly potent, but providing he is fully roused by appropriate precoital stimulation he should be able to enjoy coitus, up to his capacity.

Somewhere in the order of 60 per cent of impotence sufferers may be expected to improve significantly with the sort of superficial, practically-oriented treatment described above.

Primary impotents have been much more resistant to short-term treatment than secondary cases. Even Masters and Johnson whose therapy is applied under as near optimum conditions as is currently attainable in a western culture report a failure rate of 41 per cent (Masters and Johnson, 1970). Acknowledging their relative ineptitude they refer to the syndrome as a "major disaster area in sexual therapy". In the author's opinion the poor results in these cases are due mainly to a "constitutionally" determined low sexual drive, i.e. sexual apathy which limits positive sexual learning (masturbation, coitus) during the crucial phase of adolescent growth; without such regular outlets adult sexual proficiency may be stunted. Although "constitutional" is usually taken to imply a dominant genetic contribution, the inhibitory influence of psychosocial effects during the same period cannot be ruled out (Tanner, 1964; Johnson, 1965). Both seem largely immutable by present treatment methods.

On a clinical level, it is worth commenting on a misconception held by many primarily impotent men, even those who have suffered the condition for a decade, who almost invariably plead to be made "normal" with the implication that previously they have been "abnormal". Unfortunately this is semantic confusion. In the context of sexual activity, if it means anything at all "normal" refers to the usual or habitual way of responding for that particular individual. It is incomparably easier to restore something that used to be, than to supply something that never was. Once sexuality is laid down as a segment of personality during adolescence and early adulthood it is difficult to modify later, however well-motivated the individual is for treatment. Although the improvement rate for secondary impotence is generally much more gratifying, many men express relative disappointment that they have not been restored to their former (i.e. peak) level of competency. Many such individuals who readily acknowledge receding hair and a thickening waistline as heralding middle-age, are unable to see their declining sexual vigour in the same light. It is essential for such men to be able to accept emotionally that they will probably never be able to perform to their previous ceiling. Providing they are able to modulate often totally unrealistic expectations, significant coital and relationship improvement is possible for many. The number of impotent males who either refuse treatment or drop out within two or three sessions is high — as many as 30 per cent, with a disproportionate number being middle-aged. This observation, noted by many other workers (Ansari, 1976; Bancroft and Coles, 1976), probably reflects sexual apathy and resultant poor motivation for change: it is rarely an indictment of the therapist. In many cases they attend in the first place simply because of pressure from, or out of deference to, their sexual partner.

Problems with female sexual response, i.e. "frigidity"
This category includes reduction in response, dissatisfaction with response and absence of response. Like impotence, orgasmic inadequacy may be usefully considered as either primary or secondary: further subdivision is largely academic.
The following cases are illustrative of these problems.

Case of a female with unsatisfactory response
Mary was a delightful, if ingenuous, Irish girl aged 23, who had never reached climax during intercourse with her husband. He had told her that this was abnormal and that she should get herself treated.
Mary had lived with her husband for three years but they had married only eighteen months previously following the birth of their son. At this time she had been fitted with an I.U.D. but became pregnant again almost immediately. Having two children aged 18 months and 5 months she had been under considerable pressure at home and is constantly exhausted. She gets little or no help from her husband, who she thinks does not appreciate the stress she has been under. Mary's husband is basically much more interested in sex than she and insists on it every night. Coitus

is practised without ceremony or foreplay and Mary has never been fully roused when he penetrates. Furthermore the act rarely lasts beyond three minutes which is insufficient time for Mary to respond fully, invariably she is left high and dry and later feels frustrated and disgruntled.

The diagnostic formulation was primary orgasmic inadequacy mainly due to inadequate coital foreplay by the male, who also seemed somewhat premature. Additionally, a high level of performance anxiety had been engendered which was making things worse.

Treatment and progress. The most important steps in treatment of the couple were as follows.

(a) At a joint interview the partners were provided with factual sexual education, particularly about the importance of adequate precoital stimulation, to maximise the possibility of a full response during connection.

(b) Mary was encouraged to, and assisted in, the expression of her resentment to her husband, who, she felt, had been taking her too much for granted.

(c) Since Mary had no idea about her erotic potential, she was advised to practice self-masturbation as a means of localising her pleasure spots.

(d) Mary's husband, who acknowledged his thoughtlessness was made to see that Mary's "problem" was his "problem" and its solution demanded some attitudinal changes in him, as well as active participation and co-operation in the home assignment programme.

Equipped with sufficient knowledge the couple were then given specific behavioural goals tailored to their needs. After six home assignments, during which coitus was prohibited, Mary reported that for the first time she was getting fully roused, with good lubrication and was actually anticipating penetration. Penetration was accomplished on the tenth assignment and resulted in a climax.

Six months later, coitus had stabilised at a frequency of two to three times a week which was mutually satisfactory to both partners. Although on occasions she would not respond to climax, both felt delighted. From Mary's point of view, one of the most pleasing aspects was that her husband was now treating her as an equal and communication between them had improved dramatically.

Case of a sexually disgruntled but orgasmic female

The most noticeable thing about Margaret was how inconspicuous she looked — small, shabbily dressed, obviously anxious; she was also alone. After two or three minutes of silence in the consulting room she finally volunteered in a flat low voice that she had been told by her boyfriend she was not responding with orgasm to his love-making, that this was "abnormal" and that she should get herself sorted out.

Margaret had been dating her boyfriend for about nine months. Regular coitus had become established at a frequency of about twice a week. Initially a little unsure, she quickly came to enjoy sex which culminated in vaginal contractions (i.e. orgasm) on about 60 per cent of occasions. In Margaret's case, although pleasurable, this was a mainly introspective constrained experience. Thus, she did not "convulse", make "strangled cries", or otherwise display the standard manifestations of orgasm detailed in the popular sex magazines. Unfortunately Margaret's boyfriend was more experienced and some of his previous partners had displayed greater enthusiasm to his lovemaking. Margaret's apparent lack of involvement had got under his skin and, beginning to doubt his own virility, he demanded that she should seek help.

Physiologically there seemed no doubt that Margaret was responding to sexual stimulation with vaginal contractions of which she was well aware (i.e. the orgasm of Masters and Johnson). However, reflecting her basic character, the psychological components of her climax were decidedly muted. In her personality she was passive and emotionally flat and rarely responded with excitement to anything.

This case illustrates the interplay of personality and physiology in determining patterns of sexual response. Some extroverted women respond with an outpouring of emotion and vigorous physical activity, whilst on the other hand some introverted and controlled women may display little or no signs of involvement although, of course, vaginal lubrication is irrefutable physiological evidence of arousal. In such cases it is easy to understand how the male may begin to doubt his own virility, especially if he has had prior ego-boosting experiences with more demonstrative women. Over-compensating for self-doubt, he may counter aggressively and brand the female as inadequate. Having no frame of reference and perhaps being ignorant of the infinite variability in response patterns, she may accept such criticism at face value and be coerced into seeking help.

Treatment and progress. The most important part of Margaret's treatment was reassurance. It was stressed that she was fully responsive sexually but her orgasmic experience, in line with the rest of her personality, was "low key". Not previously aware of the fact, she was greatly heartened to hear firstly, that there was such variation in full response patterns, and that in any event the main reason for her boyfriend ordering her to seek advice concerned doubts he had about his competency. It was recommended that she make greater efforts to "let herself go" during coitus, since this would reassure her partner that he was pleasuring her.

Several weeks later Margaret attended again with her boyfriend. During coitus she had worked hard to be more active and involved and had found the experience much more enjoyable.

Margaret's case affords a perfect illustration as to how female sexuality may be influenced adversely by, on the one hand, the iconoclastic pronouncements of authority and on the other, media propagandists telling only "half the story". Thus one of the biggest drawbacks of Masters and Johnson's original work on the human sexual response was the disproportionate emphasis they put on the physiological events. Although they never intended it, the vaginal-contractions component of orgasm, so ingenuously and painstakingly recorded, became in the eyes of many lay people, and even some doctors, synonymous with that experience. In the United States some couples divorced because the wife was unable to achieve these muscular twitchings, notwithstanding the fact that she responded with great emotional enjoyment to coitus.

The "authentic-orgasm" cause has now been taken up vigorously by various "emancipated" feminist groups clamouring for equal sexual rights and full orgasms for each and every woman. In the author's view, many of these are pursuing supra-maximal responses which are probably outside their physiological capacity. Generally, fairly straightforward advice and reassurance as to the great, but entirely normal, variation in female arousal-response patterns suffice to allay anxiety and facilitate the implementation of a suitable treatment regimen, which may set rather more modest goals than the achievement of vaginal contractions.

Perhaps the most misunderstood, maligned and self-deprecating women of all are those who get no physical return whatsoever from coitus despite having a loving relationship with a sexually-responsive spouse. Bombarded by the orgasmic propagandists, they may begin to doubt their femininity. Often seeing themselves as "frigid", they may gradually grow to hate sexuality and unwittingly, or even purposefully, transmit these attitudes to their children so that, in due course, history repeats itself.

It is vital in such instances to place sexual gratification in perspective as one facet only, and not necesarily the most important, in a relationship. Indeed, providing their sexual needs are consonant, a couple may have few or even no outlets and still have a completely fulfilling partnership (Slater and Woodside, 1951). They might only become disgruntled if they heed the pundits who tell them that "normal" people of their age are performing on average twice to three times a week, with the implication that they are "abnormal". It cannot be overstressed that "normal" and "abnormal" have no relevance in this context. Couples who are only having coitus once a month, if that is what they want, are perfectly "normal" and, if therapeutically appropriate, should be told so loud and clear.

Premature ejaculation

Prematurity, for which there is no clinical counterpart in the female, is ejaculation before or immediately following penetration of the female introitus; it occurs against volition and before it is wished for by the male and usually, but not always, by the female also. The condition, which may occur either in the setting of a strong or a poorly formed erection, is a common cause of frustration, female orgasmic inadequacy, and consequent pelvic congestion.

The following case history of a young sexually active premature ejaculator and his treatment is fairly typical.

Enrique, a 23-year-old Spaniard, was ejaculating on most of his coital attempts in only fifty seconds, much to his and his girlfriend's dismay. The harder he tried to control things the more rapid his emission and his girlfriend was becoming increasingly more unhappy. Characteristic of premature ejaculators, once Enrique had reached a climax he entered a lengthy refractory period and was unable to engage in coitus again for several hours.

Enrique had been constantly precipitate during previous extensive heterosexual activity with numerous partners and was even brisk (although less so) during self-masturbation. He had lived with his present girlfriend for about one year; they seemed to be genuinely fond of each other and to think that they would probably marry if they could sort out their sexual problem. Intercourse took place about twice a week and although things had improved marginally they remained far from satisfied.

In addition to his prematurity Enrique also presented fairly obvious but not clinically disabling manifestations of general anxiety.

Treatment and progress. Management of this case included some training in physical and mental relaxation techniques and the application of "the squeeze technique" (Masters and Johnson, 1970) outlined below.

The two best training positions for the squeeze technique are either *(a)* with the partners sitting comfortably against a backrest (e.g. the bedhead), the female behind the male with her legs outside and parallel to his, or *(b)* with the male lying on his back, legs apart, knees bent, facing his partner who reclines against a backrest in a way that gives her maximum unimpeded access to his genitals. Trial and error will determine the best position for the individual couple.

When comfortable the female lightly grasps the head of the penis so that the index finger is pressing on the frenular-coronal junction and masturbates the male vigorously until he feels he has almost reached ejaculative non-return. At this point he signals and his partner interrupts her stimulation by firmly squeezing the head of the penis for two to five seconds. Providing the timing is right (and this can almost always be achieved with practice) ejaculation is suppressed. There will also be some loss of erection but this merely indicates that the method is being applied correctly. After an interval of twenty-five seconds or so the process is repeated, and then several times more, over a time interval of fifteen to thirty minutes, when if he wishes the male can proceed to orgasm.

In practice, in Enrique's case, the results were as follows.

After three weeks, during which Enrique and his partner practised the squeeze technique three times a week for up to thirty minutes a time, he was able to delay ejaculation for as long as fifteen minutes. They were advised that the time was now ripe to proceed to coitus attempted in the female superior position, Enrique lying on his back with a pillow under his head. Following several minutes preparatory stimulation and "squeezing", insertion was to be accomplished by his partner guiding his penis into her vagina. At this point both were to lie completely still and as soon as Enrique was accustomed to the sensation of vaginal containment, he was to introduce gentle pelvic thrusting, at a depth and speed such that ejaculation could be deferred, until he wished it, or at least for several minutes. If at any time during this process he began to feel he was losing control, then he was to withdraw his penis rapidly but smoothly and his partner was to use the squeeze method again until stability was re-established.

In the next six home assignments, during which his partner was encouraged to become progressively more active in coitus, despite a few mishaps Enrique achieved a significant measure of ejaculative control. Three months later he reported being able to delay emission for up to 10 to 15 minutes and both were delighted. Although with time and practice further improvement in such cases is usual, the couple were advised to retain the squeeze technique within their sexual repertoire for occasional use if and when required.

Ejaculative incompetence

Ejaculative incompetence is the inability of the male to reach orgasm and emission despite wanting to and despite technically adequate stimulation applied for a "sufficient" length of time. Primary or secondary, the condition may be specific to heterosexual activity, ejaculation being attainable during self-masturbation, or applying to all forms of sexual stimulation. Physiologically, ejaculative incompetence is probably the male counterpart of anorgasmia in the female, which occurs despite copious vaginal lubrication and other evidence of sexual arousal and good stimulation.

In the writer's experience most cases present as "sub-fertility" after several years of trying for a baby. Sometimes, however, a young male contemplating marriage seeks a consultation beforehand to get himself sorted out. The story is characteristic in outline. The male has normal libido, develops adequate erections, and up to a point enjoys coitus. However, despite prolonged thrusting, for as long as several hours in extreme cases, he fails to ejaculate. Paradoxically, since it frequently causes prematurity, anxiety engendered by "trying too hard" increases the ejaculatory threshold and may make matters worse.

In some cases detailed questioning reveals that the male withdraws his penis at a relatively early stage during coitus. Often these men are able to ejaculate during self-masturbation and it is possible that they would also be climactic if they allowed stimulation for a longer period of time. A minority admit to ambivalent or negative attitudes about sexual intercourse but most deny any reservations. Whether such inhibitory feelings are acknowledged or not, it may be conjectured that these men have no intention of ejaculating intravaginally. In such instances, premature withdrawal should probably be viewed as wilful refusal until proven otherwise, although it is probably true that in some cases (as with vaginismus) the act is involuntary. In the writer's view any male withdrawing within seven to ten minutes of beginning coitus, and who at the same time complains of being unable to ejaculate, should be viewed with clinical scepticism. A useful diagnostic ploy is to insist on prolonging intercourse for at least five to ten minutes beyond his usual time of withdrawal. To ensure maximal stimulation it is recommended that thrusting be both rapid and deep. If he is unwilling or unable to implement these suggestions, then partner masturbation of a highly demanding and relentless type for at least the same length of time should be substituted. Pseudo-ejaculative incompetence may be a manifestation of a highly egocentric and narcissistic personality who, for a variety of motives (punitive, exploitative, "emotional constipation", etc.), is unable to allow himself to ejaculate intravaginally. An examination of the relationship between the partners in joint interviews may make the dynamics clear.

True primary ejaculative incompetence may be conceptualised as a failure of learning during the crucial stage of adolescent growth, when sexual response patterns are usually laid down. It is a striking clinical fact that the majority of such cases have reached puberty late and developed slowly, having low sexual drives and few outlets. Physically they often appear younger than their years and may display features of a concomitant personality immaturity. Some are also severely inhibited. It is interesting that at some time most have experienced nocturnal emissions during Rapid Eye Movement (R.E.M.) sleep. The significance of these emissions, which tend to become less frequent with age, is not clear but there are two main schools of thought. On the one hand, analytically-oriented psychiatrists see them as physiological correlates of sexual dreaming. On the other, neurophysiologists have pointed out that these R.E.M. related nocturnal erections and emissions may simply be part of the increased mid-brain activity which is known to occur at this time. The fact that higher apes as well as neonates exhibit these phenomena points to a fundamental physiological rather than a symbolic origin.

A case of primary ejaculative incompetence is given below.

Mr. B., aged 25, attended with his wife and complained of never having ejaculated in the waking state through self- or partner-, masturbation or coitus. His only emissions had been nocturnal, occurring about once a month, usually while dreaming.

Mr. B. who ascribed his problem to his upbringing, described the latter as overly protective. He received no sexual information from his parents and was convinced that they disapproved strongly of sex. As a teenager, masturbation was infrequent and brief and never rewarding sexually. Premarital sexual activity with his wife-to-be stopped at kissing and cuddling and neither got much enjoyment out of it. They married following a five-year courtship and, despite their inexperience, did not anticipate any sexual difficulties. The honeymoon was disastrous, penetration was incomplete and the experience was unpleasant for both; there was no ejaculation. Since then intercourse had been attempted at the most once a month usually with some vague intention of trying for a pregnancy; thrusting, tentative and interrupted, had rarely exceeded two minutes. Mutual masturbation had occurred occasionally but was equally unsuccessful.

The referral seemed to have been initiated by Mrs. B. in the wake of a marital crisis. She had had a short but extremely passionate affair with another man, when she had discovered that she was fully responsive; her appetite had been whetted and she wanted more. Mr. B.'s response to the liaison (consistent with his bland, non-aggressive inhibited personality) was one of passive resignation.

The initial diagnostic formulation was that of primary ejaculative incompetence in a young male with a low sexual drive and ambivalent feelings towards intercourse. It was noted that despite a ten-year history he had apparently never been sufficiently interested to pursue a remedy.

The practical management of the incompetent ejaculator is the same whether the condition be primary or secondary. Accordingly Mr. and Mrs. B. were counselled along the following lines.

The first crucial step is for the female to force emission manually. This may have to be repeated for several days before achievement and it is important to reassure both that this is usual, and there is no rush. Once sexual tension has been generated sufficiently by prolonged sensate focus activity, the next step is direct penile manipulation. This should be provided in a demanding and relentless fashion, the female asking for relevant verbal and physical directives from her partner. The use of a moisturising hand cream by the female may be helpful in ensuring maximal comfort during what is often necessarily prolonged and vigorous stimulation. Once masturbatory ejaculations have become firmly established, by repeated practice, the next step towards intravaginal emission follows.

Again the female is required to excite her partner by compelling physical manipulation. When he begins to approach the point of ejaculatory inevitability, which all men should be able to recognise, rapid insertion of the penis should be accomplished by the female assuming the superior position. Manual stimulation should be continued until full penetration makes this impossible. Once inside, a demanding style of female pelvic thrusting should immediately begin. Simultaneously she should continue to provide any other type of genital or extra-genital caresses which the male finds exciting. If emission does not occur within a relatively short period of time and the male feels his level of arousal is declining, then coitus should be stopped and the vigorous masturbatory technique instituted once more. Again, when the point of inevitability is reached speedy intromission should be effected.

In the case of Mr. and Mrs. B. the results were as follows.

Unfortunately, Mr. B. was unable to go any further than the initial stage of masturbation which he was never able to tolerate for more than a few minutes. After two interviews it became clear that for a number of complicated motives, the most important one being an inability to "give" emotionally, the patient was committed to retaining the *status quo* and the couple later separated.

Generally, however, in co-operative subjects well motivated for treatment and able to satisfy the technical requirements of the method, some two-thirds will attain a satisfactory coital ejaculatory response within eight to ten sessions.

Sexual dissonance

Sexual dissonance refers to a disparity between the respective needs of partners which is of sufficient magnitude to constitute a relationship conflict. It does not imply impotence or frigidity but it may be a portent.

Characteristically, if the female has not been sexually active during adolescence then in the early days of marriage the male is more likely to complain of "not getting enough". However with time as the female develops sexually, her appetite and enjoyment tends to increase whilst that of her spouse often declines (Kinsey *et al.*, 1948; 1953). By early middle life, no longer pressurised by a young family, her needs may have grown to exceed those of her partner, and, becoming frustrated, she initiates a referral.

The following case is illustrative.

Mr. G., aged 42, was the Managing Director of his own very successful business. He attended alone after having cancelled several earlier appointments at the last minute. His main complaint was of being unable to match his wife's sexual appetite, but on a few occasions frank impotence had supervened during a coital attempt. Although Mr. G. acknowledged that his sex drive might have declined a little, he was also convinced that hers had increased. During the few months before his appointment things at home had gone from bad to worse. He had been under increasing pressure at work and with declining libido and his wife's apparently increasing interest, had been unable to perform as often as required. Latterly, on some occasions he had avoided coitus, pleading a headache or feigning sleep. His wife had become puzzled and apprehensive about his reticence and had begun to harbour suspicions that he might be having an affair.

Despite being asked to bring her to the interview, Mr. G. attended alone. His reasons for her absence were barely convincing and it was obvious that she did not even know that he was being seen. It was clear that he was going to have the greatest difficulty in admitting that he was no longer the performer of yester-year, and that some compromise, based on a reduced coital frequency, would need to be worked out. However, after numerous false starts, Mr. G. plucked up sufficient courage to broach the issue with his wife and arrange a joint appointment.

An important part of counselling this couple was to acquaint Mrs. G. with the biological reality that her spouse's sex drive had waned relative to hers, and, moreover, the more he was stressed by domestic and business worries the worse things would become. Once Mrs. G. was able to accept emotionally this truism and that her husband still felt the same about her, then a compromise was possible.

It was agreed mutually that they should have sex sessions initially two to three times a week. This was less than Mrs. G. would have liked but more than her spouse had been willing, and able, to provide latterly. Protracted foreplay was recommended as a means of ensuring that when coitus was attempted, Mr. G. would be fully roused and able to perform to his maximum. Once he was able to see that there was nothing to prove and he did not have to behave like a 20-year-old, Mr. G. lost much of his tension and found that he could actually enjoy intercourse, something he had not done for many months. After ten home assignment sessions the couple expressed themselves as significantly improved.

Six months later coitus had stabilised at about once a week. On other occasions when Mrs. G. became roused and her husband was not up to it, he brought her to orgasm manually. Although to her this was not as satisfactory as coitus, it was an acceptable substitute which pleasured both. Significantly, communication had improved dramatically which was benefiting their general relationship.

This type of problem was implicit in Kinsey's observation that men, much more than women, tend progressively to suffer from waning libido and potency in middle life, probably due in the main to biological ageing. Additionally, however, other influences play a part. Firstly, as a matter of empirical fact, males in a Western culture tend to be somewhat older than their spouses, this age difference tending to widen any developing libido-performance gap. Secondly, with ongoing sexual emancipation a sign of the times, women are no longer always willing to take a back seat and accept what the male decrees. These days, more and more are demanding sexual satisfaction as a right and proclaiming their parity. Although sexual dissonance can be a problem for partners of any age, in the author's experience the type illustrated is the most frequently encountered. The remedy requires the couple to understand and be able to accept the biological differences between the sexes, as a prerequisite to frank communication and a coital compromise. Much give and take is required.

In a few highly libidinous men, unable to get coitus and who for a number of reasons cannot relieve themselves by masturbation, the antiandrogen cyproterone acetate has been used to advantage.

With the expectation of a "normal" (i.e. active) sex life, Mr. D., a spritely septuagenarian, had recently married his 40-year-old housekeeper. Unhappily things had not turned out as expected. Previously accommodating and charming, his wife's personality had changed: apparently having achieved what she had set her sights on (marriage) she had locked him out of the bedroom.

Mr. D. had a much-above-average sex drive but because of religious scruples had been unable to masturbate himself. He had been troubled by nocturnal erections and emissions and increasing sexual tension. Becoming more and more frustrated and irritable he feared that he might make a sexual assault upon his wife. He was mainly seeking some means of reducing his sex drive sufficiently to ensure peace of mind. Following a full discussion of the likely effects, he agreed to a three-months trial with cyproterone acetate 50 mg b.i.d. This resulted in a virtual disappearance of his libido and nocturnal emissions and he felt relaxed and much better tempered. There were no side-effects of any sort. It is of great interest that when the drug was stopped Mr. D.'s libido did not return to its former distressing level and no further action was required. It seems probable that prolonged sexual abstinence, however induced, reduces sex-drive permanently in some, probably older, men, even if the original cause for the inactivity is reversed later.

The use of antiandrogens and other "castrating" drugs raise philosophical issues which are outside the scope of this chapter.

Finally, each practitioner in frank and full discussion with his patient needs to weigh up the pros and cons before a decision, which *must* be mutual, is taken.

Psychogenic sexual pain (dyspareunia and pelvic pain)

Non-organic dyspareunia may be found in both sexes but is much commoner in the female. Inadequate lubrication, the consequence of inexpert or insufficient stimulation, is often to blame. However anxiety, anger, disgust or other antithetic emotional states may inhibit full arousal and cause intercourse to be painful, even if stimulation is prolonged and technically adequate. In some males, in psychological terms, dyspareunia may be viewed as the counterpart of vaginismus where the symptom serves as a protection against penetration and its consequences. Careful questioning will usually suffice to reveal the underlying dynamics; common causes include various fears, ambivalence about coitus, feelings of disgust etc. As with other manifestations of sexual inadequacy, the composition of treatment is determined by the diagnostic formulation.

Pelvic as opposed to genital pain is a ubiquitous gynaecological complaint. In a sizeable minority of women in whom it is judged to be "psychogenic" it may *mask* an underlying sexual problem. Unless the practitioner is convinced that the pain has a clear emotional origin, it is probably wiser to refer the patient to a gynaecological department which has access to a suitably trained psychiatrist. Psychogenic pelvic pain must be diagnosed on positive psychological grounds and not by the absence of an organic lesion, although, of course this may be a reassuring clincher.

Characteristically, the complainant presents herself as a brave and stoical woman constantly fighting her pain; she expresses concern, even guilt, about being unable to fulfil her sexual obligations to her spouse. He is often described as "exceptionally sympathetic and understanding, never making demands if these occasion discomfort". Although often the pain is present constantly throughout the day, it fluctuates in severity, being particularly bad during sex play and attempted coitus, which may be limited in frequency or prevented altogether.

Although initially the pain might have been a "protection" against coitus, with time it may become incorporated into a life style and acquire diverse secondary-gain motives. It is not difficult in many cases to see tangible "benefits" in the shape of help around the house, or with the shopping, fostering dependency relationships, dominating or controlling a situation and so forth. The essential psychogenesis of the symptom may be clearly revealed when, despite vociferous complaints, the woman is perfectly able to continue doing something personally important, such as holding down a job, visiting socially and suchlike.

Long-standing, psychological pelvic pain is a daunting medical problem. Many such women have undergone numerous prior laboratory investigations often at the hands of many different clinicians, including in some cases laparotomy. They are usually convinced that their pain is "organic" and express a willingness to go to any (physical) lengths to seek a remedy. There is no doubt that repeated laboratory tests may give patients grounds for their conviction; they rationalise: "if there is nothing organically wrong with me why am I having so many tests?". Unwittingly, or even collusively, surgeons may perpetuate, even exacerbate, these symptoms. Indeed the invariably bulky gynecological notes of many chronic patients, full of repeated essentially normal laboratory tests have often labelled the pain as "psychological", yet more investigations have been ordered. In personal discussions it is clear that many gynaecologists are quite aware of the nature of their patient's pain, but do not know how to handle it. Sometimes patients are described as manipulative, aggressive or hysterical. For some surgeons the barely disguised threat of "trouble", i.e. litigation, should something organic be missed provides sufficient reason to order yet another test.

Unless the practitioner is especially knowledgeable about psychodynamics and personality structure, pelvic pain is best handled by an appropriate psychiatrist or psychosomatically orientated gynaecologist. Even in relatively acute cases where the precipitant is obvious, treatment may still be difficult. In chronic cases, in which the original cause has long since been forgotten, denied, or repressed and the symptom integrated into the personality, it may be impossible.

Acute or chronic, the treatment of choice for pelvic pain is appropriate psychotherapy to be followed by a sensate-focus-coital retaining programme whenever feasible.

Depending upon the circumstances and chronicity, interpretive psychotherapy may be directed primarily at the woman, with the hope of giving her insight as to the nature of her pain and a resultant desire to "relinquish" it. On the other hand, in long-standing and recalcitrant cases the psychotherapeutic aim may be simply to give the patient an opportunity of "blowing off steam" without there being any definitive treatment goal. This may suffice to ease the lot of a spouse or other dependant. Again, when indicated, interpreting the nature of the patient's symptoms to family members may be justified, even desirable. Each case must be judged on merit.

Vaginismus and non-consummation

A graphic description of vaginismus is to be found in the book *Virgin Wives:*

> When these patients are examined the mere attempt or actual touch of the labia may produce spasm and pain. The introitus may become so restricted that it entirely prohibits the entrance of the tip of the finger, or, during coitus, the penis. The spasm may involve the muscles of the perineum alone or may constrict the levators right up to the vaginal fornices. Accompanying these spasms is marked adduction of thighs, even a cramp-like spasm of the adductor muscles. These have been called the "pillars of virginity". Invariably the lumbar spine is extended in the position of lordosis; frequently the posture is one of opisthotonus with the head bent backwards. These symptoms are not only present during coitus but can be witnessed during the attempted examination.
>
> Friedman, 1962

Although vaginismus may present with varying grades of severity the condition essentially serves to protect the individual from penile penetration and its consequences, i.e. coitus and pregnancy. It is usually caused by permutations of fear, guilt and revulsion. A consensus of research findings suggests that vaginismus can often be traced to misinformation acquired during early adolescence or before. Common misapprehensions include:

(a) a belief that menstruation is unhygienic and disgusting;

(b) the assumption that sex is for men only;

(c) a conviction of "smallness" and that rupture of the hymen must inevitably be accompanied by pain and bleeding;

(d) an attitude that sex is dirty and messy.

In many cases direct questioning, or examining the fantasies of women with such misapprehensions indicates that they see coitus as exploitative, punitive and degrading. The penis is often equated with a knife or a large snake and intercourse may be visualised as painful, tearing and brutal. Commonly, such attitudes may be traced to a hostile mother, who hating sex herself, paints a frightening picture to her young and impressionable daughter. An attitude of sexual negativism acquired by contagion may persist and consolidate into the latter's adult life and in due course history repeats itself.

According to Ellison, the family constellation most frequently encountered in non-consummation is the "S.D.S." complex, consisting of a submissive father, dominant mother and submissive husband (Ellison, 1968). It seems possible that timid husbands are chosen assortatively because these women think that somebody gentle would hurt them less. Friedman, reiterating this view, also points out the subconscious collusion between a husband and wife who both fear the aggressiveness of sexuality (Friedman, 1962). Generally however, in the author's experience, the woman tends to use her symptom manipulatively to dominate the relationship and to "get her own way". It is equally true, however, that it suits some men psychologically to be "the underdog".

Almost without exception, women with severe vaginismus are convinced that they have some underlying physical abnormality. The commonest complaint is of being "too small", or having a "blockage". Some, and especially those with vaginal discharge, look for an endocrine or infective cause. Their male partners often have potency problems including prematurity, dyspareunia or impotence. Psychodynamically, both may be motivated subconsciously (or even consciously) to maintaining a sexual stalemate, i.e. non-consummation.

During the diagnostic interview a search for the origins of emotional tension underlying the defensive vaginal spasm is made. Accordingly, the patient is encouraged to express her feelings about menstruation, her own and her partner's sexual organs, love-making, child bearing and any memories of psychosexual trauma, pelvic pain etc. At an early stage a vaginal examination, preferably carried out in the presence of the male partner, is mandatory. This can be used to demonstrate to the patient the psychogenesis of the problem. Even when performed gently, with a well-lubricated little finger, muscular cramps supervene in the majority of cases; however, by retaining the finger *in situ*, even against the wishes of the woman and despite attempts at physical withdrawal, it is possible to talk most of these patients into a state of relaxation when the contractions and the pain wane. Following this initial examination, the female is set a goal of exploring and dilating her own vagina with one or more fingers whilst fully relaxed in the privacy of a bedroom. Self-masturbation is also recommended and appropriate instructions given. Once the patient has become comfortable with self-exploration, training in the use of graduated plastic dilators may hasten a favourable outcome.

The inability to carry out these simple requirements, however excused, usually points to disgust, which is an extremely bad prognostic sign. In such cases and in those with severe personality problems or when the dynamics are complex or obscure the matter is best handled by a suitable psychotherapist.

The treatment of any co-existing disorder of potency, in the male partner, will need to be integrated into an over-all programme.

The following case illustrates how involving the male at an early stage may expedite treatment.

Mrs. A., an attractive 21-year-old, married for one-and-a-half years, presented with non-consummation. Her husband elected not to accompany her, declaring that it was his wife who had the problem!

Prior to marriage she had enjoyed petting with her fiancé, but had been unable to allow penetration because of severe pain. Following marriage, despite numerous attempts, coitus had not been possible and the couple had been practising mutual masturbation as a means of sexual relief. Mr. A. was described as sympathetic, tolerant and gentle, "a perfect husband" incapable of losing his temper or hurting anyone.

The diagnostic formulation was a case of severe vaginismus due to a marked fear of, and a desire to avoid, the pain she was convinced would accompany coitus. The symptom, reflex in nature, appeared solely self-protective: there was no evidence that it was a manifestation of marital conflict, part of a personality disorder, or was otherwise serving subconscious, secondary-gain motives.

The initial treatment in the clinic consisted of vaginal examination followed by dilatation using plastic dilators of progressively increasing size, inserted while she was fully relaxed and well-lubricated. Throughout these sessions she was strongly reassured as to her patency and within a short time she had learned to examine her own vagina and also pass some of the smaller bougies. It was also demonstrated how with muscular and concomitant mental relaxation any provoked spasms could be dissipated. Additionally, she was encouraged to discuss and express her feelings towards her husband, their love-making, pregnancy and childbirth and other relevant emotional issues.

After six sessions Mrs. A. was able to accommodate the largest dilator in comparative comfort and felt sufficiently confident to attempt coitus. Accordingly she was advised to tell her husband that he must be prepared to rouse her fully with prolonged foreplay and also that he should ignore any protestations from her since, with continuing effective stimulation, she would become progressively less aware of discomfort which would ultimately dissolve into pleasure culminating in climax. But after four weeks Mrs. A. returned and in tears reported that despite great efforts from her husband penetration had not been achieved. On each occasion severe spasms had supervened and her husband had been unable to proceed further, since he could not bring himself to "hurt her".

The couple were invited to attend together when it was put to Mr. A. that he was oversensitive to his wife's complaints and, furthermore, because of his own misgivings about coitus was "colluding" with her to maintain the sexual impasse. Both were reassured strongly that full sexual arousal was incompatible with discomfiture, which would diminish reciprocally as Mrs. A. became more and more excited. It was stressed to Mr. A. that he should ignore his wife's reservations and persist with skilfully aggressive techniques to overcome her resistance to full penetration. It was pointed out that her vagina was more than able to accommodate his penis and that it was not possible to cause any physical damage through normal intercourse. At this point Mr. A. was shown the dilators and instructed to pass them into his wife's vagina. He was greatly surprised to discover she was able to take the largest, considerably bigger than his erect penis, without pain. He was also told that if muscular spasms developed during penetration, he was not to withdraw, but to stay put until the spasm and associated pain disappeared, when he should proceed to full penetration in a leisurely but relentless manner.

Shortly following this joint interview, the marriage was consummated, although the patient failed to reach orgasm. Ten months later, although coitus was being regularly enjoyed by both, Mrs. A. had still not been climactic.

This case exemplifies the submissive and gentle personality of the male partner, frequently referred to in the literature, and the collusive psychopathology that may exist between such couples which tends to maintain the *status quo*.

It should be mentioned that although vaginismus and frigidity often occur together they are different disorders both aetiologically and prognostically and require different treatments. Indeed, Friedman has pointed out that in some cases vaginismus not only protects the patient from the pain associated with the "feared object" (i.e. the penis) but also from the knowledge that they are sexually unresponsive (Friedman, 1962). Should orgasmic inadequacy coexist, this must be treated concurrently along the lines already laid down.

Sexual problems of the elderly

Reflecting a shift in emphasis of contemporary medicine, an increasing number of elderly men and women are bringing sexual problems to clinical attention. More often than not these are the consequences of physiological ageing which are not appreciated or understood by the individual, although there may be exacerbating psychological factors.

Common male complaints include not wanting coitus as often as before and requiring much longer stimulation to become erect, or wanting coitus but not being able to develop an adequate erection, having a "droopy" (i.e. flat angle) or only a partial erection and not ejaculating even after prolonged thrusting. Elderly women may similarly complain of reduced libido and enjoyment during coitus, but some who develop atrophic vaginitis may present with inadequate lubrication and pain.

Erectile failure of varying grades of severity, without a concomitant reduction in libido, which is more common in the elderly than the young, is seen frequently. There seems no doubt that with advancing years the physiological components of sexual drive, erections and ejaculations, decline faster and to a greater extent than the psychological urge, which may be retained even to the point of death (Hegeler and Mortensen, 1978). However this is normal and usual and any worrier should be so informed. To be told with conviction that he is just like the majority of similarly-aged men is often intensely reassuring.

A few elderly couples have consulted seeking nothing more than authoritative backing that sex for them is proper and to be enjoyed. Usually still physically healthy and sexually interested, they have sometimes felt intimidated by the often somewhat patronising attitude of the young that sex is their prerogative.

The management of old people's sexual problems, which incorporates an appropriate permutation of the general principles already outlined, aims to convince them that sex for them is physiologically possible and psychologically normal. They should not, however, try to match the performance of the young and providing they understand and accept the physical changes of ageing, enjoyable sexual activity remains possible. The elderly should also be strongly encouraged to view sex as conducive to health rather than as exhausting, and as contributing importantly towards delaying senility.

Women with senile vaginitis secondary to oestrogen depletion, complaining of dryness and pain on intercourse, may be helped by oestrogen administered locally as a cream or by the much more controversial systemic Hormone Replacement Therapy (H.R.T.) method.

Myocardial infarction and sexual dysfunction

Sexual apathy and lack of response are common enough *sequelae* of myocardial infarction and increasingly these days, with greater medical and lay awareness of the benefits of active rehabilitation, patients are seeking guidance about the restoration of normal sexual activity. Still a relative rarity, those who broach the subject deserve to be treated seriously.

In the writer's experience the questions most often posed are:

(a) will they be able to engage in sexual activity when recovered and how far will they be able to go (i.e. is sex likely to be safe), and

(b) will they need to observe any special precautions?

For the majority of mild to moderately severe heart attacks, providing there are no medical contra-indications, sexual activity may be integrated in a gradual fashion into an over-all programme of physical and psychological rehabilitation. It is important to stress, since many people believe otherwise, that the effects of sexual activity on the cardio-vascular system are the same as any other form of physical or emotional stress. Sex is not inherently more dangerous, nor undesirable; neither is it forbidden. As a matter of routine the subject should be discussed six to eight weeks after the acute attack. Sometimes the partners raise the matter themselves but if not the physician should introduce the topic himself in a candid reassuring manner. It should be made clear to the partners that, if sex is interesting to them, then it is a legitimate subject for concern. However, if it is not, then the matter should be dropped as unimportant. In the author's opinion it is unwise to make a patient feel that he should be sexually active against his natural inclinations, whatever the media currently say, and great circumspection is required in this delicate area. With a little experience, however, the subject can be negotiated without undue complications.

The couple should be told that, as with any serious illness, a heart attack may inhibit sexual feelings but these generally return. With recovery, and if they wish it, provided sensible precautions are observed, some degree of mutually satisfying sexual activity should normally be possible. As soon as a modest level of exercise has become stabilised as part of normal life and there is E.C.G. and clinical evidence of adequate myocardial compensation, sexual activity may be safely introduced.

Initially stimulation should be limited to mutual bodily caressing to explore the heart's capacity to cope. Providing there are no disabling symptoms such as chest pain, respiratory distress, excessive tachycardia, various types of non-orgasmic but progressively more exciting forms of stimulation should be repeated over a three-to-four week time span. Once the male has become confident that he is fully responsive and his heart is able to take it, it is permissible to proceed to more adventuresome love-making, including coitus. However, the watchword is *gradual* and in the early days it is prudent to avoid uninhibited emotional and physical exertions.

Patients may be advised that the abrupt cardiac stress of inter-course may be decreased by adopting positions that are comfortable and relaxed, and which facilitate easy breathing. For the male, the traditional superior position may be inadvisable because his weight in that posture is an isometric exertion which can raise blood pressure and cardiac work markedly. Preferable alternatives for either male or female patients include side-to-side, or vaginal entry from the rear. For male patients, the female superior position may sometimes be better. Non-specific advice may caution against sex on a full stomach or with restricting clothes.

Instructions as to the judicious use of cardiac drugs may be neces-sary. Nitroglycerine 0.5 mg sublingually immediately prior to coitus may safeguard against angina. There is some indirect evidence that points to an important role for the beta-blocker propranolol in reliev-ing myocardial hypoxia induced by elevated plasma catecholamines during coitus, independent of external cardiac work (Raab *et al.*, 1959; Levi, 1965; Gales *et al.*, 1959).

Anxiety is best treated by reassurance and relaxation training but occasionally appropriate medication may be a useful adjunct. However, since many of these preparations reduce libido as well as anxiety, great care is required in arriving at an optimal dose (*see* p. 159).

PROGNOSTIC FACTORS IN SEXUAL INADEQUACY

Approximately 60 per cent of couples presenting with sexual in-adequacy can be satisfactorily managed by relatively inexperienced therapists using the type of simple short-term practical programmes discussed. Indeed, providing the partners are honouring their side of the treatment contract, some measure of improvement should be apparent after four to six sessions, which augurs well for the final outcome. Failure to respond by this time should prompt a searching review and possible re-referral to a more experienced counsellor. Such lack of movement may suggest complex subconscious or disgused motives and diverse interpersonal difficulties which prevent optimal implementation of the practical regimen. If the sexual dysfunction has not improved at the end of the agreed number of sessions, efforts should be directed to the other aspects of the relationship which often improve dramatically when the nature of the sexual symptom is understood. Although they are perhaps not the initial treatment aims, the possibility of such benefits should never be overlooked.

Table 5 sets out the results of treatment according to diagnosis achieved in a sexual problems clinic using the type of format already detailed (Cooper, 1979), while Table 6 shows some relevant clinical variables which may have greater significance in predicting the outcome in the individual case and may be of more practical value to the therapist.

TABLE 5. PATIENTS BY DIAGNOSIS AND TREATMENT OUTCOME SEEN IN A CLINIC FOR SEXUAL INADEQUACY

Diagnosis	No. of patients	Mean age	No. with partner	Treatment Response			
				Significant improvement		No change, worse or dropped out	
				No.	%	No.	%
Impotence	50	41.5	25	28	56	22	44
Reduction of/dissatisfaction with/ absence of/sexual response in the female, i.e. "frigidity"	52	32.3	24	35	67	17	33
Premature ejaculation	10	29.6	2	6	60	4	40
Ejaculative incompetence	10	38.5	2	2	20	8	80
Sexual dissonance	23	43.4	8	14	61	9	39
Male dyspareunia	9	32.2	0	6	67	3	33
Female dyspareunia and pelvic pain	20	41.43	4	5	25	15	75
Vaginismus	11	25.5	4	7	64	4	36
Sexual problem in the elderly	4	65.8	4	4	100	0	0
Infertility	11	40.0	9	2	19	9	81
Total	200	37.7	82 (41%)	109	55	91	45

TABLE 6. SOME VARIABLES WHICH INFLUENCE THE TREATMENT RESPONSE IN SEXUAL INADEQUACY

Variable	Relationship to treatment response
Duration of sexual inadequacy	Disorders of longer duration than two years generally are more difficult treatment propositions. This is relatively less important in females.
Time of onset	Primary types of inadequacy much more difficult to treat than secondary. This is less so in females.
Developmental characteristics of of sexual inadequacy	Dysfunctions arising acutely in response to a specific psycho-physical stress, e.g. bereavement, marriage, or pregnancy, are better treatment prospects than a disorder of insidious onset. A better outcome is associated with an intermittent rather than a persistent dysfunction.
Strength of sex drive	Subjects with very low drives more difficult to treat. Relatively less important in females.

Variable	Relationship to treatment response
Direction of sex drive	Subjects other than preferentially heterosexual and coitus-oriented more difficult to treat. Same for both sexes.
Premarital experience	Physically and emotionally rewarding premarital sexual experience (masturbation and coitus) is a good prognostic indicator. Of much greater significance in the male.
Emotional feelings during sexual experience	In both sexes disgust or revulsion, very bad prognostic pointer. Anxiety and anger less so.
Personality of partners	Normal personality is associated with a better outcome. Abnormal personality and relationship problems may compromise treatment.
Emotional relationship between partners	Positive emotional feelings associated with a better outcome. This is proportionately more important in females.
Motivation for treatment	Assessed by regularity of clinic attendances and level of commitment to home assignments; a high level of positive motivation essential for a good response.

NOTE: All statistically significant at $p < 0.05$

In conclusion a few comments on the similarities and differences between prognostic predictors in male and female inadequacy are justified. Generally the degree of similarity is striking and supports those who believe that male and female sexuality, including impaired responsiveness, are in most respects equivalent (Masters and Johnson, 1970; Kinsey et al., 1948; 1953). However, a comparison of relevant findings suggests that emotional influences (especially love and tenderness, preferably within the security of a stable relationship) are proportionately more important to the female than stimulative techniques, providing some minimum requirements of potency are met.

Finally, it has been estimated that as many as one in four marriages are sexually unfulfilled. Helping these couples can be rewarding to therapist and clients alike and the shortage of experienced professionals means that there is tremendous scope to make a valuable contribution in this important segment of human interaction.

REFERENCES AND FURTHER READING

Ansari, J. M. A. (1975): "A study of sixty-five impotent males", *Brit. J. Psychiat.,* 127, 337-42.

Ansari, J. M. A. (1976): "Impotence: prognosis (a controlled study)", *Brit. J. Psychiat.,* 128, 194-9.

Bancroft, J. (1969): "Aversion therapy of homosexuality", *Brit. J. Psychiat.,* 115, 1417-31.

Bancroft, J. (1975): "The Masters and Johnson approach in a N.H.S. setting", *Brit. J. Sex. Med.,* 1, 6-10.

Bancroft, J. and Coles, L. (1976): "Three years experience in a sexual problems clinic", *Brit. Med. J.,* ii, 1575-7.

Bulpitt, C. J. and Dollery, C. T. (1973): "Side effects of hypotensive agents evaluated by a self-administered questionnaire", *Brit. Med. J.,* ii, 485-90.

Burgess, E. W. and Wallin, P. (1953): *Engagement and Marriage,* Lippincott, Chicago.

Comfort, A. (Ed.) (1975): *The Joy of Sex,* Quartet Books, London.

Cooper, A. J. (1964): "Behaviour therapy in the treatment of bronchial asthma", *J. Behav. Res. Ther.,* 1, 351.

Cooper, A. J. (1967): *Unpublished M. D. Thesis,* University of Bristol.

Cooper, A. J. (1969 (a)): "A clinical study of 'coital anxiety' ", *J. Psychosom. Res.,* 12, 143-147.

Cooper, A. J. (1969 (b)): "Factors in male sexual inadequacy: A review", *J. Nerv. & Ment. Dis.,* 149, 4 337-359.

Cooper, A. J. (1972): "Diagnosis and management of endocrine impotence", *Brit. Med. J.,* ii, 34-6.

Cooper, A. J. (1974(b)): "A blind evaluation of a penile ring: A sex aid for impotent males", *Brit. J. Psychiat.,* 124, 402-406.

Cooper, A. J. (1974(a)): "Anatomy of the female orgasm: fact and fallacy", *Brit. J. Sex. Med.,* 1, 3 25-29.

Cooper, A. J. (1978): "Drugs in the treatment of sexual inadequacy", *Brit. J. Sex. Med.,* 5, (1) 32-33.

Cooper, A. J. (1979): "Review of 215 cases seen in a sex clinic", *Brit. J. Sex. Med.,* 6, (1) 38-42.

Ellison, C. (1968): "Psychosomatic factors in unconsummated marriage", *J. Psychosom. Res.,* 12, 61-5.

El-Senoussi, A., Coleman, D. R. and Tauber, A. S. (1959): "Factors in male impotence", *J. Psychol.,* 48, 3-46.

Fisher, S. (1973): *The Female Orgasm: Psychology, Physiology, Fantasy.,* Allen Lane, London.

Ford, C. S. and Beach, F. A. (1952): *Patterns of Sexual Behaviour,* Eyre and Spottiswoode, London.

Friedman, D. (1968): "The treatment of impotence by brietal relaxation therapy", *Behav. Res. & Ther.,* 6, 256-261.

Friedman, L. J. (1962): *Virgin Wives,* Tavistock Publications, London.

Gales, P. C., Richardson, J. and Woods, E. F. (1959): "Plasma catecholamine concentrations in myocardial infarction and angina pectoris", *Circulation,* 19, 657.

Gillan, T. and Gillan, P. (1976): *Sex Therapy Today,* Open Books, London.

Gutheil, E. H. (1959): "Sexual dysfunctions in men", in Arieti, S. (ed.) *American Handbook of Psychiatry* Vol. I, Basic Books, New York.

Haslam, M. T. (1976): *Update,* April 883-885.

Hegeler, S. and Mortensen, M. (1978): "Sexuality and Ageing", *Brit. J. Sex. Med.,* 5, 16-19.

Johnson, J. (1965): "Prognosis of disorders of sexual potency in the male", *J. Psychosom. Res.,* 9, 195-200.

Kaplan, H. S. (1974): *The New Sex Therapy.* Baillière Tindall, London.

Kinsey, A. C., Pomeroy, W. B. and Martin, C. E. (1953): *Sexual Behaviour in the Human Female,* Saunders, Philadelphia.

Kinsey, A. C., Pomeroy, W. B. and Martin, C. E. (1948): *Sexual Behaviour in the Human Male,* Saunders, Philadelphia.

Kirkendall, A. (1967): *Encyclopaedia of Sexual Behaviour,* Ed. Ellis, A. and Abaranel, A., Hawthorn, New York.

Levi, L. (1965): "The urinary output of adrenaline and nor-adrenaline during pleasant and unpleasant emotional states", *Psychosomatic Medicine,* 27, 80.

Lobitz, C. W. and LoPiccolo, G. (1972): "New methods in the behavioural treatment of sexual dysfunction", *J. Behav. Ther. and Exp. Psychiat.,* 3, 265-271.

Mackay, D. (1977): "Emotional constipation", *Brit. J. Sex. Med.,* 4, 14-17.

Masters, W. H. and Johnson, V. E. (1966): *Human Sexual Response,* Little, Brown, Boston.

Masters, W. H. and Johnson, V. E. (1970): *Human Sexual Inadequacy,* Little, Brown, Boston.

Mead, M. (1939): *From the South Seas: Studies of Adolescence and Sex in Primitive Societies,* Morrow, New York.

Mellgren, A. (1967): "Treatment of ejaculatio praecox with thioridazine", *Psychother. and Psychosom.,* 15, 454-460.

Raab, W., Van Lith, P., Lepeschkine, V. and Herrlich, E. H. (1959): "Catecholamine induced myocardial hypoxia in the presence of impaired coronary dilatability independent of external cardiac work", *American J. of Cardiol.,* 19, 657.

Renshaw, D. and Ellenberg, M. (1978): "Sexual complications in the diabetic woman: Part II", *Brit. J. Sex Med.,* 5, 23-24.

Schapiro, B. (1943): "Premature ejaculation: review of 1130 cases", *J. Urol.,* 50, 374-379.

Semans, J. H. (1956): "Premature ejaculation, a new approach," *Southern Medical Journal,* **49**, 353-8.

Slater, E. and Woodside, M. (1951): *Patterns of Marriage,* Cassell, London.

Tanner, J. M. (1964): *An Introduction to Human Evolution Variation and Growth,* Clarendon Press, Oxford.

Walker, K. and Strauss, E. B. (1948): *Sexual Disorders in the Male,* Williams and Wilkins, Baltimore.

Weissman, M. M. and Slaby, A. E. (1973): "Oral contraceptives and psychiatric disturbance", *Brit. J. Psychiat.,* **123**, 513-18.

Dealing with Common Forms of Drug Dependence

Dr. Alistair M. Gordon,

M.B., Ch.B., M.Phil.(Lon)., M.R.C.P., F.R.C.Psych., D.P.M.

Medical Director, The Retreat, York. Formerly Senior Lecturer and Hon. Consultant, Department of Psychiatry, St. Mary's Hospital, London.

Dealing with Common Forms
of Drug Dependence

INTRODUCTION

It is difficult to imagine and impossible to determine a historical time when mankind was free from the use of drugs. Human curiosity has led to the discovery of natural substances which affect the body and the mind and human inventiveness has created synthetic equivalents of greater convenience and readier accessibility. Behind these human activities lie human needs — the need to escape from physical pain, the need to diminish emotional distress, the need to experience pleasure and joy, the need for magic and mysticism and the need to transcend, however briefly, the human condition.

Many of today's drugs are of ancient usage, their popularity and cultural acceptance varying with time and social custom. The borderlines between use of a drug and abuse of a drug have never been clear, shifting with individual attitudes and social perceptions. The vast expansion in pharmaceuticals in this century has dramatically increased the range of drugs and their usage. While twentieth-century man still employs drugs for the same needs as his ancient forbears, the breadth of drug use has increased awareness that social pressure, sensation seeking and social deviance may also determine drug use. Our attitudes to specific drugs can alter with time and experience and lead to their classification as dangerous to health, deviant within society or detrimental to cultural identity. In Western society, the powers to sanction, advise and curtail drug use are vested in the medical profession. Their perceptions, knowledge and experience are major determinants of the borders between appropriate use and abuse but the law, social opinion and fluctuating fashion also contribute to current concepts of abuse. The practising doctor, however, is less concerned with the complexity and vagaries of definition of drug abuse. He is confronted with the suffering and disorder which habitual use of drugs can create. The problem of drug dependency is not resolved in the surgery by a discussion of current debate about legislation of drugs, the morality of the individual, or the state of society. To begin to deal with drug dependency, the doctor needs to know how to recognise its existence, how to avoid fostering its development, how to approach its victims and how to attempt to alleviate their distress.

THE CHARACTERISTICS OF DEPENDENCE

Any substance taken by a living organism, which has the capacity to modify one or more of its functions, may be considered to be a drug. The development and use of drugs for therapeutic purposes is based on the premise that their administration to the organism in specified conditions will improve its function and well-being. All drugs carry the risk that their use may not be consistent with accepted medical practice. Drug abuse, the persistence or sporadic self-administration of a drug for non-medical purposes or use which deviates from cultural social patterns, is endemic in our society. It is most clearly typified by the wide and indiscriminate use of the vast array of proprietary preparations, particularly the salicylate analgesics, for a range of minor symptomatic ailments without referral for medical advice. Even drugs administered under medical direction are liable to abuse and practitioners are increasingly aware that patients utilise prescribed medicaments in idiosyncratic ways.

The borderlines between drug abuse and drug dependence are blurred but dependence has more clearly definable characteristics. Dependence on drugs refers to a stage, psychic and sometimes also physical, which results from the interaction between a living organism and a drug, and is characterised by behavioural and other responses that always include a *compulsion* to take the drug on a continuous or periodic basis, in order to experience its psychic effects and sometimes to avoid the discomfort of its absence. The W.H.O. defines four main features which typify dependence and these are as follows.

(*a*) A desire or compulsive need to continue taking a drug and to obtain it by any means.

(*b*) A tendency to increase the dose.

(*c*) A psychological and a physiological dependence on a drug.

(*d*) A detrimental effect on the individual and on society.

The physical dependence produced by addictive drugs is probably their most widely recognised and comprehensible feature. The addictive potential of a drug is most readily identified where the development of this physical dependence is rapid and inevitable, as with the opiate narcotics. Physical dependence refers to an altered physiological state brought about by the repeated administration of a drug, which demands the continued administration of the drug in order to prevent a characteristic group of symptoms termed the *withdrawal syndrome*. The precise nature of the biochemical and physiological alteration which results in physical dependence is poorly understood, but is generally considered to involve some metabolic adaptation at a cellular level. One familiar effect of physical dependence is the development of *tolerance* — a state in which repetitions of the same dose of a drug have progressively less effect, requiring an increase in dose to obtain the same pharmacological result. Tolerance develops at different rates with different drugs, more slowly with alcohol and more rapidly with narcotics. Although tolerance is the common precursor and concomitant of physical dependence, it may not be an essential factor and physical dependence may emerge with little evidence of escalation in drug dosage. With alcohol addiction, for example, tolerance may develop irregularly and incompletely.

Psychological dependence, rather than physical dependence, is the central factor in the development of drug dependence. Psychological refers to the sense of compulsion that requires periodic or continuous administration of a drug to produce pleasure or avoid discomfort. Certainly, some drugs which produce psychological dependence, such as aspirin or L.S.D., do so without the emergence of a physiologically-dependent state. Even with drugs like heroin, which have a marked potential for inducing physiological dependence, the addictive state probably relates more to the induction of psychological dependency. The relationship between physiological dependence and psychological dependence remains obscure. Although psychological dependence is the dominant feature of addiction, there is some evidence that physiological dependence may develop occasionally without any psychological dependence. The rapid consumption of a heavy alcohol intake over a short period of time — the drinking pattern of dipsomania — may produce a physiological withdrawal syndrome which reverses with little evidence of psychological craving.

The development of dependence relates to a variety of factors beyond the pharmacological nature of the drug itself, and includes the speed of its absorption, the route of its administration, the personality of the user, the availability of the drug and the subcultural attitudes to the drug. It is the capacity of the human mind to develop psychological dependence which invests all drugs with an addictive potential and explains the occasional appearance of an addiction to an atypical, unfashionable and physiologically non-dependent substance, as well as the non-medicinal dependencies of compulsive gambling and over-eating. In the management of drug dependence, it is the psychological dependence which is most difficult to cure and which inaugurates relapse, despite the attainment of abstinence with release from physical dependence.

THE AETIOLOGY OF DEPENDENCE

Three main factors lie behind the development of any addiction — firstly, the individual development and personality of the addict, secondly, the social and cultural environment in which dependency emerges and, lastly, the pharmacological effects of the drug itself. In each drug dependent patient the balance between these aetiological factors will vary. While some drugs, like heroin, will inevitably lead to dependence with continued use, because of their pharmacological properties, other drugs, like the hallucinogens, with less or no pharmacological addictive potential, may yet result in dependency because of the user's personality and attitude to the drug. In between these extremes are those addictive drugs, like tobacco, which have achieved such wide social acceptance in a culture that dependency may develop in normal personalities exposed to the influence and pressures of their environment and its customs.

As indicated above, certain influences, e.g. social, personal, pharmacological, play a more instrumental role in establishing dependency. Other factors act to maintain the established dependency. These include the relief of withdrawal symptoms, the development of a conditioned habit pattern, the continued association with consonant social attitudes and expectations and the disinhibiting and disintegrative effect of the drug on will and judgment. Drug dependency emerges as a disorder with no single aetiological cause, resulting from an interaction between the three influential factors discussed in more detail below.

1. The personality of the addict
Public opinion, influenced by observations of the advanced states of addiction visible in the "Skid Row" meths drinker and the hippie street-junkie, has little difficulty in formulating a generalised caricature of the addictive personality. Addicts are worthless, deceitful, immoral, unattractive, indolent, contemptuous and contemptible scourges on society. The medical profession includes many members who share such a view. Workers in the field of dependency, with experience of the full range and stages of addiction, have been unable to typify a characteristic personality which is inevitably vulnerable to drug abuse. Few would deny that the personality of the addict is the intrinsic initiating factor in the development of addiction, but no psychometric test of pre-morbid personality exists to identify with any certainty, the pre-addictive traits.

Observations of the addictive personality are necessarily retrospective, after the effects of drugs and a drug dependent life style have altered personal attributes. So we are left with a loosely descriptive, poorly defined and extremely subjective series of perceptions which make little contribution to our comprehension. Qualities of personality which appear to contribute to a vulnerability to addiction, include emotional immaturity and instability, inadequacy in response to mundane stress, low tolerance of frustration, limited capacity for delayed gratification, low endurance of the psychic distress of tension or depression, restricted tenacity in the face of life's challenges, a predisposition to escape from reality and poorly internalised behavioural control. Such personality characteristics are not unique to addicts but are familiar to the whole range of psychological illness and, indeed, in part to normal, healthy persons. The salient feature of the addict is that he chooses addiction as the symptomatic expression of his vulnerability rather than neurosis. Such a "choice" may be determined more by the opportunities of environment rather than by personal attributes.

Experimentation with addictive drugs has attracted both stable and unstable personalities alike. Young drug abusers frequently cite curiosity, boredom, rebelliousness and the pressure towards association (the group of people with whom he wishes to identify and be identified with) as the motivations behind their inaugural use. In contrast to young users, adult drug users are often introduced to drugs as medication, prescribed or self-administered, for symptomatic relief. Alcohol and tobacco hold a distinctive place in the drug spectrum because of their widespread social acceptance, and addiction to these drugs can develop without overt personality disturbance. A progression from exposure to dependency selects the most vulnerable, and certain personality types remain particularly at risk. The chronically anxious or depressive personality with low self-esteem may find escape from their affective feelings, as well as euphoria, in drug use. The anti-social personality with poor impulse control, impaired ability to sustain delay of gratification, a proclivity for illicit activity and a low sense of responsibility is readily attracted to the multifaceted stimuli of a drug life style. The schizoid personality may seek the security of a group identification without the burden of emotional demand and find acceptance of behavioural oddities in the alternative lifestyle of a junkie. Even the mature personality is not immune to the pharmacological effects of certain drugs and may find his personality qualities submerged once physiological dependence is established.

Although heavy drug users do reveal more psychopathology on formal psychological testing than the normal population, pre-morbid personality characteristics provide less useful and less definable indications than pre-morbid life events. The pre-morbid development of the addict is frequently marked by a history of parental disharmony and separation, alcoholism in the family, neurotic symptoms in childhood — particularly theft and truancy — personal or sibling criminality, educational underachievement and occupational instability. These practical indications, although reflecting personal maladaption, are probably better indicators of potential risk than subjective descriptions of personality or formal personality assessment.

2. The social setting of dependency

The conventions of most socialised cultures permit the use of certain drugs as legal and appropriate. Alcohol, caffeine, tobacco and barbiturates have all received acceptance in our society, although certain taboos such as age, religion and to some extent sex still surround their use. Exposure to legalised drugs within a culture may, itself, predispose towards dependency. The acceptance of heavy drinking in France and in certain class and occupational subcultures in Britain, fosters the development of dependency which is sociogenically rather than psychogenically determined. Sociocultural influences help to explain some of the differences in distribution and incidence of dependency within a culture. The contrasting social and religious attitudes to drinking between orthodox Jews and the Irish are reflected in the low incidence of alcoholism among Jews compared with the high incidence in the Irish. Social attitudes towards women drinking are reflected in the lower incidence of alcoholism in women, although this incidence is increasing with social changes accompanying their emancipation. The higher incidence of barbiturate and amphetamine abuse in adult women is linked with the differential social acceptance of the use of sleeping-pills and slimming-pills. The nicotine addiction of tobacco smoking is perhaps the most familiar of the socialised and legitimised drug abuses. Although no legal sanctions, apart from age, surround its use, extensive publicity to the health hazards of smoking and a distinct change in social acceptance of the habit in certain groups, particularly professional classes, has already effected a major change in the social patterns of nicotine dependence.

The ease of accessibility to drugs affects the social patterns of dependency. Certain occupations allow ready accessibility. Alcoholism is relatively more common in publicans, seamen, servicemen and journalists, all occupations where heavy drinking is expected and accepted. The high incidence of drug addiction in professional groups such as doctors, nurses and chemists reflects availability. Economic factors may also determine access to drugs, as seen in "affluence alcoholism", as well as in the drug expenditure of the affluent youth of the 1960s. The accessibility determined by the role of the "pusher" and the availability of different illegal drugs, contacts and trading are all intrinsic to the flow of drugs in the street-addict culture. The popularity of the drugs themselves is affected by the social influence of fashion and the popularity of specific drugs can fluctuate with the human need for novelty. The patterns of drug abuse in the past two decades have seen the rise and fall in fashion of amphetamines, barbiturates and hallucinogens, often linked with other social influences of the time, such as popular tastes in music. At present, cocaine, which has long waned in popularity, is on the ascendant and much in demand.

Although drug users enter the social setting of drug abuse voluntarily, youthful users particularly are influenced by the behaviour of their peer groups and are drawn towards sharing their drug experiences. Epidemics of drug abuse in localised sub-cultures are largely motivated by peer group identification. The established addict is often dependent upon the social contacts and style of the drug scene as well as the drug itself. The sub-culture may provide a peer group with shared experience, values, attitudes and friendships which are difficult to replace. Users may achieve abstinence only to relapse when they return to the drug arena in search of companionship. The illicit nature of drug abuse, also socially determined, offers a dramatic forum for the expression of adolescent rebelliousness, as well as proving immediately attractive to the established anti-social personality. Many young people have viewed their drug abuse as a social protest against a "sick society" and a rejection of its conventions, but the borderline between symbolic protest and drug dependence still tends to be traversed only by the more vulnerable personalities.

As a drug becomes more widely accepted in a society, the risk of dependency spreads increasingly to the more stable personalities. The contrast in the prevalence of alcoholism and that of heroin addiction in Britain reflects the social acceptance of alcohol and the rejection of illegal narcotic use. Many more alcoholics than heroin addicts will present "normal" personalities because sociogenic factors contribute more significantly in the development of alcohol dependency. As the effect of sociogenic factors increases in the aetiology of dependency, the prognosis for cure improves. The interaction between personality and social factors has implications for the legalisation of addictive substances in a culture. Increasing social acceptance of an addictive drug carries an increased risk of dependency for the stable personality as well as for the less emotionally resilient.

3. The properties of the drug
All drugs are potentially addictive. Because dependency develops as an interaction between the personality of the user, the environment and the drug, even drugs which may produce little or no physio-

logical dependency can create a psychological dependency in a vulnerable personality. The major drugs of dependency in current use, however, are those with *pharmacological* properties which foster dependency. Drugs which act on the C.N.S. as sedatives or stimulants and analgesic agents generally carry a high risk of dependency. A list of the commoner drugs of addiction, classified by drug type, is listed in Table 1.

TABLE 1. COMMON DRUGS OF DEPENDENCE

C.N.S. Depressants	C.N.S. Stimulants	Hallucinogens
(1) Narcotic drugs:	amphetamines	lysergic acid diethylamide (L.S.D.)
heroin	cocaine	dimethyltryptamine
methadone	diethylpropion	dimethoxymethylamphetamine
morphine		cannabis
papaveretum		
codeine		
pethidine		
pentazocine		
dihydrocodeine (DF 118)		
(2) Analgesic drugs:		
salicylates		
phenacetin		
(3) Barbiturate/alcohol type drugs:		
alcohol		
barbiturate		
methaqualone		
glutethimide		
chloral hydrate		
benzodiazepines		
hydrocarbon solvents		
paraldehyde		

Among these more common addictive drugs the pharmacological nature of the agent plays a differing role in the development of dependency. The narcotic analgesics can produce physiological dependence rapidly and will induce dependency within a brief period, even in therapeutic dosage. The personality of the user is of less importance than the pharmacological properties of the drug in the initiation of opiate dependence and even stable personalities will become addicted within a few weeks on small dosage. The pharmacological nature of the sedative-hypnotic group of drugs is less active in producing dependence. Addiction to barbiturates develops slowly, usually taking several months of regular exposure to doses above therapeutic levels. The development of alcoholism is even more insidious, usually requiring exposure to excessive drinking over several years. At the other end of the spectrum are the hallucinogenic drugs which do not evidently produce *physiological* dependence. The pharmacological nature of the hallucinogenic drugs is still important in the *psychological* dependence which may develop, because the pharmacologically-induced experience of the hallucinogenic trip contributes to the impetus for recurrent usage, despite a lack of physiological withdrawal symptoms. Some psychotropic drugs, despite their actions on the C.N.S., do not produce dependence. The phenothiazine tranquillizers, for example, lack any pharmacological properties which induce physical dependency and any abuse of such drugs appears largely dependent on the personality of the user.

The mode of administration, the dosage and the frequency of usage are all pharmacological factors which affect the development of dependency. Parenteral drug administration creates dependency more rapidly than oral usage. Dependence emerges more readily in "mainline" opiate and amphetamine users than in oral users. The rate of onset of dependency increases with increasing dosage of the drug and increasing frequency of use. The current trend of multiple, indiscriminate drug abuse suggests that the pharmacological nature of a specific drug may be less important for many users than the activity or circumstances of drug abuse, once a drug-taking pattern is established.

Addictive drugs act as positive reinforcers, producing a dependent habit as a conditioned response. Drug use may serve to relieve symptoms of tension or pain, or produce euphoria — reactions which reward the user and encourage continuation of drug abuse. The threat of development of withdrawal symptoms creates a further reinforcement towards continued use. The features of a conditioned behavioural habit pattern are also shown in the social patterns associated with the use of the pharmacological agent. Narcotic addicts can become psychologically dependent on the process of I.V. injection and experience euphoria from the injection ritual ("flushing"), using water when narcotics are unavailable. The pharmacological effects of cannabis are often minimal in the absence of the social rituals of a group experience, such as passing the "joint", atmospheric music and the special background lighting effects associated with its use. Certainly no single causative factor in drug dependence has emerged and an understanding of the development of a dependent habit requires consideration of the complex interactions between the drug, the user and the environment.

CLINICAL FEATURES OF ALCOHOLISM

Alcoholics have been defined by the World Health Organisation Expert Committeee (1952) as "those excessive drinkers whose dependence on alcohol has attained such a degree that it shows a noticeable mental disturbance or an interference with their bodily and mental health, their inter-personal relations and their smooth social and economic functioning; or who show the prodromal signs of such developments". The breadth of this definition ranging from physical, psychological and social features indicates that alcoholism is not a disorder which can be moulded to the medical model of disease with precisely definable aetiology, pathology, clinical symptoms and management.

There remains considerable controversy as to whether alcoholism should be conceptualised as a disease at all. Certainly, alcoholism is an aetiological factor in recognisable medical disease and even the most restrictive medical viewpoint could not dismiss alcoholism as a sociological problem with no medical relevance. The enthusiastic embrace of alcoholism into the arena of medical disease is all the same not without risks. Acceptance of alcoholism as a disease may allow the alcoholic to abrogate any responsibility for his disorder and may encourage the physician to assume competence beyond the bounds of his skill and training. The present trend is towards a broadening of the disease concept of alcoholism, with a recognition that the disorder encompasses multifaceted medico-psycho-sociological features. The current approach to management, utilising a multidisciplinary team including professional health workers, and social and voluntary agencies, reflects this changing viewpoint. Alcoholics are increasingly, if simplistically, seen as people who drink too much and suffer or cause suffering in consequence.

Incidence

Although nicotine addiction is the commonest addictive habit, alcoholism is easily the most prevalent of all the dependency disorders. The estimated number of narcotic addicts in the U.K. is about 4,000, the number of barbiturate addicts about 100,000 while the estimate for alcoholics reaches 350,000. The prevalence varies across the country with higher rates for Scotland and Ireland. Men are afflicted two to three times more statistically than women, though the incidence of alcoholism in women is increasing. Alcoholism generally presents as a mid-life disorder, most commonly starting in the 35 to 45 year age group but it is increasingly appearing in younger people. The young alcoholic tends to be more emotionally disturbed, has experienced more psychological disturbance in childhood and shows poorer adult adjustment than the older alcoholic. As the heavy use of alcohol is increasing in young people, youthful alcoholics are now appearing with more resemblance to sociogenic adult alcoholics, than to the psychogenic adolescent drug addicts whom young alcoholics previously resembled.

Aetiology

The general features common to the aetiology of dependence disorders have been described. Alcohol holds a unique place among the drugs of addiction because of its social and legal acceptance in Western cultures. The different rates for alcoholism between racial groups and religious groups are largely determined by the differing social acceptance of drinking and their tolerance of heavy consumption and intoxication. Class differences, regional differences and sex differences also contribute to variations in the incidence of alcoholism. Heavy drinking in men is common in the lower social classes while, in women, heavy consumption predominates in the upper social classes. Attempts to discover intrinsic *physical* factors in the individual which might predispose to alcoholism have been generally unproductive. Although some twin studies have shown higher concordance rates for alcoholism in monozygotic twins, a genetic metabolic factor specific to alcoholism is a less likely explanation than inherited personality traits. No acquired metabolic abnormality has been demonstrated and any biochemical explanation of alcoholism seems unlikely.

Psychological explanations of alcoholic development include the learning theory of a conditioned habit pattern. Heavy drinking as a behaviour may be learned by imitation from alcoholic parents or the excessive drinking patterns of a peer group. The social rewards of drinking, with its facilitation of companionship or the personal rewards of drinking with the relief of tension or anxiety, may become reinforcers in the paradigm of operant learning (*see* Chapter 1). Relief and pleasure experienced through alcohol may become linked, through a classical conditioning process, with the environmental cues attached to drinking — the pub, the party or the drinking companions — and generalisation may result in a wide spectrum of cues which trigger off or augment drinking behaviour. In the transactional analytic theory the alcoholic role is seen as the central component of a life game with the reward of forgiveness for the creation of widespread distress among the other players, many of whom have their own psychological reasons for interacting with the afflicted drinker (Berne, 1964). Both models provide a theoretical basis for approaches to psychological management.

Classification

The classification of alcoholism devised by Jellinek (1965) remains the standard descriptive classification of the range of alcohol dependencies. The five types of alcoholism described do not necessarily relate to different aetiological developments of the disorder or automatically imply distinctive management approaches, especially as one type may lead to or precipitate another. Their wide acceptance has been determined by their accurate description of the variety of syndromes of alcoholism, generally validated in clinical experience, and by their usefulness in focusing attention on the alcoholic syndromes where psychological rather than physiological dependency predominates. Jellinek's five types of alcoholism are as follows.

1. Alpha alcoholism

In this type, the *symptomatic* use of alcohol to relieve psychological or physical distress, social anxiety or environmental strain has evolved to the extent of a psychological dependence in which meeting a specific challenge is only attempted with prior or concurrent use of alcohol. Alcohol is commonly used to relieve stress in non-dependent subjects and the progress from relief drinking (alpha alcoholism) to psychological dependence evolves gradually without clear borderlines.

2. Beta alcoholism

The physical complications of alcoholism such as liver cirrhosis, gastric and nutritional disorders may develop without manifestation of overt physical or psychological dependency. Sociogenic rather than psychogenic factors predominate in this type of dependency, which is typified by the development of alcohol-induced disease in publicans, diplomats and affluent executives, this type of alcoholism being most commonly seen in sub-cultural and occupational groups, where patterns of heavy drinking are accepted as normal. Despite the absence of other features of psychological and physical dependency, social complications including financial stress and drunken behaviour incurring legal penalties may ensue.

3. Gamma alcoholism

In this type, physiological dependency is present and withdrawal symptoms occur. It is a true addictive state, differentiated by the capacity for abstinence at times but the inability to retain control over alcohol consumption once alcohol is ingested. This "loss of control" drinking is typical of spirit-drinking communities in Northern Europe. The "loss of control" drinker may be able to refrain from drinking or even restrict his alcohol use at certain times but the capacity for assured containment of alcohol use is lost and exposure may lead to uncontrolled compulsive drinking.

The history of gamma alcoholics is characterised by recurrent protracted bouts of heavy drinking, terminated by the exhaustion of the available alcohol supply or the development of withdrawal symptoms.

4. Delta alcoholism
In this form of alcoholism as dependency develops, the drinker is able to titrate his blood alcohol to his dependent metabolic needs without distorting cultural drinking patterns where periodic drinking throughout the day is normal and culturally accepted, as in the wine drinking culture of France. Bout drinking is unusual and both physiological and psychological dependency develop but usually remain hidden in the absence of enforced abstinence, unless manifested as physical complications. Minor withdrawal symptoms may develop but are relieved by "topping up" without traversing sociocultural patterns.

5. Epsilon alcoholism
In this type, episodic bouts of heavy drinking ("binges") occur, interspaced with periods of controlled drinking or total abstinence. The precipitating stimulus to "dipsomania" may be an emotional or physical stress, such as recurrent marital or familial problems or relapsing chronic illness, or social or environmental cues like the "annual reunion". Although the main determinant of dipsomania is a situational psychological dependency, "binge" drinking may be sufficiently severe and prolonged to lead to physiological dependence with withdrawal symptoms (gamma alcoholism).

The development of alcoholism
The end state of alcohol dependency is readily recognisable and characterises the picture of alcoholism perceived by the general public. Alcoholism is not an acute onset disorder but develops insidiously, though not without warning signs. It is important for the medical profession to develop alertness to the early signs of a developing addiction, so that advice can be offered and, one hopes, received before the irremediable physical consequences of dependency have developed. The development of alcoholism can be divided into a *pre-dependent* phase and a phase of *established physical dependence.*

1. The pre-dependent phase
Heavy drinking is so widely seen throughout normal populations that evidence of extensive alcohol use, even if admitted by patients, provides the doctor with little more than an index of suspicion. Alteration in the *pattern* of drinking provides a more helpful indicator. The emergence of solitary (often furtive) consumption, the symptomatic use of alcohol for emotional relief, the discovery of concealed supplies, the increased deployment of leisure time in drinking pursuits, a change of drinking companions or drinking

locations to less critical or familiar alternatives — in short, an alteration to a habit pattern characterised by the omnipresence of alcohol — all suggest a developing dependence. The early signs of dependency lie in the area of psychosocial disturbance, often without physical stigmata. The home environment is the setting where developing dependence is usually least concealed and the earliest sign is commonly marital or familial disharmony. Repeated intoxication, recurrent absences from home and a decreasing sense of priority or responsibility towards domestic matters arouse antagonism in a spouse. Although denial, concealment and duplicity are frequent early responses in the afflicted partner, rejection gradually ensues and emotional and physical alienation or separation develops within the marriage or the family. Sexual rejection of the alcoholic partner may lead to overt antagonism and physical abuse. At this stage, the emotionally or physically assaulted spouse may present to the doctor for help, often still concealing the cause of distress. Familial financial difficulties may arise from expenditure on alcohol.

The disinhibiting influence of alcohol and the disintegrating effect of dependency on personal ethics may be evidenced in increasing aggressiveness, egocentricity or grandiosity or decreased attention to personal appearance. Although initially confined to the home, this evidence of personality change later extends to public settings with a resultant estrangement from friends and colleagues. Problems may appear at work where early signs of dependency may include frequent absenteeism particularly on Monday morning, odd excuses to explain absence, recurrent absences from the workpost while on duty and a deteriorating quality of work. Frequent changes of job, often precipitated by dismissal, and a gradual decline in occupational status may occur. Developing alcoholism can, conversely, remain concealed in employment for many years, especially when the drinker holds a senior position and his colleagues collude with the developing habit or aid in concealment of its extent.

Drunkenness offences, particularly arrests for being "drunk and disorderly", indicate some loss of control in drinking. Offence behaviour like exhibitionism or theft, which is uncharacteristic of the drinker and inexplicable to him, may occur. Recurrent arrests for alcohol-impaired driving, or recurrent minor road accidents linked with drinking, are one of the important but most readily ignored signs of developing dependency in this society. Although physical symptoms are usually absent at this stage, memory disturbances after a drinking bout, gastric symptoms and neglect of food may be present.

Studies from general practice indicate that the earliest presentations to the family doctor include marital and work problems, aggressive behaviour, financial difficulties and chargeable offences, plus the important sign of the patient smelling of alcohol in the surgery. Despite general agreement among family, professional workers and colleagues, the alcoholic is likely to dismiss advice about the severity of the problem at this stage and he tends to rationalise his behaviour by blaming external events and other people for his difficulties. This dismissive attitude to drinking may alter, albeit briefly, when a social crisis such as arrest, dismissal or desertion is reached and the alcoholic may prove more amenable to advice at such times.

2. The established physical dependence phase
The appearance of true physiological dependence is heralded by changes in the drinking pattern. Early morning drinking may develop to control withdrawal symptoms like "the shakes" and regular drinking at unusual times occurs. *Craving*, the feeling of an intense need or desire for alcohol emerges as a new psychological symptom with obsessional and compulsive elements. It may be the result of a conditioned response to emerging withdrawal symptoms. Tolerance develops slowly in alcoholic dependency but may be shown in this phase by an increase in consumption to produce the same effect. As the disease progresses tolerance often declines, with an accompanying return of inebriate behaviour.

The phase of physical dependence is characterised by the appearance of the *withdrawal syndrome*. The earliest sign is colloquially named "the shakes". In its classical form, it develops on waking in the morning after drinking and comprises a bilateral rotational tremor, most marked in the hands, associated with autonomic symptoms of nausea, dry retching, sweating, *malaise* and headache. These symptoms are rapidly relieved by alcohol. Periods of transient amnesia, known as "blackouts", occur during and after drinking, and the alcoholic may wake without recall of the events or location of his actions on the previous night. In its most extreme form, alcoholic fugue states occur in which the alcoholic wanders unknowingly from his familiar environment, without recall of his activities. His general behaviour may appear normal and rational to observers during the fugue. Transient hallucinosis may appear on withdrawal without the development of complete delirium tremens. *Grand mal* epileptic fits may occur as isolated phenomena and alcoholism is an important aetiological consideration in the investigation of late-onset epilepsy. The most dramatic manifestation of the withdrawal symptom is delirium tremens (*see* p. 211).

Although these physical symptoms are precipitated by withdrawal, the withdrawal may be relative rather than absolute and the syndrome may develop while the alcoholic is still drinking. The withdrawal syndrome may be curtailed by continued use of alcohol and may appear in its fully-developed form only with enforced abstinence, perhaps following admission to hospital or imprisonment. The physical consequences of alcoholism develop slowly but may be evidenced at this stage. Even when liver enlargement is present, liver function tests may show no abnormality beyond elevated liver enzyme levels. Cirrhosis, neuropathies and cardiomyopathies are generally late developments, but gastritis, peptic ulceration, acute hepatitis and pancreatitis should alert the physician to the possibility of alcoholic dependency.

Psychosocial decline continues in the phase of physical dependency and problems in the area of marriage, work, finance and civil and criminal offence behaviour persist. Alongside the problem of decreasing physical health, the alcoholic may face divorce, unemployment, debt and homelessness, recurrent imprisonment, social isolation and suicide. The "Skid Row" alcoholic typifies the end state of this relentless decline, but many alcoholics never reach a state of total social dereliction. Recognition of the disorder must not be confined to the development of the defeated and debilitated end state.

The complications of alcoholism

Alcoholism carries with it an increased risk of disability in medical, psychological and social areas. In practice, the development of complications often precedes and inaugurates the identification of the disorder.

1. Medical complications

The various diseases associated with alcoholism include the following.

(a) *Gastric disorders.* Alcohol can induce acute gastritis, effecting ulceration and erosion of the gastric mucosa with subsequent haemorrhage and presenting as acute abdominal pain and tenderness with haematemesis. Mild gastritis may follow a bout of "binge" drinking in pre-dependent alcoholics or become manifest in its acute form as a recurrent complication of established alcoholism. Acute and chronic peptic and duodenal ulceration are commoner in alcoholics than in the general population. The psychological stress behind the drinking disorder, as well as the erosive physical action of alcohol, may contribute to its development. Certainly, the paramedian scar of gastric surgery is borne like a symbolic tattoo by many chronic alcoholics.

(b) *Pancreatitis.* Alcoholism is a major aetiological factor in acute pancreatitis. Serum amylase is often raised in alcoholics without overt pancreatic symptoms or dysfunction. Chronic pancreatic insufficiency also develops frequently in alcoholics.

(c) *Liver disease.* Acute and chronic liver disease are associated with alcoholism though the chronic disorders are more frequently and better recognised. An acute alcoholic hepatitis may be precipitated by bout drinking in the established alcoholic. It presents with anorexia, nausea and vomiting, abdominal pain with hepatic tenderness and a persistent pyrexia. Features which differentiate alcoholic hepatitis from viral hepatitis include gross hepatic enlargement, persistent pyrexia, persistent abdominal pain and less abnormal liver function tests. It is a serious disorder which may proceed to acute liver failure and death.

Chronic liver disease in alcoholics presents as a silent hepatomegaly until secondary cirrhotic complications ensue. The alcoholic cirrhotic liver shows fatty infiltration which may be reversible in the early stages. The basis of this fatty change probably involves both nutritional deficiency and a direct toxic effect of alcohol on hepatic cells. Chronic hepatic changes relate directly to the duration and dosage of alcohol use. Haemochromatosis is also more common in alcoholics.

(d) Cardiac disease. Congestive cardiomyopathy may develop in chronic alcoholics. The aetiological basis appears unlikely to be wholly nutritional and direct toxic effects of alcohol or additives to alcoholic beverages, e.g. cobalt, have been implicated.

(e) Blood disorders. Anaemias, both macrocytic and microcytic, may develop in alcoholics. In most cases, nutritional deficiencies are implicated, particularly folic acid with resultant megaloblastic anaemia. Anaemia may also develop because alcohol can interfere with the transport of iron, suppress erythropoiesis and alter erythropoietic cells in the bone marrow.

(f) Pulmonary tuberculosis. Pulmonary tuberculosis is more prevalent in alcoholics than in the general population. The association is probably indirect and related to the poor socio-economic conditions in which both disorders frequently emerge.

2. Neuro-psychiatric complications
The early neuro-psychiatric complications which include "the shakes", transient amnesia, transient hallucinations and epileptic fits have been described. Other neuro-psychiatric complications include the following.

(a) Delirium tremens. Delirium tremens is the most familiar of the major neuro-psychiatric complications of alcoholism and possibly the most serious. It is essentially a withdrawal symptom developing twenty-four to seventy-two hours after stopping drinking, or after relative withdrawal and most commonly presents in an incomplete form. Delirium tremens is an acute organic brain syndrome with clouding of consciousness, disorientation, misinterpretations and illusions, delusional ideas, hallucinations which are

usually visual and affective disturbance which usually comprises negative affects such as terror and perplexity, but may include euphoria. Motor restlessness and tremulousness are characteristic and the alcoholic may demonstrate habitual behaviour — the performance of familiar routine tasks but in an inappropriate setting. The syndrome may last from twenty-four hours to a week and generally ends in recovery, with amnesia for much of the event. In severe cases, the metabolic disturbance is extensive and hyperthermia, dehydration, electrolyte imbalance and circulatory collapse may all contribute to a fatal outcome. The mechanism of the neuropsychiatric withdrawal syndrome remains obscure but hypomagnesaemia and alkalosis which increase excitability in the nervous system have been implicated. A rebound excess of R.E.M. sleep may contribute to the nightmarish features of fear, visions and possibly disorientation.

(b) Wernicke's encephalopathy and Korsakoff's psychosis. These two alcoholic complications, originally described separately in the 1880s, appear to be closely related and mixed presentations are common. They share a similar aetiology, with deficiency of B-group vitamins, particularly thiamine (Vitamin B_1), and a similar pathology with haemorrhagic lesions and cell necrosis in the grey matter of the brain. Wernicke's encephalopathy is an acute organic brain syndrome with confusion, eye signs and ataxia. The ocular disturbance produces mystagmus, external ocular palsies and paralysis of conjugate gaze. The mental state may include a memory impairment similar to classical Korsakoff's psychosis *(see below)* but is more usually a confusional state. Ataxia may be complicated by the presence of a peripheral neuropathy.

Korsakoff's psychosis classically presents as a dysmnestic syndrome with disordered memory and disorientation in time. A more general confusional state is sometimes present with a spectrum of intellectual deficits but memory impairment always predominates. There is an impaired capacity for new learning and both short- and long-term memory are affected, although immediate recall remains intact. Peripheral neuropathy or confabulation may be accompaniments. Although some degree of recovery occurs slowly, particularly for the confusional state, if the patient refrains from alcohol and takes a vitamin-supplemented diet, the memory deficit is largely unresponsive to treatment and is probably the result of permanent structural damage.

(c) Alcoholic dementia. Some alcoholics develop a global deterioration in mental function, with general intellectual decline as well as memory loss. The clinical borderline between alcoholic dementia and Korsakoff's psychosis remains blurred, but alcoholic dementia

generally has a less acute onset and confabulation is less characteristic. The diagnosis of alcoholic dementia is commonly missed, particularly when attention is focussed on other medical complications. Electroencephalography is usually unhelpful as a diagnostic investigation. Air encephalography or brain scan, may reveal the presence of cerebral atrophy.

(d) *Alcoholic hallucinosis.* In this syndrome, hallucinations which are mainly auditory appear in clear consciousness. The content of the voices may be pleasant or unpleasant and their form usually lacks features associated with schizophrenic hallucinations. The syndrome may be acute or chronic. The acute syndrome is probably a withdrawal phenomenon and may be part of an incomplete delirium tremens. Hallucinations develop twelve to forty-eight hours after withdrawal, last up to several days and disappear with recovery. The course of chronic alcoholic hallucinosis is different, lasting from months to years during which the alcoholic often appears undistressed by his voices. The prognosis is poor, with an end state resembling dementia or schizophrenia.

(e) *Peripheral neuropathy.* Nutritional deficiency in alcoholics, particularly insufficient intake of B-group vitamins, can result in the development of peripheral neuropathies. These may be motor or sensory or combined in type. The lower limbs are more affected than the upper limbs and the distal parts are most severely involved. Pain, paraesthesia, weakness, distal muscle wasting, ankle drop and absent reflexes are common presenting features. The pathological changes involve segmental demyelination and recovery is often limited and slow.

(f) *Central nervous system degenerations.* Three neurological syndromes which affect the central nervous system are associated with alcoholism. Cerebellar degeneration, also seen with bronchial carcinoma, presents as a truncal ataxia with impaired balance although co-ordination of the limbs and speech may be preserved. Central pontine myelinolysis presents with quadriplegia and bulbar palsy. Marchiafava-Bignami disease, a degeneration of the corpus callosum, presents as a dementing disorder with epilepsy, paralysis and rigidity.

(g) *Alcoholic amblyopia.* Gradual loss of vision due to degeneration of the optic nerves may result from B-group vitamin deficiency in alcoholics. The use of methyl alcohol by methylated spirits drinkers may cause a retro-bulbar neuritis with consequent blindness.

(h) *Morbid jealousy.* A delusional conviction of infidelity in a spouse or sexual partner is the essential feature of this syndrome, which is frequently associated with alcoholism. The accused partner is exposed to repeated and unrelenting suspicions which remain unabated despite denial or forced "confession" by the partner.

(i) *Drug dependency.* The alcoholic may abuse drugs of dependency other than alcohol. Barbiturates are the drugs most commonly abused by alcoholics, as their physiological effects closely resemble those of alcohol. Barbiturate prescriptions should be avoided in alcoholics not only because of the risk of cross dependency but also because they are frequently used in suicide attempts.

(j) *Suicide.* Male alcoholics have an incidence of suicide which is eighty times greater than the expected rate. The predisposing factors which contribute to this high suicidal risk include the disordered psychogenetic influences which contribute to dependency, the physical, psychological and social decline accompanying the disorder and the disinhibiting effect of alcohol itself. Alcohol is widely used by non-alcoholics in suicidal attempts and suicidal acts are often preceded by drinking.

3. Social complications

The debilitating consequences of alcoholism are not confined to the mental and physical health of the alcoholic but extend to his immediate family and society in general. The impact of alcoholism is particularly evident in the areas of the work environment, the marital relationship, crime and accidental injury. Although it would appear likely from American studies that alcohol dependency makes an impact on industry in terms of absenteeism and lost man-hours, industry in Britain has shown little interest in determining industrial wastage through alcoholism or exploring rehabilitation programmes. Alcoholism links with crime in two main ways; firstly, it is a recurrent accompaniment of offence behaviour, probably acting as a disinhibitor and augmenting aggressive behaviour and, secondly, studies of criminal populations show a high prevalence of alcoholics, particularly among recidivists. Alcohol contributes to the accident rate in industry and in the home but most interest has focused on its association with road traffic accidents. Driving skills certainly deteriorate at blood levels of 30 to 40 milligrams per 100 millilitres of blood (the legal limit for driving is 80 mg per 100 ml in the U.K.) and alcohol is frequently and repeatedly implicated in road accidents, particularly the single motor vehicle accident. Alcohol misusers are over-represented among road traffic accident subjects and are involved in significantly more accidents per year and more traffic convictions than the general population.

Marital failure and breakdown is a major complication of alcoholism. The main stresses created by alcohol in the family include economic problems, increasing resentment by adolescent children, strains on the emotional and physical health of the spouse and fear of loss of the alcoholic spouse. The wives of alcoholics have evoked considerable interest, partly because of the surprising tenacity of some women in contending with their alcoholic husbands. Attempts to determine the characteristic personality traits of the wives of alcoholics encourage restrictive stereotyping, but recurrent personality patterns in case-work do emerge. The dominant controlling wife, the masochistic sufferer, the ambivalent protector attracted to invalidism and the aggressive career woman appear repeatedly in the marital interactions of alcoholics. The daughters of alcoholics who themselves marry drinkers or the women who make repeated marriages to alcoholics do encourage the belief that some women are positively attracted to relationships with alcoholic men. Many wives seem to find the reformed alcoholic less acceptable than their former inebriated partner. No clear patterns in the psychodynamics of alcoholic marriages emerge. Marital breakdown is common in non-alcoholic marriages and alcoholism may only serve as the stress factor which uncovers interactional marital psychopathology.

CLINICAL FEATURES OF DRUG DEPENDENCY

The disorders of drug dependency are conventionally described in relation to specific drugs or drug types. This convention is followed in this chapter but it must be stressed that the aetiological factors which lead to dependency are not drug specific. The personality of the addict and the environmental factors associated with addiction are relevant to all dependency disorders and the choice of a specific addictive drug is often random or determined largely by availability or current fashion. The recent trend in multiple drug abuse has weakened any concept of a specific drug selectivity in vulnerable, predisposed or experienced users. Drug users certainly can reveal preferences and restrictions in their choice of drugs. Some barbiturate addicts have distinct favourites among the barbiturate range, other drug users restrict themselves wholly to "soft" drugs and reject narcotics. As with any group who share generalised common features, individual differences may still emerge, but the choice of one specific drug is only one such individualistic feature. The choice of drug is not generally linked with any other associated features which might allow separation of classes of drug users into well-defined, differentiated sub-groups. The central disorder of dependency emerges as a labile entity which can attach itself to a variety of addictive substances with haphazard facility.

Multiple drug abuse has become the trend of addiction in recent years. Various drugs may be used together or in sequence. At times, the combinations appear purposeful, such as the sequential use of amphetamines and barbiturates where the latter counteracts the effects of the former, or the combined use of heroin with cocaine to potentiate the narcotic effect. More freqeuently the combination of drugs seems indiscriminate, resulting from the inter-play of need and availability. Although alcohol has been separately discussed, its use in the spectrum of multiple drug abuse is common and increasing. Even within the current jumbled miscellany of drug use, certain trends in drug combination emerge — alcohol and barbiturates which share similar pharmacological actions; marijuana, the hallucinogens and the amphetamines (the "soft" drug group); heroin, cocaine and cannabis; amphetamines, barbiturates and alcohol; sedatives, tranquillizers and methaqualone. The trend to multiple drug abuse is disheartening in its implications of loss of control and non-containment. Dependencies on a specific drug generally prove easier in management and experience suggests that wide-ranging multiple drug abuse carries a particularly poor prognosis for abstinence.

Narcotic analgesics
Opium is the dried juice obtained from the unripe seed capsule of the poppy (*Papaver somniferum*). Its use as a drug dates back six thousand years but the non-medicinal use of opiate derivatives has escalated dramatically in Western cultures over the past two decades. The narcotic analgesics include the opium alkaloids and their derivatives — morphine, heroin, codeine and papaveretum (Omnopon) — and synthetic preparation with opiate-like qualities derived from various related chemical groups — methadone, pethidine and pentazocine (Fortral). All these drugs exert a powerful analgesic action valued in medicine for the relief of physical pain. They also exert a marked sedative effect and it is this quality of euphoric sedation with dreamy detachment from reality which is most valued by the contemporary street addict. Of all the narcotic analgesics, heroin has the most powerful analgesic and euphoric effects and is the most rapidly addicting. In Britain, it is available as legally prescribed "British heroin" and in illicit forms, most commonly "Chinese heroin": British heroin comes as a small white tablet which must be dissolved before use; Chinese heroin (obtained from natural sources in Turkey, Burma, Thailand and Laos but formerly exported from Hong Kong) arrives at street level as an adulterated powder, often mixed with bicarbonate of soda, chalk or instant coffee and is usually sold in small envelopes of Chinese newspaper.

The development of dependency
Dependency can develop following continued therapeutic administration of narcotics but awareness of their addictive risks has helped to limit the extent of therapeutic addiction with the exception of

codeine available in some proprietary preparations. Occupational addiction in doctors, nurses and chemists is occasionally seen related to their propinquity to narcotic drugs but the recent epidemic of narcotic abuse has involved young, non-therapeutic users. Their first experience usually occurs at street level often commencing in teenage years. Many have considerable prior experience with other drugs and a history of anti-social traits including truancy, educational under-achievement, delinquency, promiscuous sexuality, unstable employment and poor interpersonal relationships.

Initial drug use may involve sniffing of the powdered drug ("snorting") or subcutaneous or intra-muscular injection ("skin-popping"). More established addicts rapidly progress to intravenous use ("mainlining") with its advantage of a more rapid onset of drug effects. The earliest experiences with heroin are often distinctly unpleasurable because of the drug's central emetic effect. Nausea and precipitate vomiting may override any euphoric experience. Tolerance to the emetic effect of heroin develops rapidly and the user begins to experience the relaxed euphoria known colloquially as the "buzz". Physiological dependence develops rapidly with heroin and can occur within a few weeks of regular use. Tolerance also commences early and involves the analgesic effect, the euphoria and sedation, the respiratory depression, hypotensive and hypothermic effects and the emetic effects but tolerance does not develop to the miosis, constipation or convulsions associated with drug use. Escalation of dosage follows to recapture the euphoric effect. This is succeeded by the appearance of withdrawal symptoms which foster the maintenance of dependency. Although the early abstinence syndrome is often not severe, apprehension about even mild symptoms is escalated by the street mythology, and drug-seeking behaviour ensues. With established dependency, tolerance to the euphoric effects may be complete and the avoidance of withdrawal symptoms remains the only physiological motivation for continued use.

The withdrawal syndrome
An early acute abstinence syndrome can develop within a few hours of the last use. It begins with mental feelings of restlessness and weakness, irritability and sleeplessness and in mild dependency may resolve without further symptomatic development. As dependency increases, the abstinence syndrome intensifies and includes a flu-like syndrome of rhinnorrhoea, lacrimation, sweating, muscle cramps in the abdomen and calves, nausea and vomiting, goose-flesh, chills, insomnia and diarrhoea. The symptoms increase in severity over two to three days and usually resolve in seven days without treatment. Cardiovascular collapse and death rarely occur and are commoner in street mythology than in fact.

A more chronic phase of the withdrawal syndrome may appear several months after prolonged abstinence and includes mental symptoms of hypersensitivity to stress, preoccupation with discomfort and impaired concentration as well as physiological signs of decreased blood pressure, body temperature and pulse rate.

The range of narcotic analgesics

Heroin, as the most potent euphoriant in the group, is undoubtedly the most popular street narcotic. Methadone is now second in frequency of use following its wide prescription by drug dependence centres as a substitution therapy. Methadone, prescribed either in ampoules or as a linctus, reaches the street market from the supplies of clinic attenders. Although the linctus form discourages injection, it has been used by mainlining addicts. Methadone is a less potent euphoriant than heroin and tolerance develops more slowly. Morphine and pethidine, both potent analgesics, are also less euphoriant and less common in current street use. Codeine has little euphoria-inducing property except in high dosage and pure codeine dependency is rare. Proprietary combinations, especially with salicylates, are misused though by a different social group, particularly suburban housewives. Pentazocine dependence, at least to a psychological degree, has now been reported and the drug is certainly available at street level.

The outcome of narcotic addiction

Continued self-administration of narcotic drugs leads to physical and mental deterioration but the decline is often slow, especially in users who observe sterile precautions and stabilise their dose levels. Nutritional wasting, chronic septic lesions, alopecia and chronic constipation are, however, common physical accompaniments. Indolence and apathy, loss of motivational drive, loss of libido, criminal behaviour and deteriorating self-care and personal ethics are typical mental changes. The high morbidity and high mortality are largely augmented by the serious complications of narcotic dependency, particularly the risk of overdosage, but even stabilised addicts show a shortened life span resulting from a chronic and generalised cell atrophy and necrosis.

Recognition of the narcotic addict

The habits and life style of the narcotic addict may advertise his dependency. Physical examination may reveal pinpoint pupils, needlemarks, septic skin lesions or chronic ulceration and pigmented streaking over veins. Diagnosis should not rely wholly on physical stigmata and should be confirmed by urine analysis. Thin layer chromotography will detect urinary metabolites after recent administration.

Sedatives and hypnotics

Despite the attention currently accorded to narcotic dependence, the dependence on the sedative and hypnotic group of drugs is on a considerably vaster scale. With the rapid escalation in the prescription and use of tranquillizers over the past decade, they have now probably obtained priority of place over the barbiturate hypnotics as the major drug of abuse. The sedative and hypnotic drugs comprise the two groups outlined below.

(a) The barbiturate group.

(b) The non-barbiturate group: meprobamate (Miltown, Equanil); methaqualone (Mandrax); glutethimide (Doriden); chloral hydrate (Noctec); triclofos (Trichloryl); benzodiazepines (Librium, Valium, Nobrium, Mogadon); chlormethiazole (Heminevrin).

The physiological dependency produced by these drugs parallels alcohol dependency.

The development of dependency

Two distinctive patterns of hypnotic dependence have emerged. In the first, the user — frequently a woman in middle age — has commenced use under therapeutic direction for such problems as insomnia, tension or depression. Although physical dependence is rare in therapeutic dosage, psychological dependence may develop and the patient feels unable to face the day or the night without the use of the drug. A certain number of such vulnerable patients begin to alter the pattern of administration without medical advice, escalating the dosage and frequency of administration, and changing the timing and purpose of drug use. Many women using hypnotics for stress or insomnia gradually discover that daytime administration blunts their effective responsivity to the anxieties, misery or boredom of their daily lives. Escalating dosage and the development of tolerance herald the arrival of a state of physical dependence.

A second group of users emerged in the 1960s when young street addicts added extensive barbiturate use to their spectrum of multiple drug abuse, administering the drug by intravenous injection. They obtained the drug by illicit trading or by attending various doctors as transient patients. The high risk of overdosage with intravenous barbiturate use was associated with a rise in mortality among street users. Mainline barbiturate use is now in decline but the oral use of barbiturates continues among street addicts.

Barbiturate dependence produces a state of intoxication with drowsiness and stupor, impaired cognitive function with confusion, poor concentration and memory dysfunction. Loss of behavioural control may result in disinhibition, apathy and irresponsibility. Physical signs include ataxia with staggering gait, slurred speech, nystagmus and tremor. Drug overdosage, either intentional or accidental, is a common feature. Tolerance may develop rapidly, particularly with intravenous use but it is greater for the hypnotic effect than for respiratory depression and the "safe range" is small. Tolerance disappears after one to two weeks abstinence and the risk of overdosage on relapse is considerable.

The withdrawal syndrome
Withdrawal symptoms occur from twelve hours to twelve days after stopping the drug. They include anxiety, tremor, sweating, nausea and insomnia and may proceed to an acute organic brain syndrome with confusion and hallucinations, resembling or identical with delirium tremens. The most serious withdrawal features are fits of *grand mal* epilepsy type, even leading to *status epilepticus.* These fits are often very resistant to the usual measures for reversing *status epilepticus* and render the withdrawal of barbiturates much more dangerous than opiate withdrawal.

The range of sedatives and hypnotics
All drugs in this group produce a barbiturate-like dependence although often of less severity. Methaqualone (Mandrax) which produces a mild euphoria, particularly in combination with alcohol, has proved a popular drug on the illicit market. Glutethimide (Doriden), popular as a potentiator of heroin in America, has achieved little illicit success in Britain despite its barbiturate-like dependence potential. Although chloral hydrate can produce physiological and psychological dependence with an abstinence syndrome resembling delirium tremens, serious addiction is rare in the U.K. The benzodiazepines can produce physiological and psychological dependence, although much less often, but their extensive use in the U.K. by a wide spectrum of the population has augmented the risk of abuse. The dependency is, again, of barbiturate-alcohol type and tolerance can develop. The withdrawal syndrome ranges from minor symptoms of nausea, faintness, anorexia and tremor to a major barbiturate-like withdrawal syndrome. The slower metabolism of the benzodiazepines limits the severity of withdrawal symptoms and may delay their appearance.

Psychomotor stimulants
The pharmaceutical development of drugs which rapidly lessen fatigue and enliven the dispirited appeared an immensely useful adjunct to the physicians' remedies, supplying the instant answer to the frequently requested "tonic". The realisation of the powerful addictive properties of the stimulant drugs dawned slowly, highlighted by the emerging use of amphetamines by adolescents in the 1950s. Despite a rapid decline in prescription, the stimulants remain one of the most

popular and most easily available of illicit market drugs. The psycho-motor stimulant drugs include the amphetamine group (amphetamine sulphate, dextroamphetamine, methylamphetamine), cocaine (an alkaloid from coca leaves) and diethylpropion (Tenuate).

The pattern of dependency
Amphetamine drugs were widely prescribed for depression and as slimming-drugs because of their appetite-suppressant action. Diethyl-propion (Tenuate) is marketed as a slimming aid. Therapeutic pre-scribing introduced a group of patients, largely middle-aged women, to the stimulant property of the drug and the earliest cases of depend-ency were shown by these therapeutic addicts. The drug was rapidly adopted by the street market and its illicit use expanded among young people in the 1960s. The drug is commonly used with barbiturates to counteract its stimulant effects and allow sleep ("uppers and downers") and combined preparations with barbiturates (e.g. Drin-amyl) have been popular.

Psychological dependence develops to all the psychomotor stimul-ants and physical dependence with tolerance occurs with the amphe-tamines, although not with cocaine. The stimulants produce feelings of increased confidence and self-esteem, euphoria and a sense of increased mental and physical capability. Physical effects include dilated pupils, tachycardia, anorexia and sleeplessness. The drug is usually taken orally but the intravenous use of methamphetamine (Methedrine) reached epidemic proportions among street addicts in the 1960s. This epidemic of "speed freaks" was curtailed abruptly after a voluntary ban on prescription by general practitioners. Most illicit amphetamine users employ the drug on an occasional basis and are rarely seen by doctors. Chronic amphetamine use or intra-venous administration may produce a schizophreniform psychotic reaction. Amphetamine psychosis is characterised by the acute onset, usually in clear consciousness, of paranoid delusions and hallucin-ations (mainly auditory) and stereotyped behaviour. Symptoms largely disappear within two to three days after abstinence, though vestiges may remain. Amphetamine use may precipitate schizo-phrenia in those predisposed to this illness and here the illness does not readily remit spontaneously.

Cocaine is used by intravenous injection or taken by nasal insuf-flation ("snorting"). Its effects are very transient because of its rapid metabolic destruction and the stimulant effect ("flash") lasts ten to fifteen minutes. It was commonly used with heroin, administered as a combined injection, to counteract the depressant effect of heroin and augment the euphoric effect. Cocaine produces an intense psychological dependence but no physical dependence or tolerance.

Chronic use may precipitate an acute psychosis with paranoid delusions and hallucinations, characteristically tactile hallucinations of insects crawling beneath the skin (formication). Cocaine fell out of fashion in the early 1970s but has recently reappeared on the illicit drug scene and currently holds the status of the most prized (and most expensive) street drug.

The withdrawal syndrome
In physical terms withdrawal symptoms are mild, with lassitude, lethargy, hunger and increased sleep. The psychological effects however are severe, with an intense "rebound" depression and irritability. The low rate of excretion produces a withdrawal syndrome of gradual onset but the intensity of the resultant depression, especially in contrast to the previous euphoric sense of well-being, makes withdrawal unwelcome and fosters relapse.

The hallucinogens
Drugs commonly included in this group are neither true drugs of dependency nor all hallucinogenic. True hallucinogens include natural derivates such as mescaline (from the peyotl cactus) and psilocybin (from a variety of mushroom) as well as the synthetic drugs lysergic acid diethylamide (L.S.D.), dimethyltryptamine (D.M.T.) and dimethoxymethylamphetamine (S.T.P.). Cannabis, included in this group, distorts perception to give illusions, only rarely producing true hallucinations.

The pattern of use
The hallucinogens became the hallmark of a world-wide psychodelic cult in the mid-1960s to the 1970s. The true hallucinogens, administered by mouth or injected, produce perceptual changes in all sensory modalities, particularly in visual imagery. The effect experienced varies with dosage, the environmental setting and the expectations of the user. Visual imagery may be formulated or unstructured, time perception alters, thought associations loosen with illogicality and feelings of euphoria, and changes in ego perception occur. Not all "trips" are pleasurable and many include terrifying imagery. Despite their cult-linkage with creative experience, there is no evidence of enhancement in the performance of advanced creative tasks. Physical dependence does not occur but psychological dependence and tolerance may develop. Chronic use is, however, uncommon. The usual pattern of use is the occasional "trip" and few devotees "trip" more than twice weekly. Abstinence is not associated with any withdrawal syndrome.

The lethal dose of L.S.D. is high and no deaths have occurred directly from the metabolic changes of acute toxicity. Adverse reactions do occur and include acute panic reactions, "flashbacks" and psychosis. Deaths have occurred by the behaviour resulting from panic reactions, associated with disordered perception and thought, where delusional ideas of persecution or of superhuman powers have led to reckless actions. "Flashbacks" are the spontaneous recurrence of a "trip" experience in the absence of drug use. They may occur months after the use of the drug, are usually brief, but may be repeated and frequent. Cannabis and alcohol use are associated with their appearance. It has been postulated that they result from prolonged storage of the drug. A schizophreniform psychosis with prolonged hallucinosis is a rare complication, usually following prolonged use and carrying a poor prognosis.

Cannabis, from the plant *Cannabis savita*, has been known for 3,000 years but its use escalated in Western culture in the 1960s. Initially appearing as a cult phenomenon in the young, it has spread in use to more conservative circles. The leaves of the female plant (marijuana) are commonly smoked while the more potent resin (hashish) is either smoked or eaten. The effects of the drug appear within minutes and last several hours. Reactions vary widely but mild euphoria, heightened sensory awareness, altered time perception, relaxation, disturbance of thought patterns and passivity are described. Tachycardia and reddening of the conjunctiva are among the physical effects. The general pattern is one of intermittent use and continued users rarely smoke as frequently as once a day. Heavy users do, however, form a distinctive group, involved in multiple drug use and revealing impaired social adjustment. Depersonalisation and marked sensory distortion occur in heavy users and a toxic psychosis with confusion, delusions and hallucinations has been described. An "amotivational syndrome" with loss of drive and volition has been attributed to chronic use but the evidence of serious mental illness induced by cannabis is lacking and no definite physical hazards of recurrent use have been identified.

Inhalants
The inhalation of volatile hydrocarbon solvents has been described as a habit pattern in recurrent mini-epidemics since the 1960s. Types of inhalants used include motor and lighter fuel, paint removers, plastic glues, cleaning fluid, model cement, nail polish remover and a variety of aerosol propellants. Users are remarkably young (from about seven to seventeen years) and are usually underpriviledged males with socially deviant backgrounds. Most mature out of the habit but some phase into dependency on other drugs.

The pattern of use
The inhalant is administered on a handkerchief, from a plastic bag or directly from an aerosol spray and inhaled into the mouth. It produces an intoxication of rapid onset and short duration. Inhalants

are primarily C.N.S. depressants. Their effect, like alcohol, causes delirious excitement with motor clumsiness, mental confusion, emotional disinhibition, impaired perception and cognition, slurred speech and drowsiness. The euphoric excitement may produce reckless and destructive behaviour. Additives in the solvents are often more dangerous than the solvent itself and coma and death have resulted from inhalant use. Tolerance and psychological dependence develop in chronic users but there is little evidence of physical dependence. All the symptoms of intoxication are reversible with little hangover, but side-effects may include irritation of the eyes, a chronic cough, tinnitus, nausea, vomiting and diarrhoea. Serious risks of inhalants relate to the hazard of overdosage, with the occurrence of respiratory arrest from depression of the respiratory centre and cardiac arrhythmias. Suffocation from the bag, laryngospasm and accidents from disinhibition have been fatal.

Complications of drug dependency

The complications of drug dependency include physical, neurological and social complications, and special factors in the cases of pregnancy.

Physical complications

(a) *Drug overdosage.* Drugs of dependency, particularly barbiturates, have become the major agents employed in suicidal attempts and their use for this purpose has escalated particularly among young women. Drug addicts may also overdose on drugs, sometimes with suicidal intent but more often by accident, particularly while in an intoxicated state. Brief abstinence or temporary withdrawal carries a particular risk of overdosage. Street users often enter hospital for withdrawal, with the intent of diminishing the extent and cost of their habit or losing an acquired tolerance to the euphoric effect of their drug. On discharge, they return to drug use but are no longer able to gauge their level of tolerance and may overestimate dosage levels with fatal results.

Overdosage with narcotics, hypnotics, sedatives and tranquillisers presents with coma, respiratory depression and hypotension. Pinpoint pupils and skin tracks may suggest narcotic overdosage while pupilary dilatation is common in barbiturate overdose. Acute amphetamine intoxication produces sympathetic over-activity with manic excitement and epileptic fits. Large doses of hallucinogens produce a typical L.S.D. trip but little lethal risk. The general management of drug overdosage includes the maintenance of ventilation (with intubation where necessary), the maintenance of blood pressure (with isotonic saline or 5 per cent dextrose), stomach evacuation if the patient is conscious and dialysis if coma deepens. Morphine antagonists (e.g. naloxone (Narcan) 0.4 mg by I.V. injection) may reverse the intoxication of narcotics. Barbiturate overdosage may require osmotic diuresis with urea or mannitol. Haemodialysis may be necessary when Grade III or Grade IV coma develops, when the blood level of the drug is above the lethal dose or when a combination of drugs has been used. Amphetamine overdosage may respond to parenteral diazepam. Toxic reactions to L.S.D. rarely require hospitalisation but may respond to reassurance and major tranquillisers such as chlorpromazine (Largactil).

(b) *Septic complications.* Parenteral drug users hold little respect for asepsis and rarely administer narcotics in sterile solution. Illegal heroin may contain adulterants and street addicts have a high carrier rate of *Staphylococcus aureus.* It is not surprising that septic complications occur frequently in parenteral users. Local infections are common, including subcutaneous abscesses, cellulitis and thrombophlebitis and the usual sites are the thighs and arms. Septicaemic infection may present as endocarditis, meningitis, septic arthritis, osteomyelitis or metastatic abscess. Tetanus is a recognised complication of parenteral use. Barbiturate drugs are particularly irritant to tissue and injection outside a vein may cause necrosis and ulceration. Arterial injection may result in ischaemic contractures.

(c) *Hepatic disease.* Viral hepatitis is endemic in parenteral users and commoner than toxic hepatitis. The usual infection is the Australian antigen (hepatitis B antigen) type. Recurrent episodes are common. Although acute hepatitis is the more usual and more dramatic liver disease, a chronic hepatitis with persistently abnormal liver function tests does occur and may progress to cirrhosis.

(d) *Respiratory complications.* Acute pulmonary oedema is a serious complication of narcotic addiction, associated with overdosage. A rapid onset of coma ensues with depressed respiration and cyanosis. Few patients reach hospital alive but recovery can occur in twenty-four to forty-eight hours with intubation, administration of 100 per cent oxygen and the use of morphine antagonists.

(e) *Cardiovascular complications.* Narcotic dependency is associated with endocarditis, thrombophlebitis and embolism from septic pulmonary emboli. Inhalants may produce arrhythmias which can result in cardiac arrest.

(f) *Renal complications.* Acute glomerulonephritis, secondary to septicaemia and "focal glomerulonephritis", secondary to bacterial endocarditis, occur in parenteral users. Aspirin and phenacetin addiction is a major cause of renal papillary necrosis and chronic renal failure.

(g) Other physical complications. Skin lesions including atrophy, pigmentation, keloid scars and persistent lymphoedema of the hands may follow needle use. Venereal disease is endemic in the street addict population.

Neurophysical complications
These are most frequent in alcohol dependency as previously described. Delirium tremens may occur in hypnotic or sedative withdrawal.

Social complications
Although a major aim of British prescribing policy was the elimination of an inducement to crime by free legal prescribing of narcotics, drug use and delinquency have become indisputably associated. Many street addicts enter addiction from backgrounds of proven delinquency and persist in criminal behaviour. Others adopt delinquent patterns in identification with an illicit life style. Most of the offences of street addicts involve drug offences and larceny, but the rate of serious and violent crime is high, despite the sedative effect of the administered drugs. Offence behaviour probably relates to the personality of the user and the disinhibited, anti-social attitude of their group environment and not to any direct action of narcotic or hypnotic drugs.

Pregnancy and addiction
Although narcotic use is commonly associated with amenorrhoea, loss of libido and infertility in women, pregnancy does occur in some users and presents particular problems. The question of termination or fostering should be considered in view of the risk of neglect and battering in drug-intoxicated mothers. Antenatal care is often difficult with erratic attendance. Drug withdrawal should be attempted if co-operation can be gained. Heroin, barbiturates and alcohol all pass through the placenta and babies are often low in weight. Infants may be born with narcotic or barbiturate dependence and develop classical withdrawal symptoms. In narcotic dependence, symptoms in neonates develop after twenty-four to ninety-six hours with tremors, hyperactivity, hypertonicity, tachypnoea, scratching, convulsions, fever, vomiting and diarrhoea. Camphorated tincture of opium (0.2 ml to 0.5 ml, three to four hourly) will control symptoms though phenobarbitone is preferable if seizures occur. Barbiturate withdrawal symptoms commence four to seven days after birth and resemble opiate withdrawal although seizures are rare. Phenobarbitone (10 mg/kg every twenty-four hours) is the treatment of choice, decreasing gradually over several days. Symptoms may be prolonged for several months and early discharge should be discouraged because of the delayed onset of withdrawal symptoms.

The management of drug dependency
The general principles and the major methods of management of drug dependency are described below.

General principles
The main therapeutic challenge in the management of drug dependency does not rest in the containment of physiological dependence alone. Although the major hazard of drugs of dependency might superficially appear to lie in their capacity to create physical dependency, it must be remembered that many addictive drugs (amphetamine, cocaine, L.S.D. and cannabis, for example) produce only psychological dependence. It is the achievement of release from psychological dependency which presents both patients and therapists with their greatest hurdle and accounts for the familiar pattern of recurrent relapses, despite the attainment of physiological abstinence. To withdraw addicts from their drugs is an integral but simple feat compared with the daunting problem of maintaining abstinence. The management of dependency disorders demands a long-term perspective, extending beyond the acute phase of detoxification through the chronic phase of preserving abstinence, to the goal of cured dependency and social rehabilitation. Such comprehensive treatment aims necessitate a combined approach incorporating medical, psychological and social therapeutic skills and often demand a multidisciplinary team of doctors, nurses, social workers, probation officers, employers, voluntary agency workers and the family members themselves.

Although a comprehensive treatment model might suggest a unified, contemporaneous approach, the nature of dependency usually requires a shifting therapeutic emphasis as treatment proceeds. The primary stage involves the patient's acceptance of his dependency as a problem and of abstinence as a therapeutic aim. In the next phase, the symptoms of dependency are tackled and detoxification achieved. The final stages involve exploration of the psychological and social factors behind the dependency, with development of behavioural patterns which foster psychological stability and social rehabilitation. While it might appear theoretically rational to cure dependency by resolving the underlying psychopathology directly, the presence of dependency generally prevents any capacity for response to psychotherapeutic approaches until a maintained abstinence has been achieved.

The goal of treatment remains total abstinence. Although some therapists adhere to the concept of controlled addiction as an aim (and the present British drug policy incorporates this principle), stabilised addiction remains an uncertain entity and a tenuous state. Instances of alcoholics who achieve moderate social drinking patterns have been cited but there are no known indicators which predict this outcome in individual alcoholics. Experience with "stabilised" drug addicts suggests that few can avoid escalation of dosage as tolerance develops and achievement of stable social functioning is rare even on controlled dosage. In practice, the aim of total abstinence is often forlorn, especially with drug addicts where personality disturbance is often severe, but maintained abstinence provides the only surety of cure. This aim may well be modified in some patients, particularly where dosage stability is evident and functional attainment dependent on continued administration. In elderly chronic amphetamine addicts who contain their dosage and manifest useful social functioning, it would seem inhumane to insist on attempted abstinence.

Most alcoholics continue to be treated in the medical or psychiatric units of general hospitals and drug addicts are familiar to casualty departments and medical wards throughout the country. Special facilities for dependency disorders include the regional alcoholic units and the drug dependency clinics but problems of availability, restricted capacity, or rejection by patients, may limit access. An inaugural period of in-patient treatment is usually desirable to establish abstinence and provide a drug-free environment where habit patterns may be interrupted under therapeutic surveillance. Subsequent treatment requires continuing out-patient support on a long-term basis, if relapse is to be averted. Addicts commonly reject admission to hospital, even when their dependency is acknowledged. Although the Mental Health Act 1959 allows compulsory admission on the basis of mental disturbance which threatens health, in practice compulsory admission is rarely used except where acute complications such as delirium, endocarditis or hepatitis threaten life. There appear to be considerable reservations about invoking compulsory detention for a dependency disorder which arises from the patient's active volition but it is doubtful whether addicts are really capable of exercising "free will" once dependency is established. The reluctance of the medical profession to assume a conceivably punitive role, however humanitarian in aim, has been circumvented in the management of drug addiction by the increasing use of section 4 of the Criminal Justice Act 1948. This allows the courts to impose a compulsory condition of treatment on convicted addicts for up to one year without involving the treating doctor directly in the compulsory admission procedure.

The range of therapies used in dependency include the following.

1. Drug therapy
While psychotropic drugs may relieve psychological symptoms which predispose to the use of addictive drugs, the drug dependent patient is liable to shift dependency to any pharmacological therapy

which offers relief. Drug therapy should be cautiously employed, used only briefly or intermittently for specific problems or symptoms.

2. *Psychological therapy*
A range of psychological approaches have been introduced in the management of dependency including behaviour therapy, supportive psychotherapy, group therapy, encounter therapy and psycho-analysis. All have their advocates although success lies more in the skill and attitude of the therapist than in the specific theoretical approach.

3. *Pharmacological antagonists*
Drugs which interfere with the action of addictive drugs (disulfiram, cyclazocine) or substitution with a less potently addictive drug have been used to counteract or diminish physiological dependency.

4. *Self-help organisations*
Voluntary organisations, particularly those who use cured addicts to provide identificatory models, support and examples for dependent users, have achieved considerable success. Alcoholics Anonymous, Synanon and Phoenix employ group processes with differing tech-niques to effect attitudinal and behavioural changes. Their consider-able success is undisputed although their methods and their client selection have received critical comment.

5. *Therapeutic community*
The use of a residential facility as a therapeutic community, with its stress on conjoined administration, participation and responsibility as the basis of a social group therapy, is the central therapeutic tech-nique for behavioural modification in special alcoholic units and many hostels.

6. *Community rehabilitation*
The *integration* of residential facilities, social support, occupational advice and re-training, probation after-care and the network of volun-tary and official organisations is the essential feature of rehabilitation and resettlement in the community. Although many middle-aged alcoholics have sufficient residual social attributes to utilise rehabili-tation effectively, many young drug addicts are prevented by their dependency from ever gaining formative occupational, educational and social skills which facilitate rehabilitation.

Dependency disorders are chronic, relapsing conditions. Thera-peutic failure is a common outcome in their management. Therapists require a readiness to provide long-term support, a capacity to tolerate therapeutic disappointment, an ability to exhort and admonish without moral censure, an empathy with human suffering and human failure and the flexibility to accept modification of the ideal treatment objectives, if they are to attain a sense of achievement in this exacting field.

The establishment of therapeutic contact
In most medical illness, the awareness of symptoms leads patients to seek medical advice and co-operate with treatment which could aid recovery. This familiar pattern is usually absent in dependency disorders where patient motivation is directed towards maintaining illness behaviour rather than towards cure. The rejection of therapeutic contact presents the major obstacle to treatment and alienates many health care professionals from involvement in drug dependency. The facility to tolerate and mould therapeutic rejection into a more constructive and conventional therapeutic interaction requires skill in the following areas.

1. *Identification*
Recognition of dependency disorders is the first stage in management. Dependency is under-recognised in general practice, because its developing signs and symptoms are often indirect. Psychosocial problems such as marital difficulties, aggressive behaviour, occupational instability, recurrent accidents, criminality and financial problems should alert the doctor to enquire about alcohol use. Repeated requests for drug prescriptions, particularly associated with vehement rejection of alternative drug therapy, is highly indicative of dependency. Medical morbidity in hospital practice, particularly gastrointestinal symptoms, nutritional disorders, local or systemic infections, should evoke suspicion of possible underlying dependency. Early alcoholic dementia is particularly under-diagnosed in the hospital ward, with its limited demands on social skills. Non-medical settings with which drug dependent people may make contact include specific agencies like Alcoholics Anonymous, but the courts, the police, the clergy, the social services and the Samaritans may be the recipients of the earliest signs of distress.

2. *Declaration*
Although many addicts deny their dependency, it is essential that any potential helper makes a clear, non-evasive statement of their diagnostic opinion about the cause of the disorder. Their opinion may be met with dismissal but no therapeutic progress can occur without an open acknowledgment of the disease. This opinion should be expressed unemotionally without threats, gloomy prognostications, moral censure or assurances of cure which arc unlikely to have

any lasting impact. Discussion of treatment alternatives should follow, indicating the most ideal treatment regime but leaving the patient to choose the point of entry into treatment, even when this falls short of the most promising commitment. Many patients who reject both diagnosis and treatment will reveal their ambivalence by accepting a further appointment and many interviews may be required before a positive commitment is attained. At each interview the helper should explore recent events, citing behaviour which indicates dependency and should reiterate both the diagnostic opinion and the help available. Dependent patients usually enter treatment gradually, tentatively and inconsistently and professional helpers require a non-rejecting patience to secure therapeutic contact.

3. Establishing a treatment contract
When patients accept some need for treatment, it is important to reach a mutual agreement on the terms of this contract. The purpose of the contract is to establish definite guidelines to measure achievement and clear conditions for the maintenance of therapeutic interaction. Simple early conditions may include mutual, punctual attendance and sobriety at interview with cancellation of appointments for lateness or intoxication. As treatment proceeds, the demands of the contract can be extended. Failure in the contract should not be met with total rejection but with an empathic restatement of the conditions of therapeutic interaction. Some possible avenues for future therapeutic contact must always be available when contract failure necessitates apparent rejection. The essence of the contract is the establishment of an empathic but firm and consistent interaction, in which mutual respect and responsibility can develop. An apparent barrier to this development is the need for a healthy distrust by the therapist. Most therapeutic relationships rely heavily on the establishment of trust but this only emerges slowly in the dependent patient. Over-expectations of honesty in dependent patients can result in the therapist's betrayal, with consequent dissolution of the therapy in angry rejection. Dependent patients are often experienced and skilled in manipulation. Therapists must be able to preserve empathy alongside reservations about their patients' veracity. Revealed deceits should be discussed with disappointment but rarely anger.

The therapist should recognise his role as a behavioural model for the patient and present an image which allows identification while maintaining personal integrity. The tendency in some therapists to provide easy identificatory models — by the use of addicts' argot or bohemian dress — limits the potential of therapeutic interaction. Few addicts believe that professional qualifications are achieved or maintained on regular use of heroin and have no lasting respect for such spurious self-imagery. A doctor's best aids are his own sense of personal identity, his professionalism and a genuine concern with the *distress* of dependency.

SPECIFIC MANAGEMENT

The following pages outline the specific management of problems of drug dependence, considering alcohol first separately as a special case.

Alcohol
Short- and long-term management of alcoholic dependency are considered below.

1. *The abstinence syndrome*
Symptoms of acute withdrawal may appear during planned detoxification or as a spontaneous complication of dependency. The abstinence syndrome, particularly delirium tremens, deserves hospital care. Fluid intake should be maintained to prevent dehydration, and vitamins (particularly the B-group complex) can be administered parenterally where nutritional deficits or complications are suspected. Tranquillisers will help to contain restlessness, anxiety or the acute organic brain syndrome of delirium tremens. Chlorpromazine, chlordiazepoxide and chlormethiazole have all been used effectively. Chlormethiazole (Heminevrin) is probably the drug of choice, administered in a reducing dosage schedule over seven to ten days with a commencing dosage of 1.5 gm t.d.s. With adequate hydration and sedation, gradual discontinuation of alcohol is unnecessary and abrupt withdrawal of alcohol itself is preferable.

2. *Long-term therapy*
Following acute withdrawal, a period of hospitalisation is useful to provide the alcoholic with a controlled alcohol-free environment and to allow exploration of the complex psycho-social factors which foster dependency. Although the majority of alcoholics receive such treatment in general psychiatric units, there are now about twenty regional alcoholic units in Britain which specialise in the management of the detoxified patient. In general, these units operate on the therapeutic community model involving the patient in some of the responsibilities of daily management. The use of non-directive group therapy allows problem-sharing, recognition of behavioural patterns and attitudinal change in a supportive milieu through identification and example. The average stay is six to twelve weeks and the more

advanced psychotherapeutic techniques of long-term group psycho-therapy are unlikely to be appropriate. In practice, the alcoholic units mainly attracted the better-educated alcoholics, from a higher social class with greater social stability. Supportive individual or group psychotherapy may be provided on an out-patient basis to develop insight into personal difficulties, assist with social problems and encourage the impetus of achieved abstinence. Introduction to rehabilitation agencies, particularly Alcoholics Anonymous (A.A.), may provide valuable support. Many alcoholics have relied wholly and successfully on A.A. for assistance but others find difficulty in identifying with its clients and its techniques. Treatment in a group setting is not the inviolable preserve of trained therapists and many general practitioners have found group meetings for alcoholics in their practice time-saving, educational and useful.

Two physical treatments have been used in long-term care. Aversion treatment, using electric shocks or emetic-induced vomiting to produce a conditioned aversive response to alcohol, is unpleasant, often messy and of doubtful long-term benefit. Drugs which sensitise the body to alcohol by interfering with its metabolism, such as disulfiram (Antabuse) or citrated calcium carbamide (Abstem) have been used to deter alcoholics from drinking. Despite their physiological action, any benefit probably results from their effect on psychological dependency. Their usefulness is limited by the unreliability of self-administration, occasional serious side-effects and indifferent long-term results. Care must always be exercised in the prescription of tranquilliser or hypnotic drugs to treat emerging anxiety or insomnia because of the risk of cross dependency.

3. Rehabilitation

The resolution of problems of accommodation, employment and familial adjustment are integral to successful rehabilitation. Families and employers often protect alcoholics in the early stages of their illness, until tolerance is exhausted and rejection becomes irrevocable. Recovering alcoholics are often devoid of social supports. After-care hostels, which provide a range of facilities from basic shelter to group therapy, are available in many areas sponsored by local authorities, voluntary groups, and religious organisations including the Salvation Army. Occupational retraining and resettlement may be required when former employment has been lost or occupational status has been eroded. Alcoholics Anonymous has two affiliated associations to assist the wives of alcoholics (Alanon) and the children of alcoholics (Aliteen) and involvement may help promote re-establishment of family unity. An alteration of the patient's environment, with separation from former friendships and cues which might trigger relapse, may be essential in recovery. Successful outcome is often more dependent on the recovering alcoholic's social and personal situation than on specific treatment methods. A variety of community services including social, probation and employment services make important contributions in rehabilitation.

4. The management of specific physical complications

Nutritional complications, such as Wernicke's encephalopathy, Korsakoff's psychosis and peripheral neuropathy, usually require hospitalisation and treatment with thiamine. Parenteral administration of thiamine (100 mg I.V. for seven days, followed by oral administration) may reverse the confusional states in the Wernicke-Korsakoff syndrome, although memory deficit is rarely improved. Alcoholic dementia may require institutional care to prevent further drinking and to provide nursing supervision.

Alcoholic hallucinosis usually responds to abstinence with administration of phenothiazines. Maintenance of phenothiazine therapy is necessary for the rare chronic hallucinatory states. Morbid jealousy has a poor prognosis, rarely responding to anti-psychotic medication and often only resolving with separation of the partners.

Drug dependencies

The specific management of drug dependencies is considered below, giving legal, short-term and long-term advice.

1. Notification

Doctors are required to notify a central agency, the Drugs Branch of the Home Office, about patients who are dependent on drugs scheduled in the Dangerous Drugs Act 1965. Notification is required for abuse of narcotic drugs and cocaine but not barbiturate or amphetamine abuse.

2. Restricted prescribing

Only practitioners who hold a special licence from the Home Secretary may prescribe heroin or cocaine for dependent patients. Such licensed practitioners are usually employed in drug dependency clinics.

3. The abstinence syndrome

The abstinence syndrome of the various drug groups are treated separately below.

(a) Narcotics. Withdrawal symptoms may appear spontaneously during narcotic abuse after partial or complete abstinence or occur in a detoxification treatment programme. Their spontaneous development is a common cause of self-referral to casualty departments.

Withdrawal symptoms can be alleviated by administration of narcotics. In Britain, methadone is the drug of choice and is offered to addicts on a graduated decreasing dosage schedule during detoxification over seven to ten days. Although abrupt withdrawal seems inhumane, experienced addicts may request admission for detoxification but abandon substitution therapy early, achieving more rapid physiological detoxification despite minor symptoms. Their aim is usually not cure but a lowering of tolerance with recovery of the euphoric effects of narcotics and they discharge themselves once this has been effected.

(b) Sedative/hypnotic drugs. Withdrawal requires hospitalisation and should never be abrupt because of the risk of epileptic seizures. Dependent patients should be titrated with their drug to establish the dosage level of mild intoxication. Graduated dosage reduction over two to three weeks is required to eliminate physiological dependency with safety.

(c) Stimulants. Amphetamines and cocaine may be withdrawn immediately without substitution therapy but irritability, depression and apathy can last for weeks or months. Tricyclic anti-depressant drugs can be used to relieve depressive symptoms, particularly in those predisposed to depression. Hospitalisation is often necessary for the management of the psychological dependency which presents the main risk of relapse.

(d) Hallucinogens. Acute intoxication should be managed with re-assurance, constant company and chlorpromazine (Largactil) by intramuscular injection (50 mg to 100 mg t.d.s.). Hospitalisation is rarely necessary as most "trips" resolve within twelve hours. "Flashbacks" usually disappear quickly but explanation and reassurance should be provided. The rare chronic psychoses associated with hallucinogen use may respond to phenothiazines and usually require long-term drug treatment.

5. Long-term therapy

The discussion of long-term treatment by therapy of drug dependency concentrates in the main on the treatment of narcotic dependency; for a fuller discussion of psychotherapy see other chapters.

(a) Narcotics. Few narcotic addicts accept detoxification readily. The drug dependency policy in Britain has created special treatment centres, mainly in London, where maintenance therapy and long-term support are provided with the aim of encouraging eventual abstinence. It is important to determine that a patient is actually dependent before commencing drug therapy and positive urinary chromatography should precede prescription. Methadone has been the major

drug used in maintenance therapy because it is considered less addictive than heroin. Methadone is usually prescribed as a linctus to help wean addicts from their psychological dependence on a "needle habit". Withdrawal from methadone is believed to be easier than from heroin and in-patient admission is useful when motivation towards cure increases or complications develop. Coercive measures, such as use of a probation order with condition of treatment, have proved useful in containing dependent patients in a treatment programme.

Narcotic antagonists such as cyclazocine or naloxone (Narcan) which block the effects of narcotic administration have been used to extinguish conditioned dependency. They are expensive, require high motivation and have not been widely used in Britain.

Rehabilitation is generally more difficult in narcotic users than in alcoholics. The early onset of the disorder (in youth) often results in the addict's inability to develop social skills and recovery may prove overwhelmingly challenging. A few residential units are available for detoxified addicts. They are mainly supported financially by local authorities but often run with the help of recovered addicts. They are largely designed on the Synanon and Phoenix House models which originated in the U.S.A. Group therapy, often with an aggressive encounter group approach is used, occupational retraining is encouraged and long-term residence up to one or two years is favoured. Development of a new peer group culture is important in the maintenance of abstinence.

(b) Sedatives/hypnotics/stimulants/hallucinogens. Supportive psychotherapy with attention to personal and marital problems, social difficulties and occupational skills is necessary to maintain protracted abstinence. No specific drug therapy is available and substitution therapy with other drugs should be avoided.

PROGNOSIS

Since drug dependency is a chronic relapsing disorder and the end state commonly leads to conspicuous social degradation, prognosis is often assumed to be uniformly poor. Recent British studies have indicated, however, that 60 per cent of alcoholics achieve some degree of recovery and 40 per cent of clinic narcotic addicts are drug-free five years after their first attendance. Alcoholism has a better prognosis than drug addiction, largely because sociogenic factors are more influential in its development. A stable personality and stable social adaptation may precede the development of accepted social codes. Prognosis tends to deteriorate as the social pattern of dependency deviates increasingly from cultural convention.

Prognosis in the addictive disorders is less dependent on particular treatment methods than on factors relating to the individual patient, his environment and his drug addiction. With alcoholism, young alcoholics do less well than older drinkers, women alcoholics have a poorer prognosis than men and anti-social or deviant personalities show less recovery than stable personalities. Dependency of recent onset carries a more favourable prognosis than established addiction. Although it has been suggested that dependent persons might grow out of their addiction with age and experience, there is little evidence of such effective maturation. Physical and psychological exhaustion, ensuing after chronic use, contributes more to cessation than maturity alone. Certain features such as superior intelligence, high motivation towards abstinence, the ability to evolve an alternative life style and support in marital, social and occupational areas favour good prognosis. Addicts from professional occupations, such as the medical profession, tend to do better partly because of the factors of prior selection and partly because of the threat to professional standing. Most drug dependent patients wander in and out of treatment programmes but the ability to sustain abstinence over six months in a residential setting is a good prognostic indicator. Even where prolonged abstinence involves compulsion, as in a penal setting, the prognosis remains favourable if after-care is provided and maintained. Intravenous drug administration carries a poor prognosis because of the associated morbidity and the mortality rate in narcotic and barbiturate addicts is alarmingly high.

Although the achievement of abstinence is generally easier with drugs which create a milder pharmacological dependency, the best indicators of prognostic outcome lie in the personality of the individual and his social stability. Where drug abuse develops to provide resourceful strength or energy, resolve problems or augment social skills, the outlook is unfavourable. Where basic adjustment and personal achievement are adequate, abstinence is often less challenging since the behavioural adjustments that become necessary on recovery are likely to be less extensive. Although particular treatment methods and treatment settings may not contribute specifically to prognosis, they provide at least a therapeutic environment in which the dependent patient's positive attributes may be acknowledged, fostered and strengthened. During the phase of dependency, individual capacities and motivation may be concealed, emerging only after withdrawal. The therapist should avoid an over-hasty pessimistic prognostication based on assessment of the intoxicated patient. A realistic optimism and tenacity are the therapist's greatest contribution to a good prognostic outcome.

REFERENCES AND FURTHER READING

Berne, Erik (1964): *Games People Play,* Grove, New York.

Department of Health and Social Security (1972): *Medical Memorandum on Drug Dependence,* H.M.S.O., London.

Glatt, M. N. (1974): *A Guide to Addiction and its Treatment,* MTP, Lancaster.

Hore, Brian D. (1974): *Alcohol Dependence,* Butterworths, London.

Jellinek, E. M. (1965): *The Disease Concept of Alcoholism,* Hillhouse Press, New Brunswick.

Pradnan, S. N. (1977): *Drug Abuse: Clinical and Basic Aspects,* C. V. Mosby Co., St. Louis.

Disturbances of Behaviour: A Consideration of Their Causes and Management

Dr. Henry R. Rollin,
M.D., M.R.C.P., F.R.C.Psych., D.P.M.
Visiting Consultant Forensic Psychiatrist, H.M. Prison, Brixton, London.

Disturbances of Behaviour: A Consideration of Their Causes and Management

INTRODUCTION: AGGRESSION IN "NORMAL" HUMAN BEHAVIOUR

It is a sad and sobering thought that of all living creatures man has the greatest propensity to be in conflict with himself and others. The late Sir Aubrey Lewis, Professor of Psychiatry in the University of London, implied this when he remarked, "If a baby was as strong or as powerful and decisive as a grown-up man he would be the most dangerous creature on the face of the earth." St. Augustine, according to Dr. Frank Lake's interpretation of his teachings, makes more or less the same observation: "The so-called innocence of infants is well seen to reside purely in the weakness of their bodies and in no defect of murderous intention in their wills" (Lake, 1966).

The manifestations of aggression are infinitely varied. They are to be discovered in every human situation, in each and every department in which man lives his life. In mythology, in folklore and in the recorded histories of all nations, accounts of war — a legitimatised and highly organised form of violence — take pride of place. Warriors are more highly praised than scholars: there are more public monuments to generals than there are to professors.

In times of peace, or more precisely, undeclared war, violence of a most abominable sort abounds. In the near-delusional belief in their infallibility, fanatics, religious and political, have accounted for untold misery and an incalculable number of human lives. Examples of both come all to easily to mind: in the name of religion, the iniquities of the Iniquisition and, to some extent, the seemingly endless, bloody strife in Northern Ireland can be cited. In the name of politics, men of diabolical genius like Hitler and Stalin have corrupted whole nations, some proportion of which were actively employed in, or passively permitted, the gas chambers of the Nazi concentration camps or the comparable horrors of Stalin's regime.

At a more personal and individual level, violence is omnipresent. It ranges from the anger of words to the anger of silence; from teasing and baiting to senseless vandalism and mindless hooliganism; from child-battering to wife-battering; from nagging to murder. The fuses of human aggression are constantly being lit; the resultant explosion depends only on the size of the powder-keg.

In all these manifold manifestations of disturbed human behaviour, ironically enough considered "normal", the doctor has no specific role to play. However, there may be disturbances of behaviour in individuals resulting from disease of the body or the mind in the treatment of which the doctor and, indeed, his ancillaries, play a crucial role, and it is to the consideration of these disturbances that the rest of this chapter is devoted.

DISTURBED BEHAVIOUR IN DISEASES OF THE BODY AND MIND

The romantic image of the doctor, an image relentlessly cultivated by the mass media, is one of wisdom, benignity and "unflappability", the whole framed in an immaculately cut, spotless white coat. The white coat symbolises the doctor's armour, rendering him in some magical way immune from attack. This, needless to say, is a myth. Medicine is, in fact, a high-risk profession, as the following three recent cases dramatically illustrate.

Case one

A doctor was commended at the Central Criminal Court for her bravery in tackling a former Broadmoor inmate, described as a paranoid schizophrenic, who attacked her colleague with a bread-knife. T.C.C., aged 40, was sent back to Broadmoor after the jury had decided in a preliminary hearing under the Criminal Procedure Insanity Act of 1964 that he was suffering from a disability that made him unfit to be tried.

Dr. J. H. T., aged 27, had been working in a ward with Dr. E. H., aged 56, a consultant, when Mr. C. burst in. Mr. C. had the delusion or belief that all doctors were trying to get at him or kill him and he jumped forward stabbing Dr. H. in the stomach.

(Abstracted from a report in *The Times* 3rd February 1978)

Case two

W. E. W., aged 71, was convicted in January 1978 of manslaughter and committed to Broadmoor under a Hospital Order (Section 60 of the Mental Health Act, 1959) with a Restriction Order (Section 65 of the Mental Health Act, 1959) without limit of time.

The victim was Dr. W. L., who had been W. E. W.'s family's G.P. prior to his admission to a local mental hospital in 1947, where he had continued to reside ever since. The culprit had harboured a delusion that the doctor had had an affair with his wife thirty years previously.

Case three

Mrs. J. M. C., an unemployed secretary, aged 45, of no fixed abode, was charged with the attempted murder of Dr. D. McN., consultant psychiatrist, at his hospital. The accused, a paranoid schizophrenic, had been Dr. McN.'s patient some years before. In the time since he had seen her she had harboured paranoid delusions against him. Eventually she made the considerable journey to the hospital and had lain in wait for him outside his office. She stabbed him repeatedly causing severe injuries.

She was tried at the Old Bailey and found guilty of grievous bodily harm. She was committed to Broadmoor on Sections 60 and 65 of the Act without limit of time.

In all three cases, the assaults, fatal in one case, and resulting in serious abdominal injuries in the other two, were occasioned by the paranoid delusions of deeply psychotic persons. In Case One the delusions were focussed on doctors in general and the victim was chosen at random. In Cases Two and Three they were directed towards individual doctors, and it is important to note that in both instances the delusions had been harboured for many years, illustrating yet again the fixity and dangerousness of such delusions. Indeed, it would seem that the thirst for revenge grew stronger with the years, until the culprits felt not only impelled but, in their own diseased minds, fully justified in doing what they did.

Why are doctors so particularly vulnerable? There are several possible answers.

(a) There can be no doubt that in the doctor-patient relationship, and particularly in the psychotherapeutic situation, an emotional bond great or small arises — something akin to the so-called transference/counter-transference phenomenon which is so much part of psychoanalytic theory and practice. In this complex emotional relationship elements of love and dependency are interlocked with elements of hatred and mistrust. Where the patients are psychotic as they were, for example, in all the three cases cited, inner and outer reality are confused. If delusions of persecution arise the hatred and mistrust so generated may be focused on the one person conveniently to hand -- their doctor.

(b) Doctors in the nature of their work have an intimate but innocent relationship with their patients. In a failing marriage, a rejected spouse may, in his search for a reason for the failure, come to suspect his wife's doctor. If he is the victim of a paranoid psychosis his suspicions may flower into a full scale delusion with the sort of result to be seen in Case Two.

(c) Doctors, alas, are neither infallible nor omnipotent — virtues not infrequently attributed to them. A failure in diagnosis can lead to a failure in treatment or a failure to cure or ameliorate a condition. Even though the condition may, in fact, be incurable or untreatable, failure may produce feelings of hostility in the patient or his relatives. Here again, in the setting of a paranoid psychosis, such hostility may express itself ultimately in a physical attack on the doctor or, by extension, on any doctor.

(d) By far the most common, even commonplace, explanation for the vulnerability of a doctor is that his work takes him into the front line, wherever the action is, be it the patient's home, the doctor's surgery, the casualty department of a general hospital, the acute ward of a psychiatric hospital, or a police cell. Today, doctors are being requested to advise the police on what action they should take in situations that are tantamount to a siege.

Disturbances of behaviour due to organic illness
The responsibility for human behaviour lies ultimately with the brain, an organ exquisitely sensitive to alterations in the complex checks and balances that keep it in a state of equilibrium. An imbalance may be created by a host of conditions of which the most relevant for our present purpose are as follows.

1. *Toxic confusional states or states of delirium*
These can be determined endogenously as, for example, by the toxins of hepatic or renal failure, particularly in the elderly. Or they may be engendered by exogenous toxins arising from any one of a variety of invading organisms. The delirium of pneumonia, far less commonly seen these days since the use of antibiotics became widespread, is a good example. It is noteworthy that the symptoms of pneumonia may be seriously complicated by hypoxia which in itself produces aggressive behaviour.

It is of far more than historical interest to quote Sir William Osler, an astute physician and an acute observer. Writing of lobar pneumonia, he devotes a whole section to the cerebral symptoms (Osler, 1911). Relevant passages are as follows.

One may group the cases with marked cerebral features into:

First — the so-called cerebral pneumonia of children in which the disease sets in with a convulsion, and there is high fever, headache, delirium, great irritability, muscular tremor, and perhaps retraction of the head and neck.

Secondly — the cases with maniacal symptoms. These may occur at the very onset, and I once performed an autopsy on a case in which there was no suspicion whatever that the disease was other than acute mania.

Thirdly — alcoholic cases with the features of delirium tremens.
Fourthly — cases with toxic features, resembling rather those of uraemia.

2. *Chemical intoxicants (see also* Chapter 5)

In our society the most common intoxicant by far is alcohol. There is, furthermore, irrefutable evidence that alcoholism is spreading, and what is even more disconcerting is that an even higher proportion of women and young people of both sexes are becoming victims. It is estimated that in Britain there are in excess of 300,000 alcoholics whose contribution to the totality of crime is enormous. There are as many as 75,000 convictions for public drunkenness every year, and of those otherwise convicted between 40 per cent and 60 per cent have an alcohol problem. What is more pertinent to our present theme is that alcohol disinhibits and releases aggression that can be directed outwards leading to assaults on others, or directed inwards resulting in suicidal attempts. Glatt found that at Warlingham Park Hospital nearly half the male alcoholics and more than one-third of the women conceded that when in drink they had behaved aggressively or had endangered themselves or others. Drunkenness, in one form or another, makes a major contribution to the shambles to which a casualty department may be reduced, particularly at weekends. Doctors, nurses and other ancillaries can be, and not infrequently are, at the receiving end of the flailing fists, the kicking feet and the bites of the fighting drunk.

There are other complications of severe chronic alcoholism, namely alcoholic fugue states, delirium tremens and alcoholic hallucinosis, all of which are very likely to result in disturbances of behaviour. Sufferers from these conditions may be guilty of indiscriminate assaults on those whose job it is to attend to them.

3. *Drug abuse*

Although alcohol easily leads the field as a drug of addiction there are others, more alien to our culture, which have made their appearance and are giving rise to ever-increasing concern. Each and every one of these drugs may be responsible for disturbed behaviour that can place in jeopardy the safety of those who abuse the drugs and those who are called upon to treat them.

The drugs to be considered are:

(a) Amphetamines. The ones most commonly used are benzedrine, dexedrine and methedrine. Because of the ease with which patients become addicted, doctors are prescribing alternative methods of treatment for conditions such as depression, narcolepsy and enuresis and those conditions where appetite suppressants are called for. Nevertheless, there appears to be an ample supply of amphetamine preparations readily available on the black market to which lurid names such as "French Blues" and "Black Bombers" are given.

Amphetamines are taken as euphoriants, an experience known in drug-vernacular as getting "a lift", or a "high". Because of the insomnia likely to ensue in amphetamine usage or abusage, it is by no means uncommon for sedatives to have to be taken to counteract the "high". It is easy to understand how a vicious circle of stimulants and counter-stimulants, for example, dexedrine and Seconal may be set-up.

Restlessness, irritability and confusion, so readily induced in amphetamine addicts, result in them becoming disturbed and aggressive. Where intoxication is severe, a psychotic state may develop which is clinically indistinguishable from schizophrenia. It is not particularly uncommon in psychiatric practice to come across cases of *bona fide* schizophrenia which appears to have been precipitated by amphetamine abuse. However, it is as well to bear in mind that schizophrenia and amphetamine addiction or, for that matter, any other form of addiction, are by no means incompatible. Furthermore, drug abuse is a not uncommon pursuit of the unstable including, of course, incipient psychotics.

(b) Barbiturates. The introduction of these drugs at the turn of the century was hailed as a major therapeutic advance. They very soon replaced bromides (unpleasant and toxic drugs that they are) as the most commonly prescribed sedatives. The benefit derived by their prescription to untold millions throughout the world in the treatment of anxiety and insomnia is indisputable, as indisputable as is their value as adjuncts in anaesthesia and in the control of major epilepsy.

As happens not infrequently in the history of therapeutic advances, the sting in the tail of progress becomes apparent only after the initial euphoria has worn off. In the case of the barbiturates the sting is seen in the facility with which vast numbers of patients have become addicted as the result of the legitimate, albeit unwise, medical prescription of the drugs. What is more, they have become drugs of abuse in unstable individuals who have recourse to the black market for their supplies. As an example, it is alleged that in the U.S.A., in the state of California, barbiturate addiction ranks second only to alcohol addiction and accounts for more deaths than any other drug with the exception of alcohol.

Although sedation is the therapeutic aim of barbiturates this is far from the objective of the drug-abuser. What he requires is a "lift" and this, paradoxically, is what he gets by the use of short-acting barbiturates. What in fact happens is that the drug-abuser becomes disinhibited and just because he *expects* to become euphoric, this is precisely what he experiences when drugs are taken, either orally or by injection, in the company of others of a similar disposition at a "party" or a rock concert. The state of disinhibition-euphoria is subjectively, and sometimes objectively, indistinguishable from alcoholic drunkenness. The situation is compounded when, as happens not infrequently, barbiturates are taken together with alcohol which facilitates their absorption. In these cases it is a matter of academic importance only how much of the resulting behaviour disorder is due to one intoxicant or the other. For those who have to do with them, the hazards are just the same.

Ironically, perhaps, the withdrawal of barbiturates may lead to serious consequences, the gravity of which will depend on the duration of the use of the drugs, the size of the customary dose and the susceptibility of the person concerned. The symptoms may include feelings of apprehension, tremors, insomnia, or, if sleep becomes possible, it is disturbed by horrific nightmares. Delirium accompanied by auditory and visual hallucinations, usually preceded by prolonged periods of insomnia, and indistinguishable from delirium tremens is described. In some cases *grand mal* fits are a distressing symptom.

(c) Lysergic acid (L.S.D.). L.S.D., a synthetic drug, is perhaps the most potent and sinister hallucinogen yet devised by man. It is irrelevant for our purposes to debate whether it is, or is not, a drug of addiction. Alarmingly, it requires no great expertise for the manufacture and is, therefore, relatively cheap. (In February 1978 at Bristol Crown Court the trial was concluded of thirty-one defendants accused of being involved in a worldwide L.S.D.-making network based in Britain. Drugs said to be worth millions of pounds were seized. (*The Times* 23rd February 1978.))

The drug is measured in micrograms and the effect produced is commensurate, by and large, with the size of the dose. Low doses, of, say 25 to 50 micrograms, produce a feeling of well-being and a heightened awareness of the environment which may last for several hours, although in some cases a degree of restlessness and irritation is experienced. Intermediate doses of 75 to 150 micrograms produce far more dramatic effects, particularly as the peak of the "trip" is reached. These include spatial distortions, intense and variegated imagery when the eyes are shut, and unpredictable and uncontrollable mood changes. Visual and auditory hallucinations can occur which may be unpredictably pleasant or singularly unpleasant.

High doses, i.e. 200 to 500 micrograms, produce phenomena similar to those described above. However, at the height of the "trip" there may be subjective delusions of omnipotence: to the victim there is no problem which is insoluble, no feat of physical prowess which is impossible. The belief in an ability to fly has been put to the test. In one instance, a "tripper" precipitated himself, Icarus-like, from a hotel window with disastrous results to himself and to an innocent and unsuspecting pedestrian on whom the would-be birdman landed.

There is an additional hazard of this most dangerous of drugs, the so-called "flashback". For reasons not understood, "trippers" can experience at some future time another "free trip", that is, when the drug has not been used, which may be as pleasurable or as terrifying as the one that preceded it . What is most sinister about L.S.D. is the number of instances in which those who "drop acid" begin on what is in effect a one-way journey. A "trip" is an artificially induced psychotic state akin to, if not indistinguishable from, an acute schizophrenic episode from which the victim may not recover.

The aetiological problem is precisely the same here as it is with psychotic states following the prolonged abuse of amphetamines. Are they simply brought about by the drug itself, i.e. induced psychoses, or are they psychoses precipitated by drug-abuse in those *predisposed* to mental illness?

From a behavioural standpoint, it is all too easy to see why anyone who is on a trip becomes so completely out of touch with reality and acts accordingly. One obvious manifestation could be impulsive violence, aimed indiscriminately at those, including doctors or their ancillaries, who might try to help the victim out of a bad trip.

(d) Cocaine. Cocaine, a drug of addiction, although known to the South American Indians since at least the sixteenth century, became a problem in Western Europe as recently as the last quarter of the nineteenth century. Ironically, it was first used to counter the withdrawal symptoms in morphine addiction.

Cocaine is expensive and its use is therefore restricted to the well-to-do, or to a somewhat *chic* coterie of so-called bohemians. It can be injected subcutaneously ("popped"), or taken like snuff ("snorted"). To the newcomer to the drug a stage of excitation is quickly reached. This is relatively short-lived and is followed by depression and inertia. Another dose of the drug relieves this down-phase and the ease with which it can be done tends to explain how simple it is to become habituated, or addicted.

In large doses, cocaine can produce delirium as frightening, subjectively and objectively, as delirium tremens. Both visual and auditory hallucinations are present, but what is peculiar to cocaine psychosis is the presence of tactile hallucinations, the *"signe de Magnan"*. Again, in cocaine-induced psychosis as well as other drug-induced psychoses, the difficulty is to distinguish them from a true schizophrenic episode. The tragic picture of a sufferer from prolonged cocaine psychosis is well described by Mayer-Gross *et al.* (1969).

> He appears moody and restless, at times irritable and anxious. He sleeps little, eats insufficiently, and looks pale and haggard. He is also troubled with paranoid ideas, into whose morbid nature he has partial insight. Auditory hallucinations, illusions, especially at night, which take a delusional interpretation, are common. The affective

reaction to their experiences may be extreme. The patient may wait in panic terror for his persecutors to enter his premises, to kill him or hand him over to the police: and as he is active and determined, he may be very dangerous, and trivial causes may lead to catastrophes or violence or murder.

(e) Opiates. Unlike cocaine which has little therapeutic worth, the opiate derivatives have been and continue to be of inestimable value, particularly in the relief of severe chronic pain or persistent debilitating cough. However, the benefits of opiates are seriously limited because of their tendency to produce addiction. Furthermore, together with the psychological dependence there is a bodily dependence and as the tolerance to the drug increases, so does the effective dose. The pharmacological factors present real problems to those general practitioners whose patients are in genuine need of regular doses of opiate drugs.

However, what concerns us more is the illicit use of opiates, namely morphine and heroin. Both may be smoked: that is, the vapours when heated may be inhaled; or they may be taken orally, or "popped"; or for maximum effect, injected intraveneously ("mainlined"). The last method is the most favoured among the drug sub-culture. The ritual of mainlining has in itself a sort of cachet which "sorts out the men from the boys". However, the ritual has its own built-in dangers, in that there is scant regard for the most elementary principles of asepsis or antisepsis (the lavatory pan is a not unusual source of water in which to wash needles and syringes) with dire results such as abscesses, venous thromboses, septic emboli, hepatitis, endocarditis and the like.

Such is the demand for opiates, and so enormous are the profits to be gained in their traffic, that, despite international agreements and strict surveillance, vast quantities circulate in virtually every country in the world. In the U.S.A., in particular, an unwholesome proportion of crime is concerned with the actual taking of the drugs, with the taking and peddling of the drugs, or with offences committed in order to buy the drugs.

The clinical picture presented by the addict to opiates is not uniform. However, there tends to be, in a high proportion of cases, a feeling of general malaise which is only relieved by further doses. What is far more uniform is the moral decay that ensues: that is, a growing disinclination to work, even to provide the wherewithal to buy further supplies. As a result, any subterfuge or criminal act is resorted to — lying, cheating, stealing or robbery with violence, for example. It is readily understood how the addict in desperate need of a "fix" becomes an easy prey for manipulation or coercion by criminals. Failing further supplies, the addict may suffer severe withdrawal symptoms. The state of blissful tranquillity to which he has become accustomed gives way to a state of restless irritability accompanied by a variety of physical symptoms including abdominal cramps, vomiting, sweating, general tremulousness, flu-like pains in the limbs, and insomnia. In his state of desperation, the addict sees in the doctor a source of relief from his distress. Thus the doctor becomes automatically at risk.

(f) Cannabis. Indian hemp, marijuana or hashish, perhaps the most widely abused drug of addiction after alcohol and nicotine, is included for the very simple reason that any preparation that is smoked, eaten, or drunk in tea, to produce an alteration in mood, i.e. as a euphoriant or to experience a "high", can automatically alter behaviour. The fact that there is no concrete evidence of permanent brain damage is irrelevant. What is known is that cannabis however taken can be used, like alcohol, to acquire "dutch courage" before the commission of an offence, including acts of violence.

There is one hazard to which the medical practitioner is becoming increasingly exposed as a result of the rise in the incidence of drug abuse. Doctors are authorised to prescribe controlled drugs such as amphetamines and barbiturates in the *bona-fide* course of treatment. If, however, doctors attend persons whom they consider, or have reasonable grounds to suspect, to be addicted to certain controlled drugs, they are required under the Misuse of Drugs Act 1971, to furnish in writing to the Chief Medical Officer at the Home Office, within seven days of the attendance, the particulars required by the regulations (H.M.S.O., 1973). There is, therefore, a stage-army of addicts who require controlled drugs, not for therapeutic purposes, but purely to satisfy their addiction needs, who are debarred from receiving authorised prescriptions for the controlled drugs they need. They will then employ every form of deceit in order to screw prescriptions out of gullible, or in some cases, dubiously-scrupulous, practitioners. Once it is known, that, for whatever reason, a particular doctor is an "easy touch" his or her life can become a nightmare: his surgery may be besieged by addicts prepared, if need be, to have recourse to blackmail or even physical violence to gain their own ends.

4. *Drug intolerance*

Doctor-induced disease has been well-known long before the fashionable term "iatrogenesis" was invented. To date, the most awful example is that of the thalidomide disaster, although there may be worse to come. However, it is because the aetiology of most mental illness is so little understood that empirical methods of treatment have been, and continue to be, the order of the day. There has been indeed no insult to the human body, no trauma, no indignity which has not been at some time meted out to the unfortunate victim of mental illness. Evacuation by emetics, purgatives, induced sneezing and sweating, blisters and bleeding have at one time or another in the past been considered essential treatment. In the more recent past, hapless schizophrenics have had to suffer surgical onslaughts in the search for and elimination of "focal sepsis" wherein, it was supposed, the roots of the psychosis lay hidden. Even more recently, psychiatrists still in practice may blush at the thought of the part they played in the treatment of schizophrenics with insulin-induced comas; or blush much more deeply when they recall the patients they recommended for pre-frontal leucotomy, an operation leaving the victims with their psychosis intact, but plus or minus whatever the blind, irreversible mutilation of their cortex did to them.

Today, there is a threat from another direction, that is, the abuse or misuse of psychotropic drugs. Let there be no mistake, however, these same drugs used as tranquillisers, as anti-depressants or in the control of manic states, or in the treatment of other functional psychoses, particularly schizophrenia, have revolutionised both general practice and psychiatric practice. But the object of this section is to emphasise their potency and the dramatic and sometimes frightening side-effects that psychotropic drugs may produce. The symptoms range from dryness of the mouth to a variety of extrapyramidal reactions, including oculogyric crises, agitated restlessness, dyskinesia, akathisia and, on occasion, irreversible tardive dyskinesia.

Alterations in behaviour as an expression of drug intolerance are well recognised and may resemble very closely alcoholic drunkenness. The two are all too often confused. Old people are particularly sensitive to psychotropic drugs, even the "minor" tranquillisers, such as meprobamate (Equanil) or diazepam (Valium). Their prescription for the old patient to counter restlessness and agitation may in fact aggravate rather than alleviate the symptoms and produce a condition indistinguishable from drunkenness. Such a situation arose in a case known to the author.

A lady, in her mid-80s, had been dementing over a period of years and to lessen her periodic agitation her G.P. had prescribed diazepam 2 mg t.d.s. Her husband, two years her senior, predeceased her. On the day of his funeral, which she was in no condition to attend, the G.P. with the best possible intentions, doubled the dose. When the mourners returned to the house the unfortunate widow was to all intents and purposes drunk, much to the distress of all who witnessed the tragedy.

A further example has the same moral.

A gentleman in his late 80s was given, post-operatively, promethazine hydrochloride (Phenergan) as a sedative. The result was disastrous. Instead of being sedated the patient experienced the most horrible nightmares in which, *inter alia*, he saw his wife and children put to the sword. So terrified was he of a repeat performance, that on subsequent nights he tried desperately hard to keep himself awake. It was not until the drug was stopped that, paradoxically, the exhausted old gentleman was able to sleep peacefully.

5. *Epilepsy*

The vast majority of epileptics, adequately treated, lead unremarkable and productive lives. It must be remembered, however, that epilepsy and a host of psychiatric conditions are not mutually exclusive. Thus, an epileptic, contrary to what was at one time believed, may at the same time be a schizophrenic. He may, again, be a manic-depressive, and if he is guilty of serious crime it is more than likely that this is due, not to his epilepsy, but to his functional psychosis, or to neither. It is not uncommon, however, for a period of irritability to precede a fit. More rarely, in adults the irritability can explode into anger and be accompanied by senseless aggression, particularly if they are in any way frustrated. There is a tiny minority of epileptics who from time to time experience disordered states of consciousness, automatism, twilight states and fugues. These, in turn, produce disturbances in motor behaviour which can find expression in physical violence.

6. *Brain damage*

In this context only sudden damage to the brain will be considered, although it is conceded that certain tumours, such as spongioblastoma multiforme, are rapidly growing and may first manifest themsleves in disturbances of behaviour. It is as well to remember, indeed, that cerebral tumour should always be considered in the differential diagnosis of behavioural disturbance of recent onset, particularly in the old. Sudden damage to the brain in the elderly is usually due to a cerebrovascular catastrophe. The permanent effects will, of course, depend, *inter alia,* on the extent of the damage and its location. Some degree of personality change is not uncommon, symptoms of which may be irritability, irascibility and a tendency to become verbally, if not physically, aggressive, the more so if the patient is thwarted. It is precisely this disturbance of behaviour which added to, for example, incontinence, may prove to be the last straw as far as their management is concerned. Relatives who have hitherto struggled on manfully feel that they can no longer tolerate the further disruption of their lives and demand, very understandably in most cases, that the old, demented relative be removed to hospital, or to Part III accommodation, the Local Authority "old folks' home".

In the younger age group, by far the most common cause of sudden brain damage is head injury — almost invariably sustained in road-traffic accidents. The symptoms may vary from, in mild cases, a momentary period of unconsciouness with virtually no sequel other than a short-lived headache, to unconsciousness lasting for hours or days. Disturbances in behaviour are to be seen mainly at the time when consciousness is being regained. This may range from mild restlessness and irritability to an acute state of delirium, in which violence is meted out indiscriminately to anyone who happens to be near.

Disturbances of the sort described are not infrequently compounded when the victim had been under the influence of drink or drugs at the time the accident occurred. The end result can be that an orderly casualty department is transformed into a battlefield in which members of the staff are themselves likely to become casualties.

Disturbances of behaviour due to mental disorder

In the fears and fantasies of the public, madness and aggressive behaviour are commonly linked. As we have seen already, aggression and its concomitant violence can erupt all too frequently in people considered to be "normal" as well as in people who are physically ill. Nevertheless, there are those suffering from mental disorder (using the term as defined in section 4 of the Mental Health Act 1959 (*see* p. 260)), who are undoubtedly violent and from whom the public needs maximum protection. It is as well to remember that the special hospitals (Broadmoor, Rampton, Moss Side and Park Lane) have been built in the past century to contain just such people. Furthermore, approximately one-third of those admitted to Broadmoor, which admits those considered to be within the range of normal intelligence, have been diagnosed as suffering from schizophrenia. Of them, a substantial proportion have been guilty of crimes of violence, including homicide.

There is no category of mental disorder that can claim exception from aggressive behaviour. We may now consider mental illness, one of the categories of mental disorder, first and divide it into its somewhat arbitrary component illnesses as follows.

1. *Schizophrenia*

It must be understood that this is a term applied to a group of similar, but by no means identical, mental illnesses. The difficulty has already been emphasised of differentiating between these conditions and those induced, or precipitated by, for instance, abuse of drugs such as amphetamines and L.S.D. But in practice, where the management of acute crises involves a danger to life or limb, the niceties of precise diagnosis can be overlooked.

Although there are many varieties of schizophrenia (as many varieties indeed as there are schizophrenics) it is convenient for academic purposes to divide them into three groups: hebephrenic, catatonic and paranoid. It is in the last two that violence is most likely to occur; hebephrenic schizophrenia is characterised mainly by thought disorder but there is usually accompanying inertia and apathy and explosive behaviour is unlikely.

(a) Catatonic schizophrenia. This sub-category of schizophrenia is characterised, on the one hand, by episodes of extreme apathy or inertia, intensifying at times into a state of stupor. On the other hand, there may be a short-lived period of disorganised excitement amounting to something akin to frenzy in which acts of sudden, impulsive, unprovoked violence may take place. A patient during one of these bouts of excitement may yell, smash crockery or windows or, far more seriously, make a suicidal or homicidal attempt. Once the explosion is over, the patient may retreat to his seat, resume whatever he was doing, or sink into his previous inert, apathetic state incapable — or so it seems — of explaining his outrageous behaviour. He may sometimes attempt to rationalise it, as happened in one of the author's cases.

Ian, as he is generally known, is a catatonic schizophrenic who had been continuously in mental hospitals for the past thirty-five years. For the most part he is a polite, gentle person in keeping with his middle-class, public-school and university background.

The author was present in the occupational therapy department where Ian, at his own snail-like pace, seemed content with his job of varnishing cane baskets made by other patients. Suddenly the air was rent by an ear-piercing shriek. Ian had hit a fellow patient, a girl with whom he had hitherto seemed on good terms, on the head with a wooden mallet. Fortunately he had done little harm, and the author grabbed the blunt instrument from the assailant's hand demanding to know why he had seen fit to strike his innocent friend. "Sir", he said in his polite, well-mannered way, "I have read the rules of the hospital with the utmost care and there is absolutely nothing against it".

Here is another example of the same sort of condition with, however, tragic consequences.

A 30-year-old Jamaican immigrant had been almost continuously in mental hospitals in the U.K. for the past ten years. He was considered to be "burnt out", a singularly unhappy description in this particular instance. From a state of withdrawn inertia he suddenly became restless and excited and set light to his bed. He was transferred to an "intensive care ward" from which he took his leave without permission (he was technically an informal patient) and made his way to his sister's home nearby. She allowed him to stay and the following day left the patient in charge of two children, one a mere baby. When she returned home the patient, for no apparent reason, had killed the baby.

The author examined the patient two days after the tragedy and found him once again in a state of near-stupor with seemingly no awareness of what he had done.

(b) Paranoid schizophrenia. In this sub-category of schizophrenia, usually occurring in an older age-group, the victim, almost invariably of a suspicious nature, builds up over the years a system of persecutory delusions. Hallucinations of hearing, which reinforce the delusions, are a frequent concomitant. As the force of the delusions intensifies, so is the capacity to resist the desire for revenge diminished.

We have seen at the beginning of this chapter (p. 242) how readily doctors become the focal point of such a delusional system and suffer the fatal or near-fatal consequences. There is small need to exaggerate the frequency of doctors (or nurses) as innocent victims in such attacks. Here is an example of an assault by a paranoid schizophrenic on an equally innocent victim, a workmate.

A thirty-five-year-old workman was admitted on a Hospital Order (section 60 of the Mental Health Act 1959) under the care of the author. The story was that, over a period of years, the patient became increasingly convinced that his workmates were spreading rumours in the factory and in the neighbourhood that he was a homosexual. Hallucinations of hearing reinforced the delusions. One day on the shop floor he suddenly attacked a workmate and friend with a knife. Fortunately, he was dragged away by witnesses before serious damage was done. He was arrested and charged. It is of interest that when in prison on remand he attacked a fellow prisoner in the exercise yard on to whom he had transferred his delusional beliefs.

Brief mention must be made of one variety of paranoid psychosis in which pathological jealousy, usually of the spouse, is the only presenting symptom — "The Othello Syndrome" is one appropriate title for the condition. The patient believes, in spite of lack of evidence, that his wife is unfaithful. He may brutalise her in an attempt to extract a confession of her infidelity, or she may suffer the same fate as did the hapless Desdemona at the hands of the crazed Othello.

2. *Affective disorders*
In this context, manic-depressive psychoses and other varieties of depressive illness are to be considered. In the classical bipolar form

of manic-depressive psychosis there is a phase of mania in which the mood is one of elation, or pathological happiness associated with psychomotor overactivity. This alternates with a phase in which the mood is one of depression, or pathological unhappiness, associated with psychomotor retardation. In both phases there may be disturbances of behaviour.

In mania the first symptoms to appear are sleeplessness and irritability, which in themselves tend to exhaust the patient. In addition, however, the patient may compound the effect by overactivity and indulgence in sexual or alcoholic excesses. All sense of proportion is lost and he may quite literally throw money away — more than one family has been pauperised by just this sort of totally irresponsible behaviour. However, what is more pertinent to our present theme, is the ease with which the manic patient can become aggressive and violent. No one dare thwart him or interfere with what he feels inclined to do, no matter how purposeless or irresponsible this may be. The reward for such an attempt by some well-meaning bystander is a clip on the jaw — or worse. An illustrative case follows.

N.C. was a diminutive Welshman, aged 60, charged with assaulting a policeman. It appears that the accused had accosted several women in the Strand, London, one of whom had complained to a policeman. The latter had seen fit only to caution him whereupon the accused, with considerable agility, leapt in the air and struck him in the face at the same time dislodging his helmet.

On examination when on remand in prison, he presented as a typical case of hypomania: he was fatuously cheerful, totally unconcerned about his plight, and threatening to demonstrate his pugilistic skill on any prison officer who chose to challenge him. It emerged that he was a long-standing manic-depressive. Because of his unrestrained behaviour in the manic phase his wife had felt compelled to divorce him. His children had deserted him.

He was admitted to hospital on a Hospital Order (section 60, Mental Health Act 1959) where he died twelve years later. His psychosis persisted to the end. When depressed, he was a pathetic little figure huddled silently in a corner of the ward: when in mania, he regained all his ebullience, pursued the ladies (the younger, the better) and picked fights with the men (the bigger, the better).

The great danger in depression is suicide. This is so in the depressed phase of a manic-depressive psychosis, or in other varieties of depression, particularly those associated with middle and later life. It is as well to remember that involutional depression can occur in both males and females. In the latter, however, it occurs more frequently, and is more clearly an accompaniment of the menopause. Furthermore, it is usually more dramatic in its onset and in its symptomatology.

The depressed patient may be driven to suicide by the profound feeling of hopelessness he experiences. There is, in other words, no conceivable purpose in continuing to live. Such despair may be reinforced by delusions of unworthiness and overwhelming guilt for sins, real or imagined. Hallucinations of hearing often hammer home the inescapability of the delusions. There is no greater psychiatric emergency than the threat of suicide in depression of this depth, and no method that the patient will not have recourse to (see the case given below) in order to fulfil his determination to end his life.

An even greater tragedy may ensue. The determined suicide may further consider that to leave his wife and children behind would be an act of callous indifference. He decides, therefore, that he must destroy them too. The grim irony of it is that he may succeed in killing her, or them, and then fail in his attempt to kill himself. The following case report is taken from an account in *The Daily Telegraph*, 13 December 1977.

A Fleet Street reporter who found the pressures of his job too great drowned his Japanese wife in the bath and then tried six times to kill himself, a court heard yesterday. J. K., 34, who pleaded guilty to manslaughter on the grounds of diminished responsibility, was ordered to enter F. Hospital for treatment. His plea of not guilty to murder was accepted at St. A. Crown Court.

Mr. D. H., Q.C., prosecuting, said that K., an industrial reporter, was due to become industrial editor, a job he did not feel able to hold down. While attending the TUC conference at Blackpool in September he told a colleague that everyone knew he had cracked. He said he had lost his career. Mr. H. said that on return home he discussed his problem with his wife. He and his wife had a bath together as they sometimes did, and he thinking it would be better to end it all, pushed her head under the water.

Later he told police: "Naturally she struggled, but I continued to hold her down by the throat!" Mr. H. said that K. then slashed his wrists with razor blades but did not inflict any serious injury; flung himself head first out of a window, but a plastic dustbin broke his fall; tried to hang himself with flex but could not get into the right position; drove to a bridge over the Stevenage by-pass but found it was too low to fling himself over; drove his car into the back of a parked car at 80 miles an hour but "miraculously" survived with relatively minor injuries.

3. *Dementia*
Of all the many causes of mental impairment, old age is far and away the most common. Symptomatic of dementia, whatever the cause,

is a varying degree of disinhibition, so that those afflicted tend to become cantankerous, restless, and verbally, if not physically, aggressive. The symptoms of dementia *per se* may be exaggerated by systemic illness such as congestive heart failure, hypoxia as the result of bronchitis, electrolyte upset, or dehydration and vitamin insufficiency.

The confusion, restlessness and antisocial behaviour tend to be worse at night, when the patient is weary and darkness adds to his disorientation. It is at these times that the danger of accidental fire-raising is greatest, as is the hazard of wandering out of the house lightly clad, or totally unclad.

4. Psychopathic disorder

This grave abnormality of personality is included for two reasons. Firstly, it is one of the categories of mental disorder defined in section 4 of the Mental Health Act 1959 (*see* p. 260) and secondly, in those afflicted the "unimagined strata of malignity in the human heart" are exhibited. Unfortunately, there is not a clinical definition that would meet with the approval of all psychiatrists. However, most would agree that those suffering from psychopathic disorder (psychopaths) have certain features in common, i.e. they are not insane in the generally accepted sense of the term, they are not necessarily unintelligent (some indeed are exceedingly bright) and yet they behave in a socially unacceptable way. They have no sense of morality and are therefore amoral, rather than immoral. Their lives are guided by one precept: "What is right for me, is right". They have, therefore, some of the the imperiousness and egocentricity of the child, and it is as children, albeit highly dangerous children, that they are best understood.

Although psychopaths are not of necessity drug addicts or alcoholics they may become either, or both, because of the emotional emptiness of their lives. Bouts of depression are by no means uncommon and suicide often puts an end to their destructive lives. Examples of the malignity, and in particular the casual callousness, of the psychopath are, unfortunately, not hard to come by. The following case is chosen to illustrate some of the features of psychopathy.

The man was aged 23 when he was tried at the Old Bailey on five charges of murder and a host of other charges involving violence. It was hinted that he was possibly guilty of a further five or six murders.

He showed distinct evidence of psychopathic disorder at a very tender age. As a mere infant he became known as a liar, thief and bully. Not much later his sadism was manifested in his cruelty to animals. He appeared before the juvenile court when aged 11 charged with arson and twenty-one other offences.

A career in various institutions, both penal and psychiatric, began early. He was sent in turn to an approved school, a local mental hospital, a remand centre and then to a "special hospital" from where, tragically, he was released, not once but twice, to the care of his misguided mother.

When at liberty he continued his monstrous life of drink, drugs and extreme violence. His main victims were old ladies whom he terrorised and robbed and, in at least two cases, he murdered them. His last victim, however, was a Catholic priest who had befriended him. He murdered him with unspeakable brutality.

5. *The neuroses*
By and large these minor varieties of mental illness make little contribution to the sum total of aggressive behaviour in patients. The one condition worthy of mention, however, is hysteria. The hysteric can behave in an outrageously theatrical (more accurately described as "histrionic") way and in his or her uncontrolled acting-out may become physically aggressive and cause harm to self or others.

THE MANAGEMENT OF DISORDERS OF BEHAVIOUR

As we have seen aggression and its concomitant violence, or the threat of either, can occur in an overtly psychiatric or non-psychiatric setting. There may be a real danger to the life or limb of the patient himself, or to his attendants. How to cope with such situations is outside the scope of the usual medical curriculum and it is hoped, therefore, that the following guidelines will to some degree make good the deficit.

Legal considerations
There was at one time no question that in bringing a situation, such as those sketched above, under control the good faith of members of the medical profession and their ancillaries was taken for granted. This is no longer so. The danger of litigation for assault or for wrongful compulsory detention in mental hospitals is today very real, due in large measure to the activities of certain organisations and to civil libertarians who sometimes seem to see patients' rights as more important than patients' care. However, as far as the law stands at present, a doctor in an emergency situation may use, or cause to be used, the minimum physical force necessary to render the patient harmless to himself or others. Furthermore, a doctor would be justified in administering treatment (such as a sedative injection) without

consent, to meet an emergency — or to prevent an emergency which otherwise would be likely to arise.

The guidelines given below apply to all patients, non-psychiatric and psychiatric. In the case of the latter they apply equally to those informally admitted to hospital, and to those admitted under compulsory orders. It is as well to remember that one of the progressive provisions of the Mental Health Act 1959 is to allow "mental patients" to be admitted to any hospital and not, as previously, to a registered mental hospital only. With the spread of psychiatric units attached to general hospitals it is becoming increasingly frequent to admit patients to such units, rather than to conventional mental hospitals.

The admission to hospital of patients suffering from mental disorder

The Mental Health Act 1959 of England and Wales is the most advanced instrument of legislation yet devised in this country, or in any other for that matter, for the protection of the mentally disordered and their property. Stripped of the inescapable jargon in which all legislation is drafted, the provisions of the Act are straightforward. Nevertheless, some doctors seem to regard the Act and its workings as the concern of the expert only: there are, too, bureaucrats in hospitals who would seem to derive a positive delight in discovering errors in the way in which one or the other of the essential forms have been filled up. So it is in order to enlighten the former and frustrate the latter that it is considered necessary to define terms used in the legal documentation.

The concept of mental disorder

The Mental Health Act 1959, provides for the admission to hospital (*see below*) or placement under Guardianship of persons suffering from "mental disorder" of which there are four categories (section 4 (1)).

(a) *Severe subnormality.* This means a state of arrested or incomplete development of mind, including subnormality of intelligence, which is of such a nature or degree that the patient is incapable of living an independent life, or of guarding himself against serious exploitation, or will be incapable when of an age to do so (section 4 (2)).

(b) *Subnormality.* This means a state of arrested or incomplete development of mind, not amounting to severe subnormality, which includes subnormality of intelligence, and is of a nature or degree requiring medical treatment or special care or training of the patient. (Section 4 (3).)

(c) Psychopathic disorder. A persistent disorder or disability of mind which results in abnormally aggressive or seriously irresponsible conduct on the part of the patient, and requires or is susceptible to, medical treatment. (Section 4 (4).)

(d) Mental illness. This is not further defined in the Act but is taken to mean any other form of psychiatric illness including functional psychoses, e.g. schizophrenia or manic-depressive psychosis, or organic psychoses, e.g. dementia of varying sorts.

Informal admission
A major objective of the Act is to encourage as many patients as possible to be treated as in-patients or out-patients on an informal, i.e. voluntary, basis. In this respect the Act has been inordinately successful: about 90 per cent of all admissions are on an informal basis and virtually all out-patients are informal.

Informal admission to any hospital is available to any person of any age (infants in law under the age of 16 years require the permission of their parents or guardians) who is suffering from any category of mental disorder (as above) and does not require compulsory detention in the interests of his own health or safety or the safety of others. He must be willing to accept such admission, or be unable to express a wish one way or the other. This would arise, for example, in the case of an old dement who is unaware of what he is, or where he is, or what he would like to be done for him.

A "hospital" is defined under section 147 of the Act as:

(a) any hospital vested in the Minister under the National Health Service Act 1946;

(b) any accommodation provided by a local authority and used for hospital and specialist services under Part II of the Act;

(c) any special hospital, i.e. Broadmoor, Rampton, Moss Side, or Park Lane, which are maximum security hospitals. In the nature of things these hospitals do not accept informal patients.

All that is required to secure an informal admission is to find a hospital prepared to accept the patient. The first approach is to the catchment area hospital, and it is always an advantage to have called out the appropriate consultant psychiatrist on a domiciliary consultation. He would be in a position to assess the case, to decide on the advisability of informal admission and to arrange for a bed.

Compulsory admission of patients suffering from mental disorder
It follows from what has been said that every effort should be made to avoid compulsory admission to hospital. If, however, it is considered "that informal admission is not appropriate in the circum-

stances of this case" — the official expression used in the documents for admission under sections 25 and 29 — arrangements for formal (compulsory) admission should be made without delay.

In the admission and detention of patients into psychiatric hospitals under compulsory orders under Part IV of the Act, sections 25, 26 and 29 are the ones most likely to be employed in general practice. It is as well to regard the 1959 Act as Holy Writ and it is for this reason that, as a guide to the perplexed, the sections are reproduced as Appendix II to this book.

It will be seen that the three prerequisites of a valid application for admission under compulsory orders are as follows.

(a) The first requirement is a valid application by the *nearest relative* (there is a hierarchy of precedence in descending order beginning with husband or wife down to nephew or niece), or a social worker, known as a "warrant-holder" (who has been appointed a mental welfare officer). Nowadays, the social worker is generically trained, i.e. a Jack or Jill of all trades. His training in psychiatric social work may be sketchy in the extreme as opposed to the old mental welfare officer who was an expert in this field and a tower of strength to both G.P. and consultant psychiatrist alike. Furthermore, the social worker of today may object for reasons, some clear, some decidedly unclear, to making the application. But this happens infrequently in practice. Representation to the Community Physician can be made if it is felt that a refusal to make an application is unreasonable.

(b) The second prerequisite is one medical recommendation, if practicable by a practitioner with previous knowledge of the patient in the case of section 29. In the case of sections 25 and 26, two medical recommendations are necessary, one by a practitioner approved under section 28 as having special experience in the diagnosis and treatment of mental disorder (in urban areas he is usually a consultant psychiatrist on the staff of the hospital to which the patient is to be admitted) and the other by a practitioner with previous acquaintance of the patient unless the approved doctor has such an acquaintance.

(c) A hospital willing to admit the patient is the third prerequisite. It must be emphasised that, strange as it may seem, the procedures we have discussed so far are *applications* for admission. There is no obligation on the part of the relevant area health authority to admit the patient. It is usually the consultant psychiatrist under whom the patient will be admitted who has to agree formally to accept the application. However, nurses are now demanding a greater say in who they shall nurse and they may refuse patients known to be difficult as, for example, uncooperative psychopaths.

There can be no doubt that the admission of patients can usually be facilitated if the consultant concerned is brought into the case as early as possible either as the result of an out-patient appointment or a domiciliary consultation. It is never a bad thing for a G.P. to establish a close working relationship between himself and the consultant. The pay-off may come when an admission is required as a matter of urgent necessity.

Other persons who may be involved in the admission of
psychiatric patients to hospitals
Mention has already been made of the social worker, who has been appointed a mental welfare officer, who may be required statutorily to make the application for admission of a patient under a compulsory order. In practice other persons may also be of great assistance, although their role is not statutorily determined. These are given below.

(a) The community psychiatric nurse. At one time the mental hospital operated in splendid isolation. Its staff, both medical and nursing, were like pariahs, cut off from the communities which they served. This prejudice in respect of doctors has been largely overcome, particularly since the creation of the N.H.S. in 1948. Out-patient departments manned by psychiatrists and their assistants in hospitals located in the catchment area are the order of the day as are consultations between G.P. and consultant psychiatrist in the patient's home.

Much more recently the community psychiatric nurse has come into being. He (or she) is usually on the staff of the mental hospital or psychiatric unit and his job is to act as a link-man between the hospital, the consultant and the G.P. He may be concerned, too, in the administration of long-acting phenothiazines and in the giving of support and advice to the relatives in the over-all management of the case. Moreover, he may spot symptoms of relapse at an early stage and, by alerting the G.P., timely admission or readmission to hospital could follow. This is particularly important where it is known that the patient concerned is liable to be troublesome or to become a danger to himself or others.

(b) The police. The police are of prime importance in the control of dangerous social crises. They can be of great assistance to medical practitioners faced with patients who may be a danger to themselves or others.

An excellent statement of the position of the Metropolitan Police in this context has been made and appears as Appendix I in a report on *The Management of Potentially Violent Patients* (C.O.H.S.E., 1977). The following is abstracted from that statement. There is no reason to believe that police other than the Metropolitan operate in any fundamentally different way, but G.P.s could easily find out if this is so.

It has been a cardinal principle since the modern police service was established in 1829 that police powers to act on private premises, i.e. off the public highway and away from places to which the public have access, are severely restricted and generally governed by statute.

When a person in normal occupation on his private premises finds a trespasser on his property and seeks police assistance, any officer who attends will act primarily to prevent a breach of the peace, but if his physical intervention becomes necessary to eject the trespasser, this will be given as an agent of the lawful occupier. Similarly, any assistance which is afforded to members of the National Health Service, other than that which is laid down by statute, is almost always given in accordance with the trespass principle outlined above. This means that the primary duty of dealing with the patient rests, where it properly lies, with the professional and trained medical staff.

The instruction to this Force makes it quite clear that when, for example, a mentally disordered person is on private premises and police arrive before the mental welfare officer, action should be confined to assisting in restraining the disordered person until the arrival of that officer.

A "constable" is one of a group of persons authorised by section 40 of the Mental Health Act 1959, to return patients absent from a hospital without leave.

The legal restraints which are placed on the powers of the police and other persons to enter private premises are highlighted by the fact that no right of entry exists and that section 135 (1) of the Mental Health Act 1959, empowers a magistrate's court to issue a warrant to enter premises to a named police officer on the sworn information of a mental welfare officer. Subsection (ii) of the same section enables a magistrate to issue a warrant under similar circumstances on the information of a police officer. In both of these cases police duties are quite clear as they are acting in their ancient role as "constable" under the directions of the local justices.

. . . in the case of the patient who becomes violent or difficult in the casualty department of a major accident hospital. This presents no difficulty because police are often in attendance, and well-known to the staff, and working in a place to which the public have access, and deal with problems in the same way as they would in a shop, cinema or public house.

If mental welfare officers or psychiatric social workers find themselves in difficulty with patients in a private house, the situation becomes quite different and the police officer reverts to his or her role as an agent of the trained or professional person who is attempting to deal with the problem.

. . . except where a statutory duty exists, the role of police is to act as a back-up force to trained staff, skilled in the handling of violent or potentially violent patients.

The G.P. and all the persons mentioned, i.e. the mental welfare officer, the community psychiatric nurse and the police must be regarded as a team. As with all teams efficiency can only come about when each member knows his own job and the contribution each of the other members can make. But every team must have a captain, in this instance one in whom the final responsibility for the management and disposal of the disturbed patient must rest. To the author's mind there is only one of the team qualified by virtue of his knowledge, training and experience to take the job — the doctor!

Drugs in the management of disturbances of behaviour

The introduction of a centrally-active phenothiazine amine, chlorpromazine, in 1950 heralded a new era in the treatment of psychiatric disorders, and by extension, the management of disturbances of behaviour. The French firm, Rhône-Poulenc marketed the drug under the trade-name Largactil ("large activity") in 1952, since when, under a variety of names, its use has spread round the civilised world like a whirlwind.

A host of other psychotropic drugs has subsequently come off the pharmaceutical production line in bewildering profusion. It is therefore, most important for general practitioners to familiarise themselves with a small repertoire of the new drugs in which they have confidence, whilst not forgetting the continuing usefulness of a few of the old favourites, for example, some of the barbiturates and even smelly, irritant paraldehyde. For the very same reaons it is proposed to include in this section only a tiny fistful of drugs with which the author is familiar and in which he has acquired confidence. Treatment will be discussed in accordance with the schema adopted in the consideration of the causes of disturbed behaviour, always conceding that the division between the organic and psychiatric can at times be arbitrary.

To take *organic* causes first, therefore:

1. *Toxic-confusional states (Delirium)*

These are serious conditions which are best treated in hospital, because there skilled nursing is more likely to be available.

It is, of course, of prime importance that attention is directed to the underlying cause which, as has been already indicated, can be one of many. What concerns us most here is the control of restlessness which is additionally wearing to a patient already near exhaustion. Recommended drugs which have stood the test of time are chlorpromazine (Largactil), promazine hydrochloride (Sparine) and thioridazine (Melleril) in doses of 50 to 100 mg three times a day. If it is a matter of urgent necessity to bring the restlessness under control, particularly if accompanied by aggressive behaviour, chlorpromazine (Largactil) 50 to 100 mg intramuscularly may be given (because of its irritant qualities chlorpromazine must never be given subcutaneously).

No matter which drug is selected it is essential that details of the dose and times given are included in the letter accompanying the patient to hospital.

2. *Chemical intoxicants*

Far and away the most common intoxicant to be met with in general practice is alcohol. We are concerned in this chapter only with its acute manifestations, as witness, the fighting drunk, delirium tremens and alcoholic hallucinosis, and then only with first-aid measures to bring the patient under control.

The drugs of choice in all three acute conditions mentioned are chlordiazepoxide (Librium) and diazepam (Valium). The former is given in doses of 50 to 100 mg intramuscularly repeated if necessary in two to four hours. The latter drug, diazepam, may be given intravenously in doses of 20 mg. The injection must be given slowly. There are those who remain faithful to paraldehyde, 10 ml, given orally in orange juice, or by deep intramuscular injection.

Delirium tremens and alcoholic hallucinosis are grave illnesses and are best treated in hospital, if possible in the psychiatric unit of a general hospital, where the necessary expertise is available.

3. Drug abuse

(a) *Amphetamines.* The restlessness, irritability and aggressive behaviour seen in amphetamine intoxication usually subside fairly rapidly when the drugs are withdrawn. Phenothiazines can be given if urgent control is necessary, and in particular, if it is considered that the disorganised, excited behaviour may be due to an underlying schizophrenic illness.

(b) *Barbiturates.* Barbiturates are potent depressants of the central nervous system and because of the relative ease with which they are obtained, overdoses — both accidental and deliberate — occur not infrequently. Antidotes are nowadays not considered worthwhile. It is imperative to arrange for immediate admission to hospital where intensive life-support systems are available. If there is actual or imminent failure of a vital system, the patient should be admitted directly to an intensive care unit. In a conscious patient it is permissible to attempt to make him vomit by the use of emetics, or reflexly, by sticking a finger down his throat.

There is, conversely, great danger in the sudden withdrawal of barbiturates in a patient who has long been accustomed to taking them either legally or illegally. In a planned withdrawal, for whatever reason, it is essential that cover is given by pentobarbitone sodium (Nembutal) to guard against withdrawal symptoms.

(c) *Lysergic acid diethylamide (L.S.D.).* L.S.D. "trips" are presumèd to be pleasurable and self-limiting. There are exceptions, however. Some "trips" are bad, so bad indeed that the victim is frightened out of his wits. He is brought for treatment by friends — more often than not "acid droppers" — who are themselves frightened because they have failed to "talk down" the victim. The best hope of alleviating his plight is by the use of a single intramuscular dose of 100 mg chlorpromazine (Largactil).

(d) Cocaine. The acute crisis occasioned by cocaine abuse is a state of delirium. Needless to say, the drug must be immediately and completely withdrawn. The resolution of the crisis can be helped by barbiturates, for example, pentobarbitone sodium (Nembutal) 100 to 200 mg or amylobarbitone (Amytal) 50 to 100 mg.

(e) Opiates. The treatment of opiate withdrawal is a matter for specialists, and the G.P. is urged to secure the admission of patients suffering in this distressing way to a specialised facility as soon as possible. If necessary, chlorpromazine (Largactil), given in the same way as described for L.S.D. intoxication, is useful in the control of the restlessness which is often accompanied by seriously disturbed and aggressive behaviour.

(f) Cannabis. Crises brought about by this particular drug must be relatively rare. If they do arise they too can be controlled by chlorpromazine (Largactil). As in amphetamine intoxication, the real underlying cause of the behaviour disturbance may be an emerging schizophrenic psychosis and the use of chlorpromazine is doubly justified.

4. *Drug intolerance*
As with most therapeutic advances there is so often a sting in the tail of progress. The psychotropic drugs are no exception. They are liable to produce side-effects the commonest of which are extrapyramidal in nature (*see* p. 251), symptoms that can be both, subjectively and objectively, alarming and distressing. In bringing the symptoms under control anti-parkinsonian drugs are usually effective. A well-tested drug is orphenadrine hydrochloride (Disipal) given orally in 100 mg doses, or intramuscularly (ampoules of 2 ml are marketed). The drug may be repeated in divided doses up to 300 mg in the course of twenty-four hours.

5. *Epilepsy*
Sadly there are epileptics who as a matter of course, or episodically, show disturbances of behaviour in the form of hostility, aggressiveness, agitation or restlessness. They can often be helped by chlorpromazine (Largactil), or thioridazine (Melleril) in doses of 50 mg three or four times a day.

Serious complications of epilepsy such as twilight states and status epilepticus are best treated in hospital. However, it may be necessary to begin treatment forthwith and this can best be done by the use of diazepam (Valium), or by the time-honoured method of injecting paraldehyde intramuscularly. Diazepam in doses of 5 to 10 mg is given by *slow* intravenous injection, repeated if the fits in status epilepticus recur. The dose of paraldehyde is 8 to 10 ml for adults and 2 to 6 ml in children. The injection must as always be given deep and only glass syringes may be used. If need be a further 5 ml can be given at half-hourly intervals until the fits cease.

6. *Brain damage*
Any injury to the brain merits treatment in hospital where specialist facilities for investigation and treatment are available. If it is at all possible, sedatives are best avoided because of the possibility of confusing the physical signs in a neurological examination and the probability of depressing respiration and the cough reflex. The restlessness and generally disorganised behaviour commonly seen in the transitional period between coma and the recovery of consciousness justify the use of minimal restraint until the symptoms subside.

In the management of disorders of behaviour *due to psychiatric causes* virtually the same drugs as those already described are used.

1. *Schizophrenia*
Here again we are concerned only with emergencies caused by disturbances of behaviour. In this context the catatonic variety of schizophrenia gives rise to most concern. Crises arise at the two extremes of psychomotor activity, expressed, that is, as catatonic stupor at one end and catatonic excitement at the other. In the one the patient is a danger to himself: in the other he is a danger both to himself or others.

Catatonic stupor is a major psychiatric emergency. The treatment of choice is E.C.T. and, as this is almost invariably given in hospital, no time should be lost in arranging admission, preferably to a psychiatric unit attached to a general hospital. Because of the overt dangerousness of a patient in catatonic excitement he must be brought under control swiftly. Chlorpromazine (Largactil) 100 mg intramuscularly is usually effective if, that is, the patient is prepared to submit to the injection. If it is evident that his consent is not likely to be forthcoming the doctor would be entitled to administer the injection against the patient's will. He should summon what forces he can, preferably from amongst those accustomed to such procedures, such as the mental welfare officer, the community psychiatric nurse or a police officer. What restraint is necessary must be effected swiftly, silently and overwhelmingly. Furthermore, no attempt should be made to transport the patient by ambulance, or any other form of motor vehicle, until the patient is controlled and even then only if adequate escort is available.

2. *Affective disorder*
Here too the behavioural crises arise at one or other end of a spectrum, this time from depression to mania. In the extremities of

depression the patient may become stuporose, a condition no less critical than the stupor of catatonic schizophrenia and usually demanding the same treatment, i.e. E.C.T. Early admission to a psychiatric facility must, therefore, be arranged.

In states of mania virtually the same type of emergency may arise as was dealt with above in the case of the catatonically excited patient. The same technique, the same drugs and the same caution should be used to bring an equally dangerous situation under control.

3. *The neuroses*
The one condition most likely to give rise to serious behaviour disorder is hysteria. The acting-out may pose a threat to the safety of the patient, or those around him or her. The minimum degree of restraint is allowable to control the patient. Diazepam (Valium) is the drug of choice in a 5 to 10 mg dosage. There are those, however, old-fashioned as they may be, who regard a well-directed douche of cold water as the most effective, safest and cheapest form of treatment.

4. *Psychopathic disorder*
The aberrant behaviour of the psychopath is usually a matter for the police. However, psychopaths may coincidentally abuse drink or drugs and crises attributable to these indulgences have been dealt with under appropriate headings in this chapter and in more detail in the relevant chapters.

Before leaving the subject of the control of behaviour disorders, particularly acute excitement, mention must be made of the use of haloperidol (Serenace). Experts, such as Dr. Arthur Oldham, claim that given by injection in doses of 10 to 30 mg, depending on the patient's age, sex and weight, together with procyclidine hydrochloride (to prevent extrapyramidal side-effects), the drug is speedy and relatively safe (Oldham, 1976). Its main disadvantage is the production of such extrapyramidal side-effects and the possibility in the senile or arteriosclerotic brain of irreversible tardive dyskinesia. By and large the author would not recommend the use of this particular drug as a first-aid measure of initial choice in general practice, although its usefulness in the casualty department or in acute psychiatric wards, where staff are skilled in its use, seems well established.

PRECAUTIONS AGAINST ASSAULT

In this context readers are earnestly urged to read the C.O.H.S.E. report referred to earlier. Only guidelines can be given additionally.

In his surgery, the doctor should have his desk arranged so that his back is to a wall and his face towards the door. In this way he is unlikely to be taken by surprise by an unexpected intruder. There should always be an alarm bell, discreetly hidden but easily accessible. Assistance of some sort should be readily available at all times.

In a threatening situation a "softly, softly" approach is to be recommended. Avoid any sudden movement which could be interpreted by the might-be assailant as an impending attack on him. Attempt to gain the confidence of the patient so as to try to reassure him that the doctor is on his side. But if it appears obvious that persuasion is to be of no avail the doctor, with all the help he can muster, must bring a potentially dangerous situation under control "swiftly, silently and overwhelmingly".

In every circumstance there is no substitute in general practice for an intimate knowledge, built up over the years, of the clinical histories of patients and the circumstances in which they live. This is particularly so if the doctor is called out to deal with a crisis in the home. Take, for example, an unfortunate, but hypothetical, family Brown. It is important to know that old Granny Brown's chronic bronchitis exacerbates each winter and that at these times she becomes pyrexial and hypoxic. As a result she becomes confused and aggressive and lashes out with her stick at anyone in sight. It is important to know that her son, Arthur, drinks more than he can take on a Saturday night and inevitably becomes violent, and that his wife, Mary, a diabetic, is careless with her diet and her insulin and can easily become confused and aggressive as her blood sugar fluctuates. It is equally important to know that their son, Jimmy, is a chronic schizophrenic who from time to time relapses and goes berserk. If all hell would appear to have broken out in the Brown household, it would be unwise even for the regular doctor to "go it alone". For the locum or a trainee assistant it would be sheer folly. An escort should be sought, preferably of people whose job familiarises them with the control of aggression such as the police, the mental welfare officer, or the community psychiatric nurse.

Finally, it is obviously impossible to give explicit directions for the control of every situation in which disordered behaviour may arise. There is, however, one guideline which is of fundamental importance and must never be forgotten, namely:

Discretion is the better part of valour.

REFERENCES

Confederation of Health Service Employees (1977): *The Management of Violent or Potentially Violent Patients: Report of a Special Working Party*, C.O.H.S.E., Banstead.

Glatt, M. (1972): *The Alcoholic and the Help He Needs*, Priory Press, London.

Lake, F. (1966): *Clinical Theology*, Darton, Longman and Todd, London.

Mayer-Gross, W., Slater, E. and Roth, M. (1969): *Clinical Psychiatry*, 3rd edition, Baillière, Tindall and Cassell, London.

Oldham, A. J. P. (1976): "The rapid control of the acute patient by haloperidol", *Proceedings of the Royal Society of Medicine*, 69, Supplement No. 1.

Osler, W. (1911): *The Principles and Practice of Medicine*, 7th edition, D. Appleton & Co., New York and London.

FURTHER READING

Ekblom, B. *Acts of Violence by Patients in Mental Hospitals*, Svenska Bokforlaget, Stockholm, 1971.

Scott, P. D. "Assessing dangerousness in criminals", *Brit. J. of Psychiatry*, (1977), 13, 127-42.

Stürup, G. K. "Will this man be dangerous? The mentally abnormal offender", *Ciba Symposium*, (Eds. A. V. S. de Reuk and R. Porter), J. & A. Churchill, London, 1968.

Psychological Help for Physical Illness

Professor Robert J. Daly,
M.A., M.D., F.R.C.P., F.R.C.Psych.
Professor of Psychiatry, University College, Cork and Clinical Director,
Southern Health Board, Ireland.

Psychological Help for Physical Illness

INTRODUCTION

A paradox of modern medical practice is that doctors devote a great deal of time to basic and continuous training in the physical aspects of their treatments, but give much less time and thought to that activity in which they spend most of their working lives, i.e. interacting with the patients. Yet the psychological component in the treatment of physical illness offers considerable new opportunities. Indeed some would say this traditional "art" has become even more vital with the changes which have occurred in health care delivery.

A picture of the doctor spending his day grappling with crises, in which he either succeeds in saving the life of the patient or gracefully concedes defeat and the patient dies, is now only a Victorian novelist's fantasy. Acute infectious diseases and obstetrical emergencies occupy but a small part of the average doctor's day. Instead, he is faced with the more demanding but less dramatic problems related to chronic disease. In many of these, psychological factors play an important aetiological role or even determine the outcome. It could be suggested that the main function of the doctor is to reverse illness trends, rather than to cure his patients. Of course it can be shown that "curing" is a less-than-accurate description of the work of Victorian doctors. Increasing numbers of studies have pointed to the importance of understanding the psychological and social factors affecting, not only the aetiology, but also the course and duration of the illness, the patient's adherence to treatment and the success of rehabilitative efforts. The advent of medical technologies enabling the prolongation of life have brought with them, not only a whole new range of ethical problems, but also information relating to the psychological and social consequences of these therapies. Problems have also been explored concerning patients with terminal illness and the difficulties for their families and their doctors.

Psychosomatic diseases are no longer thought of as a separate group. Instead, with all illness, one studies the relationships between psychological and social factors interacting with the physical aspects of aetiology. Unitary causation of illness is now seen as being an obsolete view and has given way to a multiple aetiological approach. Increasing technical expertise has underlined the need for a comprehensive approach to the patient. Several trends have emerged, including the following.

(a) Research in the area of psychological contributions to the aetiology of illness.

(b) Psychological aspects of the severe stress to the patient involved in the prolongation of life have been extensively researched.

(c) Psychosocial determinants of recovery from illness have been developed.

(d) Psychological aspects of the treatment of chronically ill or severely ill patients have been equally emphasised.

(e) Many groups and individuals have written about the problems of coping with terminal illness.

(f) Adherence to medical treatment has also been extensively researched.

(g) Treatment studies have evolved in the new areas of biofeedback and behaviour modification, as well as individual, group and family psychotherapies and the use of psychotropic drugs in physical illness.

This chapter concerns itself predominantly with treatment applications, but is based on information derived from many of the foregoing groups and studies.

THE SICK ROLE

Much work has been carried out into understanding the role adopted by patients who become ill. As Erikson has pointed out, basic trust in other human beings is learned during infancy through the relationship with mother (Erikson, 1963). The child understands that when it suffers discomforts such as hunger, pain and cold that mother can be relied upon to cater for these needs in a non-anxious manner and to satisfy them. Thus the infant learns that in times of difficulty he can rely upon others to help. If, on the other hand, mother is unresponsive to his needs, the infant is likely to respond by tantrums or, conversely, withdrawal and depression. Equally so, in infancy the child may learn, by mother's negative reactions to his demands, that illness is something associated with guilt and unpleasant feelings.

To a greater or lesser extent all adults respond in the sick role with a certain degree of aggression. This results from the fact that the adult experiences and resents the childlike feeling of dependency and helplessness. He also may come to believe that those looking after him are like the all-powerful parents of his early years. Psychiatrists refer to this phenomenon as transference and this encompasses all those distortions of the power of the doctor and exaggerated dependency feelings which are liable to emerge under the stress of coping with illness. Of course, early influences in the programming of the adult sick role are not confined merely to the family. Thus Zola (1966) has reported on a cultural dimension to illness behaviour in which U.S. patients of Irish extraction tended to limit and understate their complaints, whereas those of Italian origin tended to dramatise their symptoms (Zola, 1969).

PHYSICAL CORRELATES OF MENTAL STATE AND MOOD CHANGES

Engel has pointed out that mood changes are related to unpleasant mental states and enable one to cope with a problem by forcing one into activity and restoring comfort (Engel, 1971). The physiological components of these mental states may interact with the pathological physical condition of illness. This may cause worsening of the illness and it is important to remember some of the mechanisms involved. Physiological responses to changes in mental state are often undifferentiated, although there is a certain amount of correlation, as between nausea and disgust, blushing and shame and palpitations and fear. Engel has described two basic patterns of physiological response to mental states:

(a) anxiety or fight-flight reactions as described originally by Cannon (1942);

(b) depression — withdrawal with insulation against environmental change and conservation of physical resources.

With the "fight-flight" or "arousal" pattern, neuroendocrine changes occur such as the production of adrenalin and noradrenalin. Other changes include the mobilisation of free fatty acids and glucose, gastric hypersecretion, increased peripheral blood flow, hyperventilation, and alkalosis which, when marked, causes diminished C.N.S. perfusion.

In the withdrawal-conservation pattern there is a subjective feeling of displeasure correlated with hopelessness and helplessness. There is a tendency for decreased motor-activity, slumped posture and diminished muscle tone. There is a virtual absence, for example, of gastric-secretory activity with this pattern.

Numerous examples may be cited to show the psychological and social contributions to the pathophysiology of disease. Acheson showed the close interactions between social class, cultural background and the metabolic pathways of disease (Acheson, 1969). He studied the relationship between serum uric acid in social class by sex among persons in Yorkshire, Hertfordshire and Newhaven, Connecticut. Amongst the men of the Yorkshire group there was a tendency for serum uric acid to increase with decreasing social class, while in Newhaven women the same trend occurred. No trend was found amongst any of the other four sex specific groups and age did not account for the patterns observed. Bearing in mind the difference between his findings and those of several studies in the United States, we see that serum uric acid has been found to have different social class gradients in different cultural contexts. This supports the view that both serum uric acid levels and gout are under multifactorial control.

Jacobs and Nabarro examined the adrenal cortical response in acute medical illness by measuring the plasma 11-hydroxycortico-steroid (11 O.H.C.S.) concentration in 178 patients (Jacobs and Nabarro, 1969). They found that high levels occurred in patients with unstable diabetes, acute infections and severe myocardial infarctions. It has long been known that patients with primary or secondary impairment of adrenal cortical function may respond poorly to any acute illness. Furthermore, it has been found that individuals without medical illness, but under psychological stress, show similarly high levels of steroid secretion. Thus it can be seen that physiological and biochemical changes interact with psychological, social and cultural factors, not only in the production of illness, but in determining its outcome and response to treatment.

In 1942 Cannon published his classic paper on Voodoo death and numerous papers have followed since (e.g. Engel, 1971). Many authors have emphasised the importance of hopelessness and helplessness preceding sudden death. Weisman and Hackett (1961) described a predilection to death amongst surgical patients who accurately predicted their own death. Rahe et al. (1974) have emphasised the importance of an excessive number of life-changes preceding sudden death, particularly from myocardial infarction. Dimsdale (1977) has emphasised the importance of psychological intervention for those who are highly at risk for lethal emotional stress, e.g. in coronary care units. This has implications in terms of maximum presence of the doctor, prompt and appropriate use of anti-anxiety medications and more specialised techniques such as psychotherapy and behaviour therapy.

Cardio-vascular disease

The relationship between emotions and the heart is proverbial but, surprisingly, there have been few applications of modern knowledge about these interrelationships. Not only are myocardial infarction, essential hypertension, cardiac arrhythmias and angina pectoris associated with important psychosomatic mechanisms but palpitations and reduced exercise-tolerance are not uncommon accompaniments of psychoneurotic disorder. A variety of relaxation techniques may be used to combat cardiac arrhythmias, including transcendental meditation, but anxiolytic drugs are recommended only for episodes of acute anxiety. Beta-blocking agents are widely used in doses sufficient to block cardiac effects of circulating catecholamines but not so high as to interfere with neuro-transmitter function in the sympathetic nerves to the heart.

Coronary heart disease and personality

Rosenman and colleagues in their Western Collaborative Group study conducted a prospective epidemiological investigation of coronary heart disease incidence in some three-and-a-half thousand men, aged 39 to 59 years, employed in ten Californian companies. Comprehensive data were obtained over an average period of eight-and-a-half years and coronary heart disease occurred in 257 of their subjects. The incidence of coronary heart disease (C.H.D.) was significantly associated with parental C.H.D. history, reported diabetes, schooling levels, smoking habits, overt behaviour pattern, blood pressure and serum levels of cholesterol, triglyceride and beta-lipoproteins. They used their own typology of personality. Their pattern *A* patients who were coronary-prone were characterised by enhanced aggressiveness and competitive drive, with a chronic sense of time urgency. Conversely, the more relaxed type *B* subjects exhibited substantially lower coronary heart disease incidence and less atherosclerosis (Rosenman *et al.*, 1975). Keys has pointed out that the classical risk factors in coronary heart disease account for only about half of the incidence and that other variables contribute significantly (Keys, 1972). There is a widely recognised epidemiological relationship between the incidence of clinical heart disease and prospective risk factors including age, parental history of premature infarction, elevated blood pressure, cigarette smoking, serum cholesterol, triglycerides and beta-lipoproteins. Friedman *et al.* point out that the predictive relationship of any single risk factor with the incidence of coronary heart disease may be a reflection of its association with other risk factors (Friedman *et al.*, 1968).

There appear to be important clinical implications for primary prevention. Various groups in the United States are attempting to change behaviour patterns of those thought to be highly at risk for developing coronary heart disease. But such movements and such interventions do not seem to have gained any ground in the U.K. Nevertheless, for many years wise doctors working on the basis of anecdotal evidence have made serious efforts to prolong the lives of their patients by counselling, attempting to solve important personal and family conflicts and advising more time being set aside for relaxation and exercise. Men with a high energy intake, reflecting greater physical activity, have a lowered risk for C.H.D. (Morris *et al.*, 1977).

Myocardial infarction and coronary care

Interest is now developing into methods of psychosocial prevention of coronary heart disease. Nevertheless we have to accept that coronary disease remains not only a "Captain of Death" but one of the major sources of disability in our society. The sick population being dealt with is predominantly male and middle-aged, although the age of onset of coronary heart disease is diminishing (Cay *et al.*, 1976). There is a considerable controversy over the psychological impact of coronary care units and the relative mortality compared with care in conventional units or at home. Amongst the problems alleged in these units are the difficulties for a patient, with exaggerated physiological responses to anxiety-provoking circumstances, coping with such a machine-dominated environment. Undoubtedly the array of hardware in these units is intimidating and frightening, particularly for unsophisticated patients. There are also staff problems. Nurses have a tendency in intensive care units to keep their distance emotionally from their patients for fear of developing a close involvement with a person who has a high risk of dying. By contrast Cay *et al.*, (1976) found that 88 per cent of people were reassured by their stay in a coronary care unit. Nevertheless at least half of the admissions were clinically anxious or depressed. The chief problem is that the medical and nursing staff may see such acutely-ill patients as predominantly having organic problems. Staff may misinterpret the anxiety and hostility displayed by these patients. Considerable reassurance for the patient is required, together with sufficient analgesics (morphine) to reduce distress and allay the anxiety. A realistic but truthfully optimistic statement can be given to the patient about the prospects for recovery and getting back to work. Indeed early discussion of return to work is most important.

The chief psychological problems with coronary patients tend to be coping with a defensive denial of the problem and dependency. Thus the doctor must intervene psychotherapeutically, not only in a supportive context, but reflecting an optimistic reality. Later, a problem may arise in the doctor being flattered by the patient's excessive compliance with his treatment. Warm, positive feelings on the part of the doctor may develop in response to the patient's tendency to express admiration for the doctor (especially if the patient brings him presents!). This transference relationship encourages the patient to remain in the passive sick role. Such a chronic emotional relationship with the patient militates against full recovery. Many physicians themselves remark that the average age of patients tends to increase with the age of the physician caring for them. Sometimes it is difficult for both the doctor and the patient to realise that there should come a point when this dependent and reciprocal relationship may no longer be appropriate.

It is extremely helpful for the patient to start getting out of bed early to avoid organic complications especially venous thrombosis. It should be remembered that movement both physical and psychological in the direction of recovery and independence should be rewarded by encouragement and congratulations. There is the exception, of course, who will require encouragement to be "good to himself" and to depend on others for a change. Many doctors, when ill, notoriously fit into this category, because they themselves wish to look after others and resent the dependent role.

Peptic ulcer

Rutter (1963) showed that the ulcers of those patients who have persistent anxiety symptoms are more likely to become chronic than those of patients without psychiatric disability. He also found that neither physical nor social factors helped in forming a prognosis but clinical anxiety, or depression at the first attendance at hospital, was associated with poor outcome. Glen and Cox showed that poor outcome after operation for duodenal ulcer was unrelated to the type of operation, but was associated with deviant personality traits and disturbance of mood (Glen and Cox, 1968). It has also been suggested that psychosomatic disorder may in some way protect patients from more serious breakdowns. This explains the finding of Whitlock of major psychiatric disability, requiring treatment, following gastrectomy. More than half of his patients required treatment for alcoholism or drug addiction (Whitlock, 1961). Before advising gastrectomy it is most important to exclude abuse of aspirin and alcohol. Predictive psychological tests could be more widely used pre-operatively and psychotherapeutic intervention should be offered to those considered unsuitable for operation.

Respiratory disease

Many patients attending clinics for respiratory diseases are found to have psychogenic dyspnoea without a finding of organic cause for the breathlessness (Burns and Howell, 1969). Various recent social and family stresses are found in those with disproportionate dyspnoea. Such dyspnoea tends to be more episodic than in those with more severe organic disease. In addition, the dyspnoea could be more easily relieved. One of the problems in assessment is that hypoxia may cause mental symptoms confusing the test results.

There has been considerable controversy over the personality characteristics of the asthmatic. Early papers described asthmatics as suffering from "a neurosis of the respiratory tract", and Alexander

(1950) described the unresolved maternal dependence of asthmatics. Yet Aitken, in a controlled study using objective psychological testing and psychophysiological examination, failed to find other than minimal differences between asthmatics and normals (Aitken *et al.*, 1968). Undoubtedly there are psychological and emotional aspects to suffering from the illness of asthma, but once again it seems unwise to consider asthma as belonging to a group of "psychosomatic diseases" different from other diseases.

In the past, hypnosis has been widely advocated for the treatment of asthma and a controlled trial (*British Medical Journal*, 1968) was performed by the British Tuberculosis Association. The asthmatics were divided into two groups, approximately half receiving hypnosis and the other half undergoing progressive breathing exercises. Both groups showed improvement during the course of the trial but it should be noted that those who became severely ill or who received corticosteroids were withdrawn from the study and so did not contribute to the assessments. The subjective assessment by the patients and the clinical examination showed a slightly greater improvement in those undergoing hypnosis, particularly the females, but objective examinations of forced expiratory volume and vital capacity showed no difference between the two groups. The hypnotic method was thought to be of greater value in treating females suffering from asthma than was the relaxation method supplemented by breathing exercises.

Pain

The neuronal pathways for pain explain the importance of psychological factors in pain perception. Noxious stimulation of an end organ leads to an impulse along the peripheral nerve and spinal pathway to the thalamus. It must be remembered that pain is perceived at a cortical level and this involves psychological processing in all cases, regardless of the presence or absence of a noxious stimulus. Thus pain may be purely a psychological experience. In this regard it is important to remember the importance of pain in early object relations. In infancy, pain led to crying and this characteristically brought about the attention and comforting by a loved person, leading to pain relief. The mother very often "kisses it better" and this has an important corollary in that pain relief can occur merely through the attention and concern of the medical team.

Another important aspect of the early development of pain perception is the concept of pain being equivalent to punishment for many children. Pain is inflicted when they are bad. Patients often exclaim, "What did I do to deserve this?" Pain may even become the medium for relief of guilt and reconciliation with loved parents. This may lead on, in adult life, to pain as a method of reconciliation in coming to terms with those around us, or ourselves.

Understanding the interactions between the dampening effects of the reticular activating system and cortical pathways for pain throws some light on the mechanisms of powerful suggestive techniques such as hypnosis, acupuncture, and relaxation methods (e.g. "painless childbirth").

Finally, it is important to remember that pain is not simply and directly correlated with the extent of the lesion. The doctor cannot assume that because a lesion is minimal or undetectable that the pain experienced by the patient is unreal. He must also remember that his interest, manner and approach contain a tremendous potential for the relief of pain.

Intractable pain
Recurrent abdominal pain occurs in about one in every nine school children. Only 7 per cent of these have an organic cause for the pain. Apley pointed out that those children with recurrent abdominal pains tend to be more timid, anxious and tense, with the added characteristic of being fussy (Apley, 1959). They also tend to be over-conscientious and to mix poorly.

It has been found that such children grow up to be adults with a tendency to have abdominal pain (Christensen and Mortenson, 1974). Clearly more extensive psychological intervention is required in those children presenting with a psychogenic cause of abdominal pain, to avoid long-term disability. Optimistic inactivity, while an easy course to take, is inadvisable.

Some forms of refractory pain are best treated with antidepressants, e.g. atypical facial pain which is thought to be a variant of depressive illness. Other techniques such as those coming under the general category of suggestion have been reported, e.g. Mann *et al.*, have reported the use of acupuncture (Mann *et al.*, 1973). The real danger with intractable pain is that a long and futile series of physical investigations and surgical interventions may be started.

Clearly, a multidisciplinary approach to alleviatation of pain is required. Little data has yet been available on the use of biofeedback and behaviour modification, but certainly there is ample evidence to suggest that powerful suggestive techniques are effective in pain relief.

Peptides and pain
Endogenously produced opiate peptides, endorphins and encephalins have recently been discovered and the most marked effect of opiates is their ability to produce analgesia in animals and humans. It is now apparent that opiates work through at least three different analgesic mechanisms:

(a) inhibition of somato-sensory afferents in the dorsal horn of the spinal cord;

(b) inhibition of similar afferents at the level of the brain;
(c) activation of descending inhibitory pathways.

The presence of encephalinergic terminals and opiate receptors in the central nervous system areas involved in pain perception indicates that the brain contains an endogenous pain suppression mechanism. It is being suggested that analgesia induced by focal brain stimulation is mediated by the release of encephalins in the midbrain. Sweet (1980) has pointed out that the central nervous system, like advanced engineering systems, has a considerable amount of redundancy and "back-up". He points out that there are nine neuro-transmitters identified in the afferents to the noradrenaline-secreting locus ceruleus. Such multiplicity of controls means that whenever a system is moved in a particular direction, several mechanisms move in the opposite direction to produce homeostasis. He feels that such mechanisms are responsible for the tachyphylaxis to medications and the re-appearance of algesia and clinical pain which tend to follow initially successful neurosurgical procedures.

More important, the growing knowledge of such mechanisms reinforces the need for psychological, social and "human" intervention as being vitally important in the management of chronic pain.

Mutilating surgery

The psychological problems following amputation and plastic surgery, e.g. psychosis, phantom phenomena, have been well documented and the surgical teams are usually alert to these complications. It must be remembered that psychiatric illness tends also to occur after hysterectomy. Barker found that 7 per cent of 729 women who had a hysterectomy were referred to the psychiatrist at a mean of four-and-a-half years after the operation. This is two-and-a-half times higher than the incidence after cholecystectomy and nearly three times higher than the expected incidence amongst a control group. Of the psychiatric referrals 80 per cent occurred within two years of hysterectomy and the most frequent psychiatric problem was depression (Barker, 1968). There are certain patients on whom hysterectomy should be performed only after psychiatric assessment. Thus patients with complaints of menorrhagia or pelvic pain, without associated clinical or laboratory findings, or patients with a previous psychiatric history or a history of marital breakdown, ought to be referred. Depression is thought to be a not uncommon major post-operative complication of hysterectomy and it is felt that the general practitioner ought to monitor hysterectomised patients for at least two years afterwards. The doctor ought to be particularly aware of depressive illness masquerading as somatic symptomatology and particular attention ought to be paid to complaints of exhaustion or the recurrence of symptoms. Once diagnosed, the problem of treatment with antidepressants and supportive psychotherapy is relatively easy.

Similar problems occur after mastectomy (Maguire *et al.*, 1978). They conducted a controlled study of the incidence of psychiatric symptoms amongst women who presented with suspected breast cancer and who had a mastectomy. One year after surgery, 25 per cent of the mastectomy cases required treatment for anxiety or depression, or both, compared with only 10 per cent of controls. Of the operated cases 33 per cent, compared with 8 per cent of the controls, had moderate or severe sexual difficulties. Perhaps the most serious aspect of their report is that women who asked for help from the medical team appeared not to get it. In many cases this was due to the inability of the doctors to recognise and treat these emotional disturbances. The authors suggested once more that careful monitoring of such cases would help with earlier identification and treatment. The usual response of the G.P.s who were asked for help by these women, was to prescribe tranquillisers in low dosage, and the surgeons, while concerned about their patients, had apparently failed to enquire explicitly about their emotional well-being.

Accidents

Accidents constitute not only a major cause of mortality in our society, but they also pose an increasing problem of hospital management and, more recently, prevention. Many doctors have been preoccupied with the psychological *sequelae* of accidents and a great deal has been written about "compensation neurosis" (Miller, 1961). It is also common knowledge that *sequelae* of accidents include — as well as accident neurosis — post-concussional syndrome, depressive illness, occupational disability and rehabilitation problems.

The cognitive aspects of psychological precursors to accidents have been amply dealt with by Russell Davis (1958, 1966). Hirschfeld and Behan dealt in a more comprehensive way with the accident process. They showed that the physical injury resulted from a psychological process which was defined and documented. They claimed to identify this process in almost every case they examined. They saw the physical disturbance being used as a solution to the problems of the patient. This attractive hypothesis explains the unwillingness of patients to give up their illness following an accident, and the chronicity of disability and the litigation which follows. Hirschfeld and Behan indicated that when chronicity supervenes the patient actually seeks out doctors who will not cure him, but rejects others who appear capable (Hirschfeld and Behan, 1963). It seems more likely therefore that the depression noticed so often in accident wards may have *preceded* the physical injury rather than arisen as a complication of it. Certainly, with road accidents, the victims have often (in perhaps as much as a half of all cases) incurred their injuries under the influence of alcohol (Bofin et al., 1975).

It may thus be seen that psychological treatment is of prime importance in many cases seen in accident wards. Patients who have suffered from alcohol addiction must undergo a physical examination and have their history taken with this in mind. Chronic alcoholics usually show stigmata such as a reddened face or palms, palpable or painful liver, tremor and scars from old accidents. As with most cases, a history taken from a relative can be invaluable in establishing the diagnosis.

Depressed patients in accident wards must be diagnosed and treated. In a minority of cases failure to do so can result in further accidents or suicides. It has been suggested that there is an unconscious and even conscious motivation towards suicide in many road accidents (Selzer and Payne, 1962). Retrospective psychological "post mortems" carried out in the United States (Finch, 1970; Schmidt et al., 1970) claim that a majority of drivers in single car fatalities were observed by relatives, friends and workmates to have been suffering from symptoms of treatable depression just prior to their accidents.

In any event, depression seen following an accident should be vigorously treated and it is most important that all the doctors and nurses concerned understand the objectives and support one another in doing so. Most cases suffering from psychiatric illness will require follow-up after their discharge from the accident department and this is best undertaken by the primary surgical team obtaining, where necessary, consultation with the psychiatrist.

Mental function after anaesthesia

With the tendency to earlier post-operative discharge from hospital, the immediate and long-term mental effects of anaesthesia become more important. These effects are marked and constitute an acute organic brain disorder with confusion. Simpson et al. (1976) suggest that the minimum acceptable level for discharge from hospital is 60 to 90 per cent of mental functioning and this implies seven to nine hours stay in hospital following general anaesthesia. It is extremely important to remember that this level of mental functioning associated with delirium can produce an emotionally traumatic situation for the patient, the effects of which may persist long after full recovery of organic mental functioning. This ought to be borne in mind when considering day-care surgery for individuals.

Intensive care units

Intensive care units (I.C.U.s) have become an essential part of most general hospitals and as with other new developments in medical technology, such as maintenance haemodialysis, the initial attention is focused on mastering the technology. Later, we have time to look more closely at the more comprehensive effects.

Kornfeld has been amongst those who have reported psychiatric problems from such units. He discussed the psychiatric reaction produced by the serious medical and surgical illness which brings the patient to the unit (Kornfeld, 1969). The major problem is the acute organic brain syndrome or delirium and this can be serious, with the confused, agitated patient pulling out infusion sets, catheters etc. There is also a threat to the cardio-vascular status in such a patient and the need for immediate treatment with phenothiazines is indicated. These should be administered intramuscularly and should be established on a maintenance regime rather than "P.R.N." doses. It is also imperative that the cause of the psychotic state is quickly established and wherever possible remedied.

Kornfeld also reported the psychiatric reactions produced by the unusual environment of the unit. In these units the patients are surrounded by modern electronic equipment designed to produce optimal care. It is easy to lose sight of the impact of this on the patient. Sometimes, observers have been worried about the effects of psychological responses in the cardio-vascular state of patients with life threatening illness. Many intensive care units do not have orienting clues in the environment. Thus without an outside window, patients do not know whether it is day or night and are liable to be confused by the incessant round-the-clock activity. In addition, in some units all the staff are masked and there is constant noise from the air-conditioning and other apparatus. Not surprisingly, this combination can lead to delusions and hallucinations occurring in a large proportion of patients, particularly where the brain has been insulted by anaesthesia, analgesia or open-heart surgery. It has been shown that the delirium usually clears within twenty-four to forty-eight hours of the patient's being transferred to a standard hospital environment. Patients interviewed by Kornfeld complained of lack of proper sleep and were in a general state of apprehension.

Sensory deprivation and sleep deprivation with normal subjects in laboratories have led to similar abnormal states. It is therefore suggested that those involved in intensive care units should follow the recommendations given below.

(a) Nursing procedures should be modified to allow uninterrupted sleep. Furthermore patients should be enabled, wherever possible to sleep at night and remain awake during the day.

(b) Wherever possible, patients should be in individual compartments where rest is improved and they are not subjected to the psychological trauma of seeing emergency procedures performed on neighbouring patients.

(c) Monitoring equipment should be outside of these individual compartments. This helps to avoid the monotony of constant rhythmic signals of sound or light. It also minimises the dangers of emotional reactions to feedback of physiological signals.

(d) Wherever possible, telemetry should ideally be introduced to allow increased mobility which is so hampered by wires and tubes from extremities.

(e) The constant noise from oxygen equipment and air-conditioning should be reduced wherever possible.

(f) The patient should be given plenty of meaningful stimulae such as that provided by radio, television, and conversation with relatives and staff. It is also important that the patients themselves control the radios and televisions since outside control increases their sense of helplessness.

(g) Each room should be equipped with a large clock and calendar which is visible to patients and which may help with orientation.

It is also important that staff should be trained in the origins of the emotional symptoms developing in patients in intensive care units and how they can be minimised, e.g. by the staff carefully explaining to the patient at every step what is happening.

Psychiatric follow-up of I.C.U. patients

Follow-up studies have shown that the sights and sounds which can be truly horrifying to laymen visiting intensive care units are even more horrifying to the layman who is a patient in such a unit. Nevertheless, some patients develop a psychological dependence and feel anxiety after leaving these units, feeling safer in the atmosphere of a high level of technical expertise. This can usually be dealt with by careful discussion by the doctor. Unfortunately, one sees reactions of depression and marked irritability in some patients following their terrifying experiences in this environment, compounded with the threat to life which they have experienced. Such reactions are similar to those which follow psychological trauma in other circumstances, e.g. war or other disasters. There is no limit to the improvement which can be brought about by increased awareness in the medical and nursing staff. It is extremely important that all staff are willing to discuss the problems with their patients.

Staff working in such units are particularly exposed to stress themselves. These are unusual environments both for working in and for being patients in. The rapid turnover rate of nursing staff in many units bears witness to this phenomenon. Sometimes the difficulty is rationalised by rotating staff through such units, so that the ordeal is minimised and shared. Nursing staff must work harder than in other units and must be willing to face death occurring amongst their patients more frequently. In some units, the permanent nursing staff are far more knowledgeable and experienced than the junior doctors, who find it hard to ask for help when they are inexperienced in dealing with the complicated equipment. Sometimes, in emergencies, there is no clear delineation of the areas of responsibility for each staff member and such ambiguity can give rise to anxiety in the staff and even risk to the patient.

It is most important that the everyday working conditions in intensive care units are maintained at a good level. Secretarial and other help should be provided for the nursing staff and both doctors and nurses should keep to their regular meal times and off-duty periods. Loss of sleep in junior medical staff occurs frequently and can seriously impair efficiency. Regular meetings between the nursing staff and the medical staff are important to improve channels of communication and also to provide emotional support.

Isolation units

Bacterial isolation (gnotobiotic treatment) has been introduced in a wide range of illnesses to reduce the incidence of infection, e.g. during cytotoxic treatment, organ transplants, burns, etc. Gordon has described the psychological aspects of isolator therapy for acute leukaemia. He examined patients suffering from acute leukaemia treated in such isolators over a two year period and concluded that treatment in such situations could augment the stress of adaptation to leukaemia. He felt it was very important to identify the problems experienced in such environments. He also found that individual patterns of adjustment and defensive manoeuvres were related to the characteristic psychological mechanisms employed by these patients to cope with the dependent position. He felt that psychiatric assessment was very important in order to plan management and he emphasised that some maladaptive coping mechanisms in patients may even appeal to, and be welcomed by, their physicians. He felt that psychiatrists could alert the staff to the problems of managing, e.g. the patient putting a brave face on things or the apathetic, withdrawn patient. He also underlined the importance of using psychotherapy as opposed to depending on psychotropic drugs (Gordon, 1975). Nevertheless, anxiolytic drugs could be beneficial over a short period of time, e.g. on admission and discharge and over times of physical deterioration. He pointed out the dangers of psychiatrists taking over the domination of the group during consultation; instead the psychiatrist ought to encourage those in closest contact to the patient to assume the leadership in such roles.

GRIEF AND SERIOUS ILLNESS

Expanding literature on this subject stems largely from the initial work of Freud (1917) on mourning and melancholia. He pointed out that grief and depression were essentially similar processes, except that in the latter case the loss is usually a more symbolic one. When a person is faced with an "object loss", as with the death of somebody near and dear, or the loss of one's physical health or functioning, or when coping with more symbolic loss, such as the loss of an ideal, one has to undertake a certain amount of psychological rearranging. Such coping Freud called "grief work". Freud's proposition was that both grief and depression contained an element of hostility originally directed against the lost object, or dead person, but now turned back on oneself.

Later workers have tended to de-emphasise this hypothesis. Erich Lindemann (1944) studied the grief reactions which occurred following the disastrous Coconut Grove fire which killed many people in Boston. Lindemann showed that acute grief was a definite syndrome with psychological and bodily symptoms. Furthermore he showed that the syndrome may appear immediately after the crisis or might be delayed or even exaggerated or absent. Sometimes, in place of the typical syndrome, distorted pictures may occur. In normal grief there is a tendency to somatic distress including sighing respirations, exhaustion, loss of taste, dry mouth and so on. The sensorium may be altered to give a sense of unreality and there is a preoccupation with the image of the deceased. Thus hearing and seeing the dead person, which occurs so commonly in the bereaved, may lead to a fear of insanity. Guilt reactions are common. Hostile reactions may also occur, with loss of warmth and irritability. The bereaved person tends to lose the normal patterns of behaviour. Customary routines are hard to perform and there is a loss of initiative and ability to converse easily. Sometimes, there is an identification with the deceased with a tendency to adopt the mannerisms of the deceased person.

The chief task in normal grief is emancipation from attachment to the lost object, with readjustment to the environment no longer containing that lost object. The formation of new relationships is also a part of this work. The danger is that many patients try to avoid the intense distress connected with grieving and to avoid any expression of it and in this respect the doctor can provide considerable help.

Morbid grief
Delayed grief reactions are not uncommon and in fact grief reactions are frequently seen on the anniversary of the loss. One sees many

self-poisoning cases being admitted on the anniversary of the death of a loved one. Another aspect is that one death may reawaken the grief over another past bereavement, and grief reactions sometimes occur on reaching the same age as a deceased relative.

Distorted reactions of various kinds frequently occur, such as hypomanic activities with overactivity in the absence of a sense of loss. During such time, expansive activities may occur. Another common problem is the acquisition of the symptoms of the deceased person with increasing hypochondriasis. Even the medical symptoms of a deceased person may appear (Parkes, 1969). A progressive social isolation, with increasing distance from relatives and friends, may bring about the classic picture of the reclusive widow or widower.

Many doctors and nurses are dismayed to find themselves the object of furious hostility by the grieving relatives who may accuse them of neglect or inadequate treatment. Because of the difficult coping task they face, the bereaved persons may show flattening of emotional life, hiding their feelings in case they show their overwhelming hostility. This often leads on to loss of patterns of social interaction, so that the relative cannot initiate activity and depends very much on others to help him organise his life. It is in this area that Widows' Clubs and other groups can help considerably with preventive action. A danger is that the bereaved or grieving person may take action detrimental to his own social and economic welfare, with protracted self-punitive behaviour, such as giving away his belongings, and being lured too easily into economic follies. Depression with agitation is a frequent severe grief reaction during which time the person develops, as well as agitation, insomnia and feelings of worthlessness, with a very high suicidal risk. Another distorted reaction is denial and many people recall cases of the deceased's clothes kept hanging in the closet and the relatives listening for their footsteps even years after their loss.

Anticipatory grief

When family members are faced with the news that their relative has a fatal illness or has to undergo a difficult and dangerous operation there is a danger that they may pass through all the phases of grief in anticipation of the loss of that person. They may, inappropriately and prematurely, develop symptoms of depression, fantasising the different forms of death that will befall their relative, and (more seriously) anticipate ways of adjusting to the loss. When the operation turns out to be successful, or the person with carcinoma is alive for many years afterwards, there are very considerable psychological problems since the grief work has already been done. The loved ones, to a greater or lesser extent, have lost their attachment to the patient. The medical team must avoid any such inappropriate anticipation by realistic advice and support. As always, appropriate and designated communication is necessary.

Serious illness and acceptance of loss

When following careful examination and laboratory investigations, the doctor decides that his patient is suffering from a chronic disabling or terminal illness he has to form an opinion of the patient's ability to co-operate with treatment. In addition, consciously or unconsciously, he forms his own feelings for, and opinion of, the patient — an opinion which can have important consequences for the future doctor-patient interactions. At this stage it is normal for the patient to be depressed and even hostile and rejecting, if he is realistically dealing with his altered physical state and changed family and work relationships. Paradoxically, the doctor may prefer those patients who enter into a manic defence and appear full of good cheer or who, in one way or another, practise the psychological (usually maladaptive) defence of denial. Such distorted grief reactions by the patient are more often than not a precursor of later maladjustment and inability to co-operate with treatment. Furthermore, such patients' families have a more difficult task ahead of them. The doctor who fails to understand normal grief responses often cannot cope with the normal grief and rejection of such patients. These must be expressed by the patient in order to maximise his prognosis and to improve his long-term prospects for quality of life.

Ideally, the doctor must give the patient the opportunity to vent his disappointment and sadness and feelings of loss. The doctor must also learn to cope with his *own* feelings of despair when patients hint at his inadequacy and failure to bring about a cure.

Grief and selection for special treatment programmes

Some modern treatments are so expensive, economically and in terms of staff provisions, that selection for suitability has to be made by the medical team. Maintenance haemodialysis falls into this category as does transplant surgery and to a lesser extent such treatments as hip-replacement surgery. A paradox arises when doctors see the normal grieving and depressed patient as being most unsuitable for their specialist treatment, while patients practising maladaptive defences such as hypomania and denial are chosen as being most suitable for the treatment.

Because of this, it is most important for those engaged in such selection to understand the psychological mechanisms involved. Furthermore, it is of considerable assistance to use objective psychological testing in order to assess suitability for treatment and avoid distorting emotional doctor-patient interactions (Daly (b), 1969).

Such tests as the Hostility and Direction of Hostility Questionnaire of Foulds (1965) and the Sixteen Personality Factor Questionnaire (Cattell, 1970) are very useful in this regard.

Environment and terminal illness
Rees used a simple method to assess the distress of dying patients in a way that could be charted routinely by nurses (Rees, 1972). He found significant differences between deaths at home and in hospital for three factors. Patients dying at home were:

(a) more likely to be fully alert shortly before death;
(b) less likely to be suffering from vomiting, incontinence and bed sores;
(c) less likely to have unrelieved physical distress.

He found no significant difference in the distress of patients dying in general practitioner hospitals compared with other hospitals, though the numbers compared were small and he felt that a larger study should be carried out.

Agate felt that patients who are dying but cannot remain at home should be cared for as near as possible to their friends and relatives. He also felt it was important that no particular ward should be marked out as the ward for the dying, because of the disastrous effect on the morale of the patients and staff. He felt, instead, that there should be a high proportion of single rooms as close as possible to nurses' observation points with plenty of glass panels, so that the patients could easily see and be seen. The single rooms should be used for treating the very ill, the noisy and disturbed or the dying, according to the needs of the moment, so that no particular room earns the stigma of being "the place for the dying". He felt that there should be ready access of relatives visiting the dying patients. Furthermore, he felt it was important that all grades of staff should meet regularly in case-conferences (including medical and nursing staff and chaplains), so that the policy being adopted is known to all and in particular, "Who has said what, and to whom" (Agate, 1974).

Psychotherapy for the dying
Various authors have dealt with the problems of treating patients who are facing death and coping with the problems they and their families are facing (Hinton, 1967; Cramond, 1970). The classic problem is that facing death is as uncomfortable for the doctors and nurses as it is for the patient and his family. Hinton pointed out that 80 per cent of dying patients know that they are dying and would wish to talk about it, but that 80 per cent of doctors deny

this and believe that the patient should not be told. Dying patients tend to be avoided by the consultants and senior nursing staff. Talking with the dying patient is often left to the most junior staff members who, perforce, become evasive and uncertain while facing the patient. Thus the patient's suffering is compounded and he may even feel like a leper.

The controversial decision of whether "to tell or not to tell" is in fact a false dichotomy and very much exaggerated as a dilemma facing the team. Most doctors who have done research in this area agree that forming a trusting personal relationship with the doctor enables those patients who are ready to do so to ask about their condition. The doctor may need to indicate to the patient that he is prepared to talk about the situation by referring to the topic of his prognosis in general terms. It seems advisable to give the patient the most optimistic but truthful account of his prospects in terms of their probable outcome. This is important because of the tendency of patients to distort their prospects one way or another, or to misunderstand simple anatomy and physiology. To find out in detail from the patient what he really thinks is wrong may be a salutary experience. The doctor who takes time to do this will often be amazed at some of the misunderstandings shown by the patient. Clarification in this way will improve the patient's trust in the doctor and his ability to co-operate with the treatment. It is also important to give the patient the understanding that the distressing accompaniments of terminal illness such as dyspnoea, nausea and pain will be vigorously and adequately treated.

As already pointed out, patients must be enabled to express their sadness and disappointments, their fears and feelings of loss. In turn the doctor must be enabled to cope with the patient's occasional expression of hostility and disappointment, together with his own feelings of inadequacy at being unable to prevent the progress of the illness. The patient's feelings of shame and guilt over regressing to infantile dependency on nursing staff or at being incontinent, must be dealt with by simple reassurance in a calm accepting manner by all concerned.

Those with firm religious beliefs or who are confirmed atheists are better able to cope with the idea of death than those who are lukewarm half-believers. This latter category may need more emotional help than those of stronger faith.

COMING TO TERMS WITH SERIOUS ILLNESS

Multiple sclerosis

Based upon their personal experience of the illness the Burnfields have described the common psychological problems in multiple sclerosis (Burnfield, A. and Burnfield, P., 1978). They explain that a person is very often shocked on learning the diagnosis even though they might have suspected it previously. Reactions of fear, anger and denial may occur as in other serious illnesses. This is usually followed by a normal expression of grief and depressive symptoms with feelings of loss. Following this there comes a period of slow adjustment in establishing a new identity, based on a feeling of acceptance of their limitations. They point out that the process is similar to bereavement, is normal, and must neither be discouraged nor over-indulged. Lack of expression of these feelings may lead to later symptom formation and poor adjustment. They point out that the widely-reported euphoria in multiple sclerosis may mask underlying depression and is a cover against an intolerable situation. Various C.N.S. lesions interacting with emotional problems lead to increasing degrees of handicap and may be particularly disabling unless the patients receive adequate counselling and support. This may be carried out by the family doctor if he feels confident to do so, or by a specialised counsellor or a member of the psychiatric team.

Surridge and Jambor investigated the intellectual loss associated with multiple sclerosis and showed that two-thirds of the patients with multiple sclerosis showed the typical patchy dementia, with impairment of conceptual thinking and perseveration. They suggested that classical euphoria was very significantly correlated with intellectual loss and denial of disability (Surridge, 1969; Jambor, 1969).

Mental problems arise in a variety of chronic progressive diseases such as rheumatoid arthritis whose victims often show feelings of resentment and hostility (*British Medical Journal*, 1969). It has been suggested that in such cases, when doctors are untrained in psychiatry, psychological symptoms are more easily elicited by the use of standardised questionnaires to detect anxiety, depression and aggression. It has been pointed out that, unless psychiatric symptoms are treated in these cases by psychotherapeutic and other measures, worsening of the disease process occurs with rapid deterioration.

Maintenance haemodialysis

New technologies bring with them new problems to the medical team. It must come as something of a surprise to many doctors that their patients are far from being grateful, initially, for being put on the life-saving programme. On the contrary, they are very often depressed, hostile or practising denial of their illness. Further reflection shows, of course, that it is normal to become depressed when facing the real and symbolic losses entailed in the illness and the arduous treatment regimes involved. Patients must be encouraged to work through this initial period of mourning. It was found that patients with high levels of hostility have somewhat poorer prospects of survival than those with lower levels of hostility (Daly, 1969 (a)). Similarly, many patients undergoing such treatments are markedly depressed and as such require treatment since the suicide risk is extremely high.

Early reports of dialysis focused on the obvious psychiatric difficulties of the patient undergoing treatment. With more prolonged and careful observation, it has been seen that the emotional reactions of families and the dialysis team itself are also of great importance to the outcome of the treatment. It appears that in order to survive or regain a reasonable level of rehabilitation, the patient must have a satisfactory relationship with both the social system (encompassing doctors, nurses, changed family and work relationships) and the biological-mechanical system which ensures his basic survival. Dialysis may be the prototype of many similar mechanically-based and life-saving chronic treatment methods and deserves particular attention from psychiatrists. The physician tends to have as the focus of attention the patient undergoing treatment. For this reason the family and the entire social environment are in danger of being neglected.

Amongst other writers, Engel (1962) has described the tendency of doctors to view disease in the archaic conceptual frame of a bad influence from without taking possession of the patient. The "badness" is implied in concepts such as that of the germ theory of disease which surprisingly still governs the thinking of many doctors. It is comforting for both patient and doctor to think that everything unpleasant comes from without. Perhaps more pertinent to dialysis is the mechanistic concept that views the body as a machine and disease as a condition due to a defective part. Contributing to this limited approach towards patients has been the attitude of many psychiatrists that their role in a general hospital is merely to treat patients who happen to fall ill with a psychiatric illness.

The difficulties for psychiatrists of working with other specialists should not be minimised. Hawkins attempted to unravel the causes of misunderstandings between psychiatrists and other doctors, one of the chief of which is vocabulary (Hawkins, 1962). Doctors acquire an empirical and intuitive understanding of behaviour and much of the difficulty merely lies in transmission of information. Also, there is a natural tendency to be defensive and antagonistic towards someone who claims to have more knowledge about an area that one feels one understands quite well. Thus it is sometimes easier for a physician to collaborate with a statistician, who clearly has another field of competence, than with a psychiatrist who is often unwilling to declare the limits of his territory: and psychiatrists often have their own need to appear competent in general medicine. Therefore it is not surprising that many psychiatrists are only willing to give advice or become involved when patients have clear-cut psychiatric syndromes, thus avoiding territorial disputes. Unfortunately, unified concepts of health and disease no longer permit the "cobbler to stick to his last". And the lethality of emotional maladjustment which is indicated in various studies is by no means a new concept.

The use of denial in patients undergoing chronic life-saving treatment methods is generally thought to be highly maladaptive and I found this to be so in the case of dialysis. The use of denial was significantly associated with less satisfactory outcome of treatment. It seems that patients do vary in their ability to accept an arduous role of enforced dependence on a mechanical life-support system and the experts who operate it.

The effects on the spouse of an ill person are often underestimated. The family involvement in treatment is especially important. For a long time it was thought that the physical aspects of haemodialysis treatment led to the sleep deprivation known to be associated with this illness. A paradoxical finding was that the spouses of patients on home dialysis suffered significantly more sleep deprivation than the patients themselves (Daly and Hassall, 1970). Thus psychological aspects of illness are of grave importance not only for the patient but for his family. Similarly, studies of those bereaved have shown them to be more susceptible to lethal illness (Parkes, 1969).

One must look carefully at the possibilities for prevention of emotional problems in families of those undergoing dialysis, particularly in the case of children. Very often the spouse is devoting all the time to the patient and the emotional strain on the children is marked. The need for considerable help from social workers is indicated, both for the spouse and for the children, if disability and unnecessary suffering are to be avoided.

TREATMENT METHODS

Psychopharmacology

With the current widespread over-use of psychoactive drugs there seems little point in encouraging further use of such medication. Through the activities of advertisers and because writing a prescription is an easy way out for some doctors, the fallacy has arisen that treatment in psychiatry is equated with the use of medications. But, generally speaking, personal intervention by setting aside time for discussion and support and allowing the patient to talk, meeting with the family, or referral to those who are prepared to conduct psychotherapy in more detail, are better courses of action than the prescription of psychoactive drugs. Nevertheless the fact remains that, appropriately used, psychoactive drugs are of considerable assistance when psychological symptoms arise during the course of physical illness.

There are several clear indications for the use of phenothiazines (or equivalent major tranquillisers). Thus where brain function has been impaired through systemic disease, or C.N.S. lesions, or where there has been any gross insult to the C.N.S., an organic brain syndrome may develop. In these situations it is important to prescribe phenothiazines on a regular, planned basis with appropriate adjustments in dosage. Unfortunately, too often in these situations the phenothiazine is used on a "one-off" basis. Phenothiazines should also be prescribed whenever psychotic symptoms develop, as often happens when the subjective stress of the illness combines with direct organic effects.

Most doctors nowadays are trained to recognise depression in all its forms. Nevertheless, many patients with physical illness suffer from undiagnosed and untreated depression. It is essential in these cases to make a careful diagnosis and to institute treatment where required. In those cases of severe depression which have not responded to psychoactive medication or where there is a crisis such as risk of suicide it may be appropriate, following a consultation between the various specialists concerned, to institute E.C.T. With careful anaesthesia, seriously ill, depressed people, even after myocardial infarction, may be given E.C.T.; and in some cases it may be life-saving, restoring the will to live.

Sleep and physical illness

Pain, or nausea of themselves account for only a small part of the insomnia experienced by patients undergoing physical illnesses. Hospital environments are often noisy and anxiety provoking. It is to be hoped that improved staff training, together with variable lighting and carpeting of medical and surgical wards, should improve this position. Very often there is a wish to have hypnotic medications prescribed when simple discussion and reassurance, or even a glass of milk, would suffice. Allowing the sleepless patient to read, but preventing his taking naps during the day are similar common-sense expedients.

Psychiatrists are increasingly concerned over the problems of dependence (and even addiction) diminishing long-range effectiveness, self-poisoning and withdrawal problems involved in the use of hypnotic drugs. Occasional short-term prescription of hypnotic medication is indicated during physical illness; and for various reasons, but especially because they are safer, benzodiazepine medications are generally preferred. Following withdrawal of many hypnotics there is a rebound of paradoxical or R.E.M. sleep (Priest, 1978). During this stage of sleep there is an increase, with greater variability, in heart rate, respiration and blood pressure. Thus the physician who prescribed hypnotics for his physically ill patient, say with myocardial infarction, must bear in mind the dangers during withdrawal of that medication.

Sleep disturbances occur in various physical illness. Hyperthyroidism for example causes fragmented short sleep with excessive amounts of delta. The recovery of sleep after successful treatment of thyrotoxicosis is very gradual and it may take up to a year before normal sleep patterns are achieved (Dunleavy et al., 1974). The sleep of uraemic patients has been known for some time to be grossly disturbed and many pharmacological agents commonly used for the treatment of physical illness cause insomnia. One must not forget of course that caffeine-containing beverages are very effective disturbers of sleep. Finally, it must be remembered that sleep disturbances are often the chief sign of the depressive illness accompanying physical disability.

Biofeedback

Biological feedback (biofeedback) is a technique which has developed largely on the basis of the advances in electronic technology which have taken place over recent decades. It is based on the idea of relaying physiological information back to the patient so that he is enabled to alter autonomic responses not normally subject to conscious control. The parameters used are E.E.G. (alpha waves), skin conductance, heart rate or E.M.G. Patients can be trained via these techniques to achieve muscular relaxation, decreased arousal etc. A large variety of units are now being marketed at a reasonable price. Unfortunately, there is a considerable need for more controlled clinical studies. Nevertheless there have been reports on the treatment of such problems as migraine (Sargent, 1977), arrhythmias (Weiss and Engel, 1971) and hypertension (Benson et al., 1971). Other areas involved in studies included gastrointestinal problems such as irritable colon syndromes.

Behaviour therapy

Relaxation techniques are also widely used in behaviour therapy. Most behaviour therapists reject psychodynamic considerations involving unconscious conflicts. Instead they base their treatment on alteration of learned behaviour. There has, unfortunately, been the tendency to mutual hostility and criticism between the exponents of psychotherapy and behaviour therapy. Nevertheless, a combination of psychodynamic and behaviour therapy principles can be used successfully (Aitken et al., 1971).

Doctor-patient co-operation

Very few doctors are so naive as to assume that their patients take the treatment which is prescribed in a uniform or standard way. It is known that adherence to treatment may be either exaggerated or conversely there may be non-adherence. There are extensive problems in estimating the degree to which patients comply with treatment, but one study (Park and Lipman, 1964) revealed that significant omission of medication occurs in about 50 per cent of out-patients although it is less common among in-patients. Adherence is affected not only by the nature of the illness but by its duration and the consequences of stopping medication. Hence those illnesses (such as diabetes) in which the consequences of decreasing medication are immediate and disastrous tend, not surprisingly, to promote a high degree of compliance. Obviously, the ability to pay for medications and the degree of supervision and attitudes towards illness (such as that of seeing it as God's displeasure) are as important as negative feelings about the doctor prescribing the medication. Reynolds and colleagues found that those doctors who enquired more often about improvements, gave reassurance about side-effects and were optimistic about the benefits of treatment, produced a high degree of adherence (Reynolds *et al.*, 1975). Sometimes very simple but practical expedients are important. Thus it has been found that once-daily regimes for medications increase adherence (Blackwell, 1976). Clear and comprehensible labelling is important and for the treatment of hypertension and other diseases the use of calendar packets has been shown to increase compliance.

Obviously it is essential to detect non-adherence to treatment. It is important wherever possible for the doctor to monitor adherence and to educate and motivate his patients. But there is a confounding paradox of the doctor excessively exhorting his patients to adhere closely to his advice, producing increased anxiety and fear. These patients then often tend to deny their illness and to not adhere to treatment. It is important to use non-threatening, open-ended questions to enquire about treatment adherence. The doctor can only increase his patient's compliance by educating him about his illness and its treatment. An obvious point also is that, wherever possible, treatment regimes should be adjusted to minimise side-effects and discomforts.

One example of excessive compliance with treatment is supplied by Liddell and Cotterill who reported habituation to occlusive dressings. The patients had been treated many years before for either gravitational ulcers or eczema of the skin. Although the skin of all the patients had returned to normal it was impossible to persuade them to abandon their initial therapy. They felt that several factors motivated their lonely patients. Particularly, they regarded the behaviour as attention-seeking and sympathy-seeking. Also, four of their patients were males who had successfully avoided work on the grounds of their skin disease (Liddell and Cotterill, 1973).

Groups and physical illness

The early protagonists of group psychotherapy were quick to notice that those surgical wards in which patients indulged in group inter-action in day areas had faster post-operative recovery rates. It is also well established that voluntary and self-help groups associated with a particular illness are of considerable help to both the patients and their families. Into this category would fall the British Diabetic Association established in 1934 by Dr. R. D. Lawrence and H. G. Wells. There are now groups concerned with wheelchair victims, muscular dystrophy, cystic fibrosis and mastectomy, as well as the well established groups for the deaf, the blind, epileptics, spastics, etc. Such voluntary groups provide mutual help via newsletters, advice, social friendship and helping patients to obtain specialist opinion. They also, to a lesser degree, perform the somewhat altruistic function of channelling money for research and rehabilitation.

Formal group psychotherapy is also widely reported for particular physical illnesses and some of these have been reviewed by Sclare (1977). Bastiaans and Groen described good results in the treatment of bronchial asthma with group psychotherapy and A.C.T.H. (Bastiaans and Groen, 1955). Group psychotherapy has also been used for the treatment of obesity, anorexia nervosa and other conditions but at present is used for only a small part of the spectrum of physical illness.

Similarly, formal, individual psychodynamic psychotherapy is used only to a very limited extent; and because of the doctor's time and the protracted training involved this is likely to change very little. Nevertheless for some special cases, and where the resources are available, intensive long-term individual psychotherapy can be highly effective (Bastiaans, 1977).

PSYCHOLOGICAL ASPECTS OF THE DOCTOR'S BEHAVIOUR

The physical examination should not only be thorough and pain-staking but be seen to be so by the patient. Although some patients distort the advice of the doctor, most patients will be considerably helped by a careful examination followed by suitable reassurance where appropriate. No careful history is complete without a detailed account of the psychological and social factors contributing to the ill-ness and, contrary to the belief of many doctors, patients do not take exception to, but rather welcome, enquiries in these areas. Traditionally the doctor's behaviour towards his patients has been based on intuition, but it is important to realise that the doctor too, like all other human beings, is beset with problems related to inhibitions, resistances, apprehensions and prejudices. Most doctors develop a characteristic "bed-side manner" or professional style during their training years. While this may suffice for the majority of patients, invariably occasions will arise when this rigid attitude becomes inappropriate. For this reason, to reach his maximal functioning, the doctor requires self-awareness and to understand his own emotional needs and conflicts, often originating in his own family relationships, e.g. with his parents, and sometimes having had an important motivational influence in his career choice.

Self-observation should not be a source of anxiety for the doctor. He should know, in particular, the categories of patients he tends to dislike or to avoid, e.g. elderly people, self-centred young women, or men about his father's age. If, in achieving this task, the doctor is reasonably kind and tolerant towards his idiosyncrasies then no undue anxiety may arise. By bringing them into consciousness, he thereby avoids unconsciously-motivated negative influences in the treatment situation.

With regard to "sympathy" or identifying with the patient's difficulty and distress, it is widely accepted that one must not enter into the feelings of another to the extent of becoming similarly depressed. This is particularly important in those dealing with the very seriously ill or terminal cases. Failure to maintain one's objectivity may lead to feedback of feelings of hopelessness and depression between the doctor and the patient. Some doctors once having tried this, may thereafter withdraw to a cold aloofness which is equally distressing for the patient. It is important that he understands fully the difficulties of the patient and explains this understanding to the patient, but at the same time not identify with any pessimistic feelings of the patient. Doctors who do not have a satisfactory family and recreational life of their own may experience difficulties in this task of achieving empathy.

REFERENCES

Acheson, R. M. (1969): "Social class gradients & serum uric acid in males and females", *Brit. Med. J.*, iv, 65-7.

Agate, J. (1974): "Care of the dying in geriatric departments", *Lancet*, i, 364-6.

Aitken, R. C. B., Zealley, A. K. and Rosenthal S. (1968): "Psychological and physiological measures of emotion in chronic asthmatic patients", Paper to the Annual Meeting of the Psychosomatic Research Society, 2nd November, Royal College of Physicians, London.

Aitken, R. C. B., Daly, R. J., Lister, J. A. and O'Connor, P. J. (1971): "Treatment of flying phobia in aircrew", *Amer. J. of Psychotherapy*, 25, 530-42.

Alexander, F. (1950): *Psychosomatic Medicine; Its Principles and Applications*, W. W. Norton, New York.

Apley, J. (1959): *The Child with Abdominal Pains*, Blackwell Scientific Publications, Oxford.

Barker, M. G. (1968): "Psychiatric illness after hysterectomy", *Brit. Med. J.*, ii, 91-5.

Bastiaans, J. and Groen, J. (1955): "Psychogenesis and psychotherapy of bronchial asthma", in O'Neill, D. (Ed.): *Modern Trends in Psychosomatic Medicine*, Butterworth, London.

Bastiaans, J. (1977): "Psychoanalytic psychotherapy", in Wittkower, E. D. and Warnes, H. (Eds.) *Psychosomatic Medicine*, Harper & Row, Hagerstown, Maryland.

Benson, H., Shapiro, D., Tursky, B. and Schwartz, G. E. (1971): "Decreased systolic blood pressure through operant conditioning techniques in patients with essential hypertension", *Science*, 173, 740-2.

Blackwell, B. (1976): "Treatment adherence", *Brit. J. Psychiat.*, 129, 513-31.

Bofin, P. J., O'Donnell, B., Hearne, R. and Hickey, M. (1975): "Blood alcohol levels in road traffic fatalities", *J. Irish Med. Assoc.*, 68, 23, 579-82.

British Medical Journal (1968): "Hypnosis for asthma – a controlled trial", iv, 71-6.

British Medical Journal (1969): "Mental Problems in Rheumatoid Arthritis", Leading Article in *Brit. Med. J.*, iv, 319.

Burnfield, A., and Burnfield, P. (1978): "Common psychological problems in multiple sclerosis", *Brit. Med. J.*, ii, 1193-4.

Burns, B. H. and Howell, J. B. L. (1969): "Disproportionally severe breathlessness in chronic bronchitis", *Quart. J. Med.*, 38, 277-94.

Cannon, W. B. (1915): *Bodily Changes in Pain, Hunger, Fear and Rage*, Appleton-Century-Crofts, New York.

Cannon, W. (1942): "Voodoo Death", *Amer. Anthropologist*, 44, 169-81.

Cattell, R. B., Eber, H. W. and Tatsuoka, M. M. (1970): *Handbook for the Sixteen Personality Factor Questionnaire (16PF)*, I.P.A.T., Champaign, Illinois.

Cay, E., Philip, A. and Aitken, C. (1976): "Psychological aspects of cardiac rehabilitation" in *Modern Trends in Psychosomatic Medicine 3*, Hill, O. (Ed.), Butterworth, London.

Christensen, M. S. and Mortenson, O. (1974): "Long-term prognosis in children with recurrent abdominal pains", *Arch. Dis. Childh.*, **50**, 110.

Cramond, W. A. (1970): "Psychotherapy of the dying patient", *Brit. Med. J.*, iii, 389-93.

Daly, R. J. (1969 (a)): "Psychiatric aspects of maintenance haemodialysis", *Proc. 4th Int. Congr. Nephrol., Stockholm 1969*, **3**, 121-30. (Karger, Basel/Munchen/New York, 1970).

Daly, R. J. (1969 (b)): "Hostility and chronic intermittent haemodialysis", *J. Psychosom. Res.*, **13**, 265-73.

Daly, R. J. and Hassell, C. (1970): "Reported sleep on maintenance haemodialysis", *Brit. Med. J.*, ii, 508-9.

Dimsdale, J. E. (1977): "Emotional causes of sudden death", *Am. J. Psychiat.*, **134**, 1361-1366.

Dunleavy, D. L. R., Oswald, I. and Brown, P. (1974): "Hyperthyroidism, sleep and growth hormone", *Electroenceph. clin. Neurophysiol.*, **36**, 259-63.

Engel, G. (1962): *Psychological Developments in Health and Disease*, Saunders, London.

Engel, G. (1971): "Sudden and rapid death during psychological stress", *Ann. intern. Med.*, **74**, 771-82.

Erikson, E. H. (1963): *Childhood and Society*, W. W. Norton, New York.

Finch, J. R. (1970): "Vehicular suicides", Paper read at 123rd Annual Meeting of American Psychiatric Assoc., San Francisco.

Foulds, J. A. (1965): *Personality and Personal Illness*, Tavistock Publications, London.

Freud, S. (1917): "Mourning and melancholia", *Collected Papers*, Hogarth Press, London, 1925.

Friedman, M. and Rosenman, R. H. (1959): "Association of specific overt behaviour patterns with blood and cardiovascular findings: Blood cholesterol level, blood clotting time, incidence of arcus senilis and clinical coronary artery disease", *J. Amer. Med. Assoc.*, **169**, 1286-96.

Friedman, M. *et al.* (1968): "The relationship of behaviour pattern A to the state of the coronary vasculature: A study of 51 autopsy subjects", *Amer. J. Med.*, **44**, 525-37.

Glen, A. I. M. and Cox, A. G. (1968): "Psychological factors, operative procedures and result of surgery for duodenal ulcer", *Gut*, **9**, 667-71.

Gordon, A. M. (1975): "Psychological aspects of isolator therapy in acute leukaemia", *Brit. J. Psychiat.*, **127**, 588-90.

Hawkins, D. R. (1962): "The gap between the psychiatrist and other physicians. Causes and solutions", *Psychosomatic Medicine*, 24, 94-102.

Hinton, J. (1967): *Dying*, Penguin Books, Harmondsworth.

Hirschfeld, A. H. and Behan, R. C. (1963): "The accident process", *J. Amer. Med. Ass.*, 193-9.

Jacobs, H. S. and Nararro, J. D. N. (1969): "Plasma 11-hydroxy-corticosteroid and growth hormone levels in acute medical illness", *Brit. Med. J.*, xx, 595-8.

Jambor, K. L. (1969): "Cognitive function in multiple sclerosis", *Brit. J. Psychiat.*, 115, 765-76.

Keys, A. (1972): "The epidemiology of coronary heart disease", *C.V.D. Epidemiology Newsletter*, 2-5.

Kornfeld, D. S. (1969): "Psychiatric view of the intensive care unit", *Brit. Med. J.*, i, 108-10.

Liddell, K. and Cotterill, A. A. (1973): "Habituation to occlusive dressings", *Lancet*, i, 1485-1486.

Lindemann, E. (1944): "Symptomatology and management of acute grief", *Amer. J. Psychiat.*, 101, 141-8.

Mann, F., Bowsher, D., Mumford, J., Lipton, S. and Miles, J. (1973): "Treatment of intractable pain by acupuncture", *Lancet*, ii, 57-60.

Maguire, G. P., Lee, E. G., Berugton, D. J., Kuchemann, C. S., Crabtree, R. J., Corneel, C. E. (1978): "Psychiatric problems in the first year after mastectomy", *Brit. Med. J.*, i, 963-5.

Miller, H. (1961): "Transport accidents", *Brit. Med. J.*, i, 919-25.

Morris, J. N., Marr, J. W. and Clayton, D. J. (1977): "Diet and heart: A postscript", *Brit. Med. J.*, ii, 1301-68.

Park, L. C. and Lipman, R. S. (1964): "A comparison of patient dosage deviation, reports, pill count", *Psychopharmacologia*, 6, 299-302.

Parkes, C. M. (1969): "Effects of bereavement on physical and mental health – a study of the medical records of widows", *Brit. Med. J.*, ii, 274-9.

Priest, R. G. (1978): "Treatment of sleep disorders" in Gaind, R. and Barbara Hudson (Eds.): *Current Themes in Psychiatry*, Macmillan, London.

Rahe, R., Floistad, I. and Bergan, T. (1974): "A model for life changes and illness research", *Arch. Gen. Psychiat.*, 31, 172-7.

Rees, D. E. (1972): "The distress of dying", *Brit. Med. J.*, iii, 105-7.

Reynolds, E., Joyce, C. R. B., Swift, J. L., Tooley, R. H. and Weatherall, M. (1965): "Psychological and clinical investigations of the treatment of anxious out-patients with three barbiturates and placebo", *Brit. J. Psychiat.*, 111, 84-95.

Rosenman, R. H., Brand, R., Jenkins, D., Friedman, M., Straws,

R. and Wurm, M. (1975): "Coronary heart disease in Western collaborative group study", *J. Amer. Med. Ass.*, **233**, 872-7.

Russell Davis, D. (1958): "Human errors and transport accidents", *Ergonomics*, **2**, 24-33.

Russell Davis, D. (1966): "Railway signals passed at danger: the drivers, circumstances and psychological processes", *Ergonomics*, **9**, 211-22.

Rutter, M. (1963): "Psychological factors in the short-term prognosis of physical disease: (1) peptic ulcer", *J. Psychosom. Res.*, **7**, 45-60.

Sargent, J. D. (1977): "Biofeedback and biocybernetics" in *Psychosomatic Medicine*, Wittkower, E. D. and Warnes, H. (Eds.), Harper & Row, Hagerstown, Maryland.

Schmidt, Chester W. Jn., Perlin, S. and Dizmang, P. (1970): "Vehicular suicides and driver fatalities, single car accidents", Paper read at 123rd Annual Meeting of Amer. Psychiat. Assoc., San Francisco.

Sclare, A. B. (1977): "Group therapy for specific psychosomatic problems", in *Psychosomatic Medicine*, Wittkower, E. D. and Warnes, H. (Eds.), Harper & Row, Hagerstown, Maryland.

Selzer, M. L. and Payne, C. E. (1962). "Automobile accidents, suicide and unconscious motivation", *Amer. J. Psychiat.*, **119**, 237-40.

Simpson, J. P., Glynn, C. J., Cox, A. G. and Folkard, S. (1976): "Comparative study of short-term recovery of mental efficiency after anaesthesia", *Brit. Med. J.*, i, 1560-2.

Surridge, D. (1969): "An investigation into some psychiatric aspects of multiple sclerosis", *Brit. J. Psychiat.*, **115**, 749-64.

Sweet, W. H. (1980): "Neuropeptides and Monoaminergic Neurotransmitters: their relation to pain", *J. Roy. Soc. Med.*, **73**, 1955.

Weisman, A. and Hackett, T. (1961): "Predilection to death", *Psychosom. Med.*, **23**, 232-56.

Weiss, T. & Engel, B. (1971): "Operant conditioning of heart rate in patients with premature ventricular contractions", *Psychosom. Med.*, **33**, 301-21.

Whitlock, F. A. (1961): "Some psychiatric consequences of gastrectomy", *Brit. Med. J.*, i, 1560.

Zola, I. K. (1966): "Culture and symptoms: An analysis of patients presenting complaints", *Amer. Sociol. Rev.*, **21**, 615-30.

FURTHER READING

Psychosomatic Medicine, Wittkower, E. D. and Warnes, H. (Eds.), Harper & Row, Hagerstown, Maryland, 1977.

Modern Trends in Psychosomatic Medicine 3, Oscar W. Hill (Ed.), Butterworth, London, 1976.

Dying, Hinton, J., Penguin Books, Harmondsworth, 1967.

Coping with Mental Handicap

Dr. Alexander Shapiro,
C.B.E., M.D., F.R.C.Psych.
Senior Lecturer in Mental Handicap, Middlesex Hospital Medical School, London.
Formerly Consultant Psychiatrist, Harperbury Hospital and Consultant in Mental Handicap, Middlesex and Royal Free Hospitals, London.

Dr. Marian Leyshon,
B.Sc., M.B., B.Ch., D.P.M., M.R.C.Psych.
Consultant Psychiatrist in Mental Handicap, Harperbury Hospital, Radlett, Herts., England.

Coping with Mental Handicap

INTRODUCTION

Mental handicap is caused by a multitude of disparate conditions having in common the fact that they produce social inadequacy. As children are incapable of social independence, a somewhat different definition is used and the ability to learn, instead of the social capacity, becomes the criterion for assessment. It is usually assumed that the social inadequacy is produced by low intelligence, yet this is not the whole story, as personality disorder and psychiatric disturbance can affect social competence profoundly, and it is the additive effect of these deleterious factors that determine whether the individual is capable of functioning competently within the social group in which he lives. The social matrix in which the individual lives can markedly affect the success or failure, as different cultures make different demands upon their members and have different expectations of minimal skills and abilities. For example, a primitive, illiterate community makes much less demand on academic abilities, but makes greater demand on other abilities to ensure the survival of the individual, whereas our culture expects its members to be literate so that the inability to acquire this skill constitutes a grave disadvantage. The immediate environment in the same culture may also affect success or failure: an individual living in an accepting and caring family can adapt to the demands and expectations within the community much more easily than if struggling to maintain himself alone.

There is a further limitation to the concept of mental handicap: and that is for a condition to be considered as causing mental handicap, it should have been acting upon the mind before it stopped growing and developing. The limit for this period is said to be up to the age of 18.

Intelligence is a concept, which, although well understood pragmatically, has defied strict definition. Definitions have varied from: "It is the quality that intelligence tests test", to Spearman's "Capacity for eduction of relations and the eduction of correlates"

(Spearman, 1911). Perhaps more helpful definitions are those of Burt: "Innate all round intellectual ability" (Burt, 1937), or Wechsler: "Intelligence is the aggregate or global capacity of the individual to act purposefully, to think rationally and so deal effectively with his environment" (Wechsler, 1958). There are still discussions as to whether intelligence is a single faculty or whether there is a number of intelligences such as verbal, mechanical, mathematical and so on.

Low intelligence can be produced through two different mechanisms. The first is poor intellectual endowment, and the second is due to some pathological factor which interferes with mental functioning. Non-pathological, poor intellectual endowment is due to the fact that intelligence being a normal biological characteristic (just like height, weight or strength etc.) is distributed normally along a Gaussian curve. The measure of dispersion (or variability) of a natural characteristic is a statistical measure known as Standard Deviation (S.D.) from the mean. It is so chosen that roughly two-thirds (68 per cent) of a normal population fall within + 1 S.D. and − 1 S.D. from the mean. With one-sixth lying above and one-sixth below these measurements, 95 per cent (95.5 per cent) fall within ± 2 S.D., and practically the total population falls within ± 3 S.D. (99.73 per cent), so that effectively there is a limit beyond which normal variation does not exceed. As will be seen later (p. 314), modern intelligence tests have a S.D. of 15 points of intelligence quotient (I.Q.), so that to all intents and purposes intelligence due to normal variation does not fall below an I.Q. of 55 points. Furthermore, the more the intelligence deviates from the mean, the fewer affected persons there will be (there will be 34 per cent with intelligence from normal to I.Q. 85, 13.5 per cent with intelligence from I.Q. 85 to 70 and only 2.5 per cent with an I.Q. below 70. Such limits do not operate when the intelligence is depressed by a pathological lesion which, if severe enough, can reduce intelligence virtually to zero. Hence in cases of very severe intellectual defect, we may suspect the presence of pathology. Stature is a good analogy. Short stature may be due to normal height variation, particularly if the individual comes from short stock — or it may be pathological dwarfism. The shorter the stature the more it is likely to be due to pathology, and extremes of dwarfism are almost invariably due to pathology such as achondroplasia.

INTELLIGENCE TESTS

Intelligence is measured by intelligence tests. The function of intelligence tests is to measure innate ability, and to assess the individual's potential rather than his achievement. They were originally developed by Binet to measure the educational potential of Paris school children in the first decade of this century.

Ideally, therefore, an intelligence test should be free of any measurement which depends on educational attainment or where cultural or social factors influence the score. Such an ideal has proved to be unattainable, but in practice, when testing persons with the same educational and cultural backgrounds, the tests do give acceptable results. A useful test should be both *reliable*, i.e. show little fluctuation in results when the test is administered on successive occasions, and also a *valid* measure of intelligence, and not of some other irrelevant factor such as dexterity or acuity of vision. It is important to keep in mind that test results are easily influenced by such factors as motivation, fatigue, emotional state, practice effect on retesting, and so on, and, therefore, no test has absolute reliability. Validity is even harder to establish, and in the final count amounts to the correlation between the test results, the theories held by the test designer, and also on the standardisation to which the test has been subjected during its developmental states.

The daunting catalogue of potential errors may put the clinicians completely off intelligence tests. In practice, however, provided one uses regularly the same test, that one is aware of the variability of the results and that one does not use test results as absolute measurements, but rather as approximations and indications of function, they can be of very great value in helping with the total assessment of an individual's potential. In this connection the highest results (if not due to errors of technique in administration, or to practice results) are much more significant than low results, which may have been occasioned by irrelevant factors which impair performance (e.g. apprehension, emotional disturbance and psychotic episodes). As the test constitutes an interview under very standardised conditions, the test situation can also furnish the experienced test administrator with a considerable amount of information on the emotional state and personality of the patient.

The unit of measurement of intelligence is a point of I.Q. which is equivalent to a percentage. This is derived from the fact that Binet's pioneer tests were designed to test children, and that children were assessed as having a certain "mental age", i.e. being able to answer questions and solve problems that a normal child of that age can do. Obviously the mental age of a child is meaningless unless its real (or chronological) age is taken into account. The intelligence quotient is calculated by dividing the mental age (M.A.) by the chronological age (C.A.) and multiplying by 100 to get rid of decimals. Thus a child with a M.A. of 5 when he is 5 will have an I.Q. of 100 (M.A. of 5 divided by a C.A. of 5 and multiplied by 100. A child of 10 with the same M.A. of 5 will only have an I.Q. of 50 (M.A. of 5 divided by a C.A. of 10 and multiplied by 100).

Such a measure is accurate enough when dealing with children up to the ages of 10 to 11. With older children, and especially with adults, considerable adjustment to the score is necessary, due to the fact that after this age the development of intelligence slows down and stops completely at the ages of 15 to 18 years on attaining the adult level. After that a slow decline occurs which increases with the years, and regresses to senile intellectual deterioration (though this process is a very variable one). The analogy with height of children gives a visual illustration of this process.

Another problem with tests for adolescents and adults is to ensure the evenness of measurement. If a test is too easy most people will get the results right, and if it is too difficult most will fail, and in either case the test will not discriminate between people of varying abilities.

It was to get round these difficulties that modern tests such as the Wechsler Adult Intelligence Scale (W.A.I.S.) were designed so as to have a standard deviation (S.D.) of 15 points I.Q. (This means that, as has already been stated, 16 per cent of the total population have an I.Q. below 85 (which equals 1 S.D.) and 2.5 below I.Q. 70 (which equals 2 S.D.). There is a negligible number of people who fall below an I.Q. of 55 (which equals 3 S.D.).

The practical consequences of all this are: firstly that the lower the I.Q. the greater is the probability that there is some pathology at work; and below an I.Q. of 50 the probability is that all cases are due to pathological causes. Secondly, and this is very important, that there is no cut-off point which divides the normal from the subnormal I.Q. For as intelligence diminishes the affected individual enters a zone of vulnerability in which unaided social survival becomes progressively less likely and more dependent on optimal environmental conditions, which include social support and supervision. To draw an arbitrary line at I.Q. 70, as has been suggested in the past because it is a convenient statistical point (equalling 2 S.D. from the mean), is highly unrealistic when dealing with individuals rather than defining categories. This is all the more so when it is considered that social competence, with which we are concerned, is the cumulative result of the effect of a number of factors of which intelligence is but one, albeit an important one.

In dealing with individuals we need an approach which can perhaps be best described as a "clinical" one, in which each case is treated as if it were unique rather than a member of a category. When assessing a handicapped person, and deciding on the optimal action to be taken in his, his family's and in the community's interests, the clinician would have to weigh carefully all the relevant factors at work and be aware that the claims of the different people concerned may be conflicting. It is also important to realise that the decision taken may be valid at the time when it is made, and may have to be altered as the circumstances vary, for the circumstances may affect markedly the social adjustment.

Thirdly, it is important, therefore, to realise that mental handicap is not a permanent and immutable condition as has been claimed by the early workers such as Doll (1941) but on the contrary, a variable condition dependent on external environmental factors, as well as on internal ones such as the presence or absence of personality disorder or of psychiatric symptoms etc., so that in one person widely varying performances can occur all in the presence of the same level of intelligence. The concept of "being liable to be dealt with" which was written into the Mental Deficiency Acts, but dropped from the Mental Health Act 1959 is a very useful one.

Although intelligence tests proliferated in the twenties and thirties, the number of tests now in clinical use is limited. This is an advantage, as the clinician has the same comparable yardstick, and has not to make allowances for the varying effects of different tests. The test used most constantly was the original Binet test in its English adaptation by Burt, and then in the standard versions produced by Terman and his successors at Stanford University in the U.S.A. The latest revision of the Stanford-Binet was published in 1960. Like its predecessors, it measures the mental age from 2 to 18 years, and at each age there is a number of items to be solved (these are called subtests — the whole integral test is referred to usually as a "battery" of tests or as a scale). These vary from such items as obeying simple commands, repeating digits, pointing to objects on a picture and stringing beads (at the age of 2) to a measure of vocabulary pointing out verbal absurdities, defining abstract words, and completing sentences (at the age of 18). This test is still very widely used for children.

The universal test used for adults is the Wechsler Adult Intelligence Scale (W.A.I.S.) which, as has already been pointed out, was devised and standardised on adults. The subtests are classified as being "verbal" or "performance" and conclusions about emotional and personality disturbances can be drawn from the imbalance of the two parts of the test (or scale as it is officially called). One problem is that this division does not correspond to any of the theoretical factors or types of intelligence. The test was designed for clinical use, and was developed in the Bellevue Hospital in New York, and the balance between the different subtests can be a useful measure of intellectual deterioration. In mental handicap practice this test has become established as the standard test, with the advantage that results obtained in different places, and at different times, can be easily compared, and improvements and deterioration assessed over the years. When compared to the results obtained on the Stanford-Binet test the W.A.I.S. usually yields a result which exceeds the former by 5 to 10 points I.Q.

Psychologists using the W.A.I.S. as routine, have tended to use the Wechsler Intelligence Scale for Children (W.I.S.C.) in preference to Binet, as it gives a comparable result to the Adult Scale, and provides a continuity in longitudinal studies. This scale too gives a somewhat higher result than the Stanford-Binet test.

In individuals in whom there is a language difficulty, there are so-called non-verbal tests of intelligence, of which the commonest in use are the Raven Matrices. They are most useful in testing people of normal or near normal intelligence, who do not speak English; they are too difficult for those patients where inability to communicate is not a linguistic, but an intellectual problem.

Young babies below the age of 2 years present special problems as there are very rapid changes in physical development at the same time that the intelligence is insufficiently developed for direct measurement. One resorts, therefore, to total developmental assessment and results are expressed as developmental quotients (D.Q.s) on the assumption that the normal development of the locomotor or sensory systems will be consistent with intellectual development when this can be measured direct. The pioneer of developmental studies was Gesell with his Developmental Scale (Gesell and Amatruda, 1947). Since Ruth Griffiths introduced her Developmental Scale (Griffiths, 1955) which was standardised on British babies (Gesell worked in the U.S.A.) the tendency in the United Kingdom is to use her test. There is still no firm agreement about the predictive value of developmental scales for the ultimate attainments of adults, but like other tests this one gives measurements that are of great value for longitudinal assessments.

Usual tests such as those that have been described cannot be used in the presence of physical or sensory handicap. Special tests have been designed for testing the blind, the deaf, and those afflicted by cerebral palsy. The testing of these handicapped people is fraught with special difficulties, and reliable results can only be obtained by specially trained and experienced testers.

There has been a tendency of late for some psychologists to decry the use of tests, because of theoretical considerations and their occasional unreliability. The authors, however, tend to agree with those of their psychologist colleagues who consider that, as long as one is aware of the fallibilities of tests, and as long as one is not likely to assume an unrealistic accuracy just because the result is given as a number, psychometric testing in skilled hands is a very valuable ontribution to the full clinical assessment of an individual with handicaps.

Scales of social attainments are of particular value in measuring the progress of the mentally handicapped. The Vineland social maturity scale is such a measurement (Doll, 1953), presenting eight sets of items to determine social ability. These measure general self help, occupation, communication, socialisation and motor ability. Gunzburg also developed scales of social ability in the form of a set of circular charts exhibiting social skills in sectors (Gunzburg, 1963).

These are referred to as "Progress Assessment Charts of Social and Personal Development".

Before a brief consideration of clinical aspects, a note on nomenclature is given below to clarify the terms in use.

NOMENCLATURE OF MENTAL HANDICAP

In the early years of the 19th century, when modern scientific study of mental handicap can be said to have begun with the pioneer work of Itard and Seguin, the term "idiot" was used loosely to denote all grades of mental handicap. This was the term used in the first legislation on mental handicap in this country in the 1886 Idiot's Act and it survives anachronistically in the professional term *"Idiot Savant"* (a mentally-handicapped person who has an extraordinary ability in one isolated area, e.g. remembering dates, quick calculations) and in common usage in the term "village idiot". By the end of the century the term "mental deficiency" had become the established term in the United Kingdom and in the U.S.A. The terms "feeble-minded", "imbecile", and "idiot" became used to designate the severity of mental handicap (or defect), so that the term feeble-minded (or moron in the U.S.A.) referred to the less severely affected, imbecile to moderately affected and idiot to the profoundly affected person. As these terms acquired pejorative meaning in common parlance, and were disadvantageous to the handicapped, the nomenclature was changed. The Americans used the term mental retardation, and the people affected have tended to be called "retardates" — this term was adopted by W.H.O. In the context of mental handicap it was an unfortunate choice as the word *retardation* is already used in general psychiatry to describe a symptom of depression and, in the field of mental handicap, to describe backwardness in development due to the stunting effect of an adverse environment.

In the U.K. the terms "subnormality" and "severe subnormality" have been introduced by the Mental Health Act of 1959. These terms, too, are unsatisfactory as, apart from the fact that many mentally handicapped persons are abnormal as well as subnormal, "subnormality" is confusing, as it can either refer to the whole subject of mental handicap or, as a distinction from "severe subnormality", refer only to the less severely affected. Because of this terminological confusion the late Richard Crossman, when he was Secretary of State for the Department of Health and Social Security, introduced the much more satisfactory term "mental handicap" which has been used since on all official documents, and has come to be generally accepted.

In addition to these terms, the medical profession uses occasionally the term "amentia" usually in a context which distinguishes it from dementia — the difference being that in amentia the mind never reached its normal development, whereas in dementia there has been deterioration in an individual who had in the past been of normal intelligence. As has already been stated the term mental handicap or any of its synonyms are applied to those conditions where the damage was caused to a developing brain, which in consequence had not reached normal development. Very occasionally the term is used in naming a syndrome or a nosological condition as in "naevoid amentia". On the European continent the term "oligophrenia" is in common medical use, and has on occasions been used in English speaking countries.

CLINICAL ASPECTS OF MENTAL HANDICAP

It is not within the frame of reference of this chapter to discuss classification and clinical manifestations of the various conditions producing mental handicap: so the authors restrict themselves to a few basic comments and refer the reader to standard texts on the condition such as Hilliard and Kirman (1965) or a short introductory text, such as Heaton-Ward's (1975).

Mental handicap is caused by a large number of conditions some of which are relatively rare and, therefore, not by a unitary condition. As the developing mind is more vulnerable to disease and injury, most of the conditions operate in early childhood and a considerable number prenatally. Genetic and intra-uterine factors play a very important part. Perinatal conditions are still important in spite of improved antenatal care. Postnatal conditions are equally important and range from trauma and infection to those conditions which interfere with the development of intelligence such as malnutrition and adverse environment which produces inadequate stimulation; or interference with learning and communication through disease such as cerebral palsy, or epilepsy, sensory handicaps or emotional deprivation.

For human intelligence to develop fully, the child must be given full opportunity to explore his world, and to learn from contact with adults and his peers. If these opportunities are denied or interfered with, intellectual development is stunted. Sensory handicaps, particularly if unrecognised, can interfere powerfully with this process, and can be disastrous. High tone deafness deserves special mention in this connection. Some children do not appear to be deaf as they respond to loud noises, but as they cannot hear the higher tones, which are essential to the intelligibility of consonants, they cannot understand the meaning of speech. These children, therefore, may be thought to be mentally rather than sensorily handicapped. Cerebral palsy also can affect adversely the development of intelligence, in addition to the effect of any cortical lesion, which produces primary disability. This occurs because the paralysis and extensor spasms interfere with the baby's normal exploration of his own body and surroundings, and development of a correlation between tactile, visual and other sensory modalities. It is for these reasons that the accurate assessment of the sensory and motor state of a young child suspected of mental handicap is of extreme importance.

The disastrous effect of maternal deprivation upon a young baby has been known for a long time now, and evidence has been accumulating for the last couple of decades that poor material environment and lack of stimulation in disadvantaged families can have a very severe and adverse effect on children, especially if associated with maternal deprivation. Although the severe malnutrition that has been shown to affect physical as well as mental development in the third world (Cravioto *et al.*, 1966) is not normally operative in the U.K., studies in this country and in the U.S.A. have shown that intellectual development is impaired in greater degree as one descends through the social classes. There is good evidence that this effect is not a genetic one as had been supposed in the past, but rather the effect of a dreary, unstimulating environment, social and intellectual, to which such children are subjected. These facts hold out hope that the manipulation of the social environment and educational stimulation may prevent, in a considerable number of people, the development of mild handicap, and thus make them capable of functioning as normal individuals.

There is a hierarchy of aims in the treatment and management of the mentally handicapped as follows:

(a) prevention;
(b) treatment;
(c) management.

It is obvious that one has to have recourse to treatment only when prevention fails or preventive measures do not exist or prove unavailing. By the same token, management becomes necessary only if treatment is incapable of curing the pathological conditions. The fact that so many of our activities are concerned with management is a measure of our ignorance about mental handicap and our inability to prevent and cure. The ignorance which still exists about mental handicap is a challenge for study and research.

Prevention
Preventive measures fall under several headings as follows.

1. *Immunisation*
This concerns the creation through general public health measures of a population which is immune to the effect of agents that can produce mental handicap.

Immunisation against rubella of women before child bearing age, and the use of anti D immunoglobulin in Rh-negative pregnant women, are examples of such measures. Prevention of exposure to infection of women in the early stage of pregnancy — and active treatment if any infections do occur — are also important. It is hoped that the development of anti-cytomegalovirus vaccine will be the next important step in the prevention of handicap due to intra-uterine infection.

2. *Genetic counselling*
Recent developments that have made it possible to diagnose with a considerable amount of confidence heterozygote carriers of recessive inborn errors of metabolism have made the genetic counselling more certain. Conditions where this is possible include phenylketonuria, galactosaemia, and hepato-lenticular degeneration. The setting up of "at risk" registers can be of great value in ensuring that potential heterozygotes can be offered diagnostic help without waiting for the birth of an affected child to draw attention to the existence of a genetic hazard.

3. *Antenatal diagnosis*
An increasing number of conditions can be diagnosed by examination of maternal serum. In addition to obvious investigations such as that of Wasserman reaction it is now possible to detect alphafeta proteins in the maternal serum, and this makes possible the diagnosis of spina bifida.

The development of amniocentesis has proved a great advance in prenatal screening. This is a procedure in which a specimen of amniotic fluid is withdrawn from the uterine cavity at the fourteenth week of pregnancy. The fluid is investigated for enzyme deficiencies such as that found in Tay-Sachs disease, and for the presence of alphafeta proteins signifying a neural tube abnormality such as spina bifida. The foetal cells are cultured and examined for chromosome abnormalities such as those found in Down's syndrome (mongolism), and karyotyped for sex chromosome abnormalities. If such a procedure could be offered to all pregnant women over 40 — or ideally over 35 (when owing to the effects of maternal age the liability to have affected babies rises sharply) — then it has been calculated the incidence of conditions of mental handicap due to chromosome disturbance could be very considerably reduced.

The prevention is achieved by termination of pregnancy. Here as in other fields of medicine, advances of scientific techniques bring in their wake problems of medical and general ethics. The decision whether a pregnancy is terminated or not must be left to the parents. Any other course of action is an infringement of personal freedom, and not tolerable in our society. The fact that the community at large has to bear the cost of the handicapped if the parents decline to avail themselves of the possibility of termination of pregnancy, is a small enough price to pay for having a free society, which respects the individual. It may, however, be very difficult for the prospective parents to make their minds up, especially as they may be suffering from emotional stress caused by the realisation that they are about to have a mentally-handicapped child. It is essential that they should be given full information on the situation in terms intelligible to a lay person. They should be encouraged and supported to form their own judgment, rather than have a ready made decision thrust upon them, no matter how clear the issue may appear to professional eyes. Such help must include the discussion of the unconscious meaning of the situation, and their emotional reaction to it, as well as the objective facts of the case.

4. Obstetric factors

Careful attention to maternal health during the antenatal period, skilful management of labour, and the management of neonatal crises has a considerable result on the incidence of handicap due to perinatal causes.

One aspect, however, needs special mention and that is the relationship of low birth weight and mental handicap. Modern advances in intensive care of premature and low weight babies have resulted in survival of a large number of these babies who not so long ago would not have been considered viable. As prematurity and low birth weight in a number of cases are the consequence rather than the cause of abnormalities, it means that there is an increased survival of handicapped children. The latest figures indicate that if the low birth weight is not extreme, i.e. below a birth weight of 1½ kilograms, then prognosis is not as bad as it originally had been feared. However, this is an area that requires, and is receiving, due attention from obstetricians and neonatal paediatricians.

5. Social and economic factors

It has been shown conclusively that the correction of early adverse environment can reverse the damage that has been done, and it would appear that correction of handicap due to the influence of these factors should be relatively easy. Unfortunately, however, children who have been placed temporarily in a favourable environment, relapse fairly rapidly when they return to their families, if the families continue to live under conditions of poverty and deprivation. The cure obviously is the general improvement of living conditions of a large proportion of the world's population, a need which so far has taxed the ingenuity and goodwill of all the national and international agencies. However, within the framework of the local scene, careful and intensive work by social and educational agencies can minimise considerably the educational and intellectual retardation which still occurs even in the countries which are economically more favourable.

Treatment

Treatment of the mentally handicapped is also progressing and developing. The criterion of incurability proposed by some early workers and responsible for much therapeutic nihilism (Doll, 1941) is no longer tenable. Either complete cure, or a close approximation to normality, is now possible with many of the inborn errors of metabolism, such as phenylketonuria and maple syrup urine disease. This is at present achieved by dietary control, but it is hoped that in the future the preparation of the missing enzymes will make the unpleasant and stringent diets no longer necessary. This is already possible in cretinism. Medication is also effective in hepatolenticular degeneration which responds to treatment by penicillamine.

Epilepsy is another condition which responds to medication although it cannot be said to be permanently cured. However, controlled medication not only affects the incidence of seizures, but also secondary manifestations such as personality disorders and capacity for learning. The latter is particularly important in the cases of children in whom the presence of seizures, and particularly of *petit mal* seizures, can seriously interfere with the development of intelligence.

Cerebral palsy is another area where recent developments have been of great help. Physiological methods of treatment such as those developed by the Bobaths (1956) can effect considerable improvement in control of movements and mobility. Although physiotherapy cannot cure completely, it can produce enough improvement to free a child sufficiently from the constraints of its neurological lesion to allow it to develop mentally. It must be realised that the limits of neurological and intellectual improvement are set by the severity of the cerebral lesion, but that the intellectual state is independent of the severity of the neurological condition; so that severely incapacitated children who appear to function on a very restricted intellectual level are capable of showing surprising increases in ability following successful treatment. It goes without saying that the cerebral palsied child requires a "total push" approach: mental stimulation and training in social skills must proceed *pari passu* with physical treatment.

Mentally handicapped people are subjected to mental illness as are people of normal intelligence. The clinical features are sometimes modified thus making identification of the illness a diagnostic challenge. Diagnostic problems arise particularly amongst the severely subnormal who may have little or no powers of verbal communication. Both psychoses and neuroses occur in the mentally handicapped, and may often be the precipitating factor in the need for hospitalisation.

Treatment of the illness is essential, as the presence of mental illness will limit considerably the level of functioning of the individual. Medication is proving very effective especially in the treatment of depressive illness and schizophrenia in the mentally handicapped.

Management

Management is the provision of facilities to those people whose disability cannot be cured, but can be alleviated. The fact that management looms so large in the field of mental handicap is a reflection on our therapeutic impotence at present. In its widest context, it includes education and training specially devised for the handicapped, which although particularly important in the case of children, must be prolonged into adult life because of slower maturation, and slower learning processes of the mentally handicapped. There is, however, an unfortunate tendency among those involved in the provision of services to the mentally handicapped only to think and talk in terms of training at all ages. It is essential to realise that an adult mentally-handicapped person has the social and emotional needs of an adult and not of a child, and that when dealing with adults our concern should be the creation of a pattern of life which should be as satisfying and as stimulating as possible.

It is hoped that the period of training and education would have adapted the handicapped person to function as well as he is able, and sufficiently adequately to do so in the community. Should the disabilities prove to be too great, then it becomes our task to create a special environment which should be supportive, and which should minimise the patient's disabilities as much as possible; such a process has been described as social splinting. In a word our aim is to adapt the handicapped to his social and cultural environment, but should this be impossible then we have to adapt the environment to the individual.

When organising management the following considerations are relevant to the planning and provision of optimal systems of care, and should be discussed before describing the available provisions.

(*i*) There is a wide range in the severity of the disabilities requiring vastly different provisions of care.

(*ii*) There are radical differences between the needs of, and therefore, the services required for adults and children.

(*iii*) In deciding the best course to take, it is important to consider the family and the community at large, as well as the handicapped person.

(iv) The handicapped need a very wide range of services which necessitate the involvement of a large number of disciplines. It is essential that they should be integrated to ensure their optimal effect.

(v) Disabilities fluctuate — the services should, therefore, be flexible enough to accommodate themselves smoothly and rapidly to changing needs.

(vi) There is still no consensus of opinion on the best type of care, and this question is still the subject of much discussion and argument.

1. *Wide range of disabilities and needs*

There is a very wide variation in the severity of handicap from persons of borderline intelligence who have succumbed temporarily owing to the concatenation of adverse circumstances, to the profoundly handicapped whose abilities are those of a baby in the first months of life, and who are unable to communicate and who are completely dependent on others for the most basic care.

In general, one can divide the handicapped into three major groups the moderately affected, the profoundly handicapped and an intermediate group.

(a) The moderately affected. The first group have their intelligence mildly or moderately affected, and could live in the community more or less as normal individuals, although their contribution to the social group in which they live would be only a modest one. In these patients low intelligence alone is insufficient to cause the social breakdown, so that it is only a small minority of all people with moderately low or borderline intelligence who require therapy or other forms of help, and who come to the attention of medical and social agencies. The breakdown when it does occur is commonly due to the concurrent effect of a number of factors, some intrinsic and some external and beyond the control of the individual. In such cases the prognosis is good and, unless complicated by extraneous factors, the provision of the necessary treatment and rehabilitation, and if need be the manipulation of the social environment, should result in the return of the patient to the community as an acceptable member of society. In dealing with these cases, the aim is the adaptation of the mentally handicapped person to his social role as an acceptable and contributing member of the group to which he will belong. This includes familiarity with the expected modes of behaviour, in work and leisure situations. In rehabilitating this type of patient, it is important to ensure his assimilation into the social group and if the social group within which the patient lives only partially accepts the handicapped person then there may be serious consequences stemming from this partial rejection; this matter will be discussed later on in this chapter.

(b) The profoundly handicapped. At the other extreme, we have the profoundly handicapped, often suffering from multiple handicaps, for the conditions which produce such extreme damage to intelligence, either through a lesion or maldevelopment, are bound to affect other systems – in particular the central nervous system producing severe neurological conditions. Such people are completely isolated by their profound handicap, and will require total care throughout their lives; they will have but a tenuous awareness and contact with their environment, both social and material. Their isolation will continue wherever they are, and beyond giving them the care they require such as feeding, toileting and dressing, the most one can hope for is to achieve habit training and the communication of their basic needs. (An interesting new development is the attempt to teach signs indicating basic needs to non-communicating patients, i.e. who are incapable of speech.) This gloomy prognosis is given advisedly, for too sanguine expectations of progress by parents and staff can lead to heart-break and feelings of guilt. On the other hand, these patients may be capable of emotional response, and their very helplessness can forge a rewarding emotional link between them and those who care for them.

(c) An intermediate group. Between these two groups, we find an intermediate group, which is very important from the point of view of management. It consists of individuals who are capable of self-care, such as dressing, washing, attending to their toilet, and feeding; their speech usually is sufficiently well developed to allow them to communicate freely, although their ideation is limited and their interests restricted. They lack usual items of knowledge and information, which are taken for granted in normal individuals, and what they have is usually limited to awareness of events in their immediate environment; and their conception of the world at large is limited and nebulous. They are usually illiterate and have very limited capacity to deal with numerical concepts, and normally cannot go beyond counting on their fingers, and adding or subtracting single digits. They are thus incapable of planning their future, tend to be very unrealistic in assessing their life situation, and are unable to take decisions which necessitate any abstract thinking. They show the social and intellectual development of children within the end of the first decade of life, and require considerable supervision and guidance in their day-to-day life. On the other hand, they are capable of normal emotional and social responses, and are capable of productive and gainful employment as long as their assignments do not overtask their limited comprehension, and as long as their work does not involve complicated processes or the need to take rapid decisions. Given a sufficiently supportive and non-demanding environment, they are capable of managing their day-to-day activities.

These people will need to be under some sort of supervision or in-patient care for the rest of their lives. It is over the best type of care for them that there exists still considerable disagreement, as the type and aims of training and therapy will depend on the type of care provided. The matter is obviously a fundamental one, and deserves special detailed consideration (*see* section 6, p. 332).

2. *The different needs of, and criteria applicable to children and adults*

All children are socially incapable, hence the diagnostic criteria are bound to be profoundly different from those of adults. From a psychometric point of view, as children's minds are plastic and developing, it is the stage of development and the capacity to learn that are the relevant pointers to the presence of handicap, and it is the developmental retardation that is the measure of the handicap. In consequence, the criteria of mental handicap as applied to children are not those of social adequacy, but rather the ability to meet the demands made upon them by the educational system. Children who fail to do so are described as being educationally subnormal (E.S.N.) either mildly or severely so; the abbreviations E.S.N. (M) and E.S.N. (S) are in common use, especially by the Education Authorities, for the mild and severe respectively. The difference in criteria used for children and adults has had the interesting consequence that the more mildly affected children who have educational difficulties usually have less social disabilities when they grow up, especially after they have had special teaching. Follow-ups of children who had attended schools for the E.S.N. (M) have demonstrated that the majority of them have made satisfactory adjustment as adults, and are living lives as normal individuals in the community. The numbers of E.S.N. children are thus greater than the number of overtly mentally-handicapped adults.

Recent studies have indicated that scholastic abilities are very sensitive to an unfavourable material, social and emotional environment, and that very careful screening, both physical and social, is needed when assessing E.S.N. children.

The needs of mentally-handicapped children are the same as those of normal children, and are now well-known and recognised. In babyhood the need is for a good and permanent relationship with parental figures. Babies need attention, consistent care, and a loving relationship to be able to grow and develop in comfort and security. The growing child's emotional needs can be met within the family circle, but as the child grows up, living within a small, accepting, caring group is not enough. The older child has wider needs of contact with children of his own age and level of intelligence. He also has needs concerned with education and training to ensure that he develops to maximal potential and is prepared for adult life, equipped with the necessary skills to function to his full potential in the appropriate social setting.

Although such concentrated attention and care is normally given within the biological family, it does not necessarily follow, as is frequently supposed, that family care is the only way of attaining these aims. One sees fairly frequently insistence that the mentally handicapped child should remain in the family. Should family conditions be adverse (and the incidence of mental handicap is much greater in families of low social status with superadded social and emotional problems) or if the child is rejected by the family, then provision of alternative care presents better prospects if it will ensure consistent and loving care.

The needs of adults are quite different, and this fact is not adequately realised in the present planning and provision of services. As the child grows up and passes through adolescence to adult status its needs for social interactions grow and extend. This is equally true of the handicapped as of the normal. People need to live among their peers and interact with them, and to feel that they participate in the group's decision making, and contribute as members of their society. This is necessary for self-respect and self-reliance. Meaningful work which is seen to have relevance and importance is an essential part of such living patterns.

These truisms have not been realised by the providers of present-day care, who still plan on the assumption that the needs of the adult handicapped are an extension of the needs of children. Hence the insistence on continuing training *ad infinitum* (without specifying what is the purpose of this training) and on living in small family groups, or on the handicapped adults remaining to live with their family whenever possible. There is, unfortunately, little or no concern for the quality of life and the encouragement of meaningful participation in social activities among one's peers.

Clinical experience has demonstrated that the handicapped living in small groups and in their families become easily bored and frustrated. Those living with their families are frequently overprotected and infantilised. There is almost complete ignorance of the structure and organisation of social groups which encourage independence, self-reliance and contentment, and there is urgent need of fact-finding research in this area of social psychiatry.

3. Factors affecting the choice of care
When considering the wide number of options and deciding on the most advantageous, a large number of factors must be taken into account.

It is obvious that no professional agency can give as much attention and affection as an accepting, loving family, and that if such a family wishes to keep their handicapped child at home then that is the best solution. In order to be able to cope with the greater demands which a handicapped child makes on its mother and family, there is need of professional help and support both in clinics and at home. Parents need help in knowing how much to expect from the child, so as not to have unrealistic expectations and on the other hand not to over-protect and under-stimulate. Such support for parents will be discussed later in this chapter.

There are circumstances when consideration must be given to caring for the child away from home. This may be due to rejection of the child by either or both parents. When this occurs, and it is liable to happen most frequently when the handicap is diagnosed at birth, insistence on the child remaining at home may subject it to poor care and even neglect and ill-treatment. It may be the cause of marital dissension (the birth of a handicapped child may trigger off the breakdown of a marriage, though in such cases marital disharmony has usually existed beforehand, and the handicapped child is less of a cause than an excuse). On the other hand commonly shared problems may bring the parents closer together. Any involvement in the marital situation which may be indicated must be professional and skilled. Multiple handicaps in the older child may impose a physical burden on the mother which may necessitate its removal to alternative forms of care, and also single-parent families may be taxed beyond their resources by the handicapped child. In such cases, it may be possible to alleviate the burden by providing day-care facilities, and this is at present a fashionable solution, while letting the child live at home.

Such an arrangement may solve the problem or it may temporise and put off the need to take a decision. The older child, by needing constant supervision, may be very burdensome to the mother, and studies have shown that families with mentally handicapped children are in all social respects worse off than control families (Tizard and Grad, 1961). In all these cases the family's feelings and wishes must be paramount, and advice and persuasion only resorted to when it is obvious that the parents are overtaxing themselves, or unable to give adequate care.

A severely handicapped, disturbed, noisy and hyperkinetic child may be totally disruptive to the family, particularly to any siblings. Not only do they find their possessions destroyed, and are prevented from studying, but the disruption of a normal home atmosphere may interfere very severely with their social activities and friendships, and be responsible for emotional disturbances. Some parents, motivated by guilt or by the unconscious need to make reparations to the affected and afflicted child, may subordinate to this the needs and interests of normal children in their unrealistic devotion to the handicapped child. Such a situation must be watched closely, and needs skilled clinical handling.

Such very disturbed children can exert influences *beyond* the immediate family circle, and night screaming, noisiness and destructiveness may cause complaints from the neighbours and insistence that the authorities should remedy the situation. This may be the deciding factor that leads to taking the child into care.

When the handicapped child grows up quite different problems emerge. For normal people, growing up means severing the close maternal bonds even though the emotional bonds may remain as strong as ever. A grown-up child normally leaves home, establishes social and emotional relationships which are external to the family, and usually marries and sets up a family of his own. In cases when an adult son or daughter remains living with both or one parent, this usually results in social isolation and frequently is associated with emotional problems. The same is true of the handicapped. Those left at home will usually be the group of higher intelligence and good social adaptations, since the more severely handicapped with disturbed behaviour should have left home earlier for the reasons already discussed, unless they are manageable, when they will remain at home as over-grown children.

As has already been discussed, the adult handicapped person needs the company of peers, and their living in a sheltered community may widen their interests and lead to a more stimulating and active life. The intermediate-grade handicapped person often is of happy and compliant disposition and may not be aware of his needs and deprivations. In such situations it is not uncommon for the parents to become emotionally dependent on the handicapped child, particularly if the spouse is dead or no longer a member of the family. The parent having spent a considerable part of his or her life caring for the handicapped child feels deprived on losing this life-long association and may go through a period of mourning when the adult leaves home.

Quite a different problem can be encountered in very mildly affected individuals who are members of an intellectually superior family. Such people of borderline intelligence would be considered normal had they been members of an unintelligent family. As it is, the gap between their family's intellectual status and attainment and theirs is so great that, by the family's standard it constitutes marked intellectual handicap. Such people are perfectly viable in the community but in a much humbler setting than the family occupies, and the problem is to get the family to accept a marked lowering of expectations, as far as achievement and occupational status goes, and also the acceptance of a much lower social status for their handicapped members.

It cannot be repeated too often that the decision to allow the handicapped to leave home (often a heart-rending one) must be taken by
the family, but that the family must be given a considerable amount
of support both to reach a rational decision and to help come to
terms with the distressing emotional situation.

4. Wide range of disciplines involved and their formal interrelationship

Mental handicap, being a global condition affecting a human individual, raises questions of interest to a wide range of biological and
behavioural sciences from molecular biology to sociology, and a
large number of disciplines become involved in the treatment and
management of the mentally handicapped. Foremost among them
are medicine (and especially psychiatry), psychology, education and
social work. It is obvious that a large number of disciplines impinging
in an uncoordinated manner upon a handicapped person would not
have an optimal effect upon the subject of their endeavours, and
would even be harmful if they were at cross purposes with each other.

Over a very long time, the traditional psychiatric team consisting
of psychiatrist, psychologist, social worker with the nurse, especially
in the case of in-patient care, and the teacher (if children and adolescents were involved), has provided an integrated and co-ordinated
care with considerable success. Obviously a single service being
concerned with all the manifestations of mental handicap is in a
position to deploy its resources most effectively. What can be
achieved by such a unified service is demonstrated by the very
successful organisation provided by the Northern Ireland Authority.
In the rest of the United Kingdom the services for the mentally
handicapped have always been split, from the days of the inception
of the National Health Service.

At the time of the inception of the N.H.S. the purveyors of services
were the hospitals and, in the community, the Medical Officer of
Health acting on behalf of the Local Authorities. The only other
authority involved was the Local Authority education service since
the passing of the 1944 Education Act, but they were concerned
with children deemed to be normal except for having learning problems. Thus the responsibility of providing and administering services
for the mentally handicapped fell upon the medical services. Since
then, following the setting up of large departments of social services
under the Local Authority, the responsibility for the provision of
care in the community has been taken over by these social services.
Soon after, the Education Authorities took over the training and
education of all children including those in hospital. The result has
been a fragmentation of services, and a considerable strain imposed
on keeping the channels of communication open between all the
workers concerned with the same person.

The reasons for this shift of responsibility, with emphasis on the contribution of the different disciplines, are quite complex, but it may be sufficient to say that the revolt against the pre-eminence of medicine, and strivings towards professional independence of the other disciplines involved, have exerted a powerful influence. The theoretical rationale has been that because many of the mentally handicapped are affected by a stationary condition, and because many are handicapped purely as a result of biological variation in intelligence, their condition is, therefore, not an illness nor the result of an illness. The "medical role" is not applicable, it is argued, and the condition should be of no interest to medicine, besides being outside its competence. Such a view shows a grave misconception of medicine and its functions. Medicine is not limited to the consideration of pathology, it is concerned with health and optimal functioning, and becomes involved whenever the existence of the handicap interferes with adequate adjustment.

The present change of responsibilities for the provision of care has had an unfortunate effect. The Department of Social Services had an enormous burden of welfare provisions laid upon it from its inception. The care of the mentally handicapped constitutes only a small part of its duties, so that some authorities have been unable to fulfil their obligations; meanwhile the hospitals have been run down with a resultant diminution of their capacity to help. The situation is aggravated by the fact that the capacity of community services to deal with disturbed and even strange behaviour is less than had been anticipated and the hospitals have been under pressure to meet the burden of the more difficult cases. The suggestion that the whole of the services for the mentally handicapped should be taken over by the social services would have disastrous consequences. There is some evidence that the pendulum has begun to swing back as the problems of providing community care have become more glaring.

It is true that alternative types of care are possible, but in this country the running down of existing medical services at a time of financial crises is fraught with grave danger.

5. Flexibility

Whatever the organisation of services it is essential to ensure that the patients' needs are met without any time lag. As has been pointed out, changing circumstances may alter radically the social adjustment and the need for a different type of care. Illness and death of a parent, a psychotic episode, the loss of employment or even the need of the family to have a break make it necessary for the individual to pass from one type of care to another as his needs dictate with the minimum of fuss and bureaucratic interference.

The majority of mentally-handicapped people have always lived at home with their relatives, and this proportion will increase in the future. They usually attend adult training centres during the day, unless they are multiply-handicapped or have behaviour disorders when they are catered for in day hospitals. If the behaviour disorder becomes unmanageable or there is a breakdown in the caring capacity of the relatives, hospital admission may be sought, and should be readily provided.

Some mentally-handicapped adults in the community live in hostels provided by local authorities. These house usually between twenty and twenty-four people and are supervised by the social services. The residents are encouraged to become progressively more independent, and when a reasonable degree of independence has been achieved they may move into a group home where they live with three or four other mentally-handicapped people in a relatively unsupervised setting. It is not easy for them to cope with unpredictable events, and it may be necessary occasionally to move back to the hostels for further training or help with emotional difficulties. Hospital treatment may be needed from time to time for psychotic episodes or neurotic illness.

Movement from one type of care to another always should be accomplished with the minimum of disturbance.

6. *Discussions on the best forms of care*
The last twenty years or so have witnessed a considerable debate on the advantages of different types of care. The issue is whether it is better for the mentally handicapped to remain at home as long as it is humanly possible, or whether they should be cared for elsewhere; and more particularly, if they are to be housed away from home, whether it should be in the traditional large hospitals or whether they should be cared for in small units in the community. According to one point of view, the role of hospitals should be restricted to looking after multiply-handicapped people who need continuous nursing care and medical attention, and treating those mentally handicapped who have superadded psychiatric disorders, such as psychosis, personality disorder, and behaviour disturbances. Such hospitals should be small and set up close to and, if possible, within the areas they serve. Some people even go beyond this and take up the extreme position that there is no place at all for hospitals in the care of the mentally handicapped, and that all existing hospitals should be pulled down.

A historical approach may help to clarify the issues involved. The traditional method of care of the mentally handicapped between the wars was in large institutions. The majority of the hospitals for the mentally handicapped in the U.K. were built in the twenties and thirties for, although the Mental Deficiency Act was passed in 1913, its provisions could not be implemented till later owing to the war and its aftermath. It is indicative of attitudes to care that a large number of institutions for the mentally handicapped were called "colonies" and that it was only after they had been taken over by the National Health Service, at its inception, that they were renamed "hospitals". This double nomenclature underlines the dual functions of hospitals for the mentally handicapped.

In the first place, they were planned as places of shelter where the patients should be given support and care — in fact granted asylum from the stresses of the outside world. They were conceived as colonies, which would be as self-supporting as possible, whereas much of the running of the institution would be done by the patients themselves under supervision and with help from staff, and this cooperative endeavour would give a meaning and aim for life there. It is interesting to note that the latest developments of care by voluntary bodies have gone back to this idea. Organisations such as Cottage and Rural Enterprises for the Mentally Handicapped (C.A.R.E.) exist with the explicit purpose of settling the handicapped in small, cooperative though supervised settlements, which are usually of a farming nature. The fashion in this respect has now gone the full circle as farms, until their closure by the Ministry, were an integral part of the colonies for the "mentally defective".

It has become fashionable to represent hospitals as places where the inmates are impersonally regimented into a dreary conformity, and it is not denied that some of the institutions' care was poor and that abuses did occur. In fairness, though, the majority of colonies laid great stress on the quality of the patients' lives and showed great concern for their happiness and well-being. It is not realised, for example, that insistence on training and education was a regular feature of hospital care at a time when the educationists had rejected the more severely handicapped children as being ineducable.

Shortly after the Second World War, and in the U.K. largely through the influence of Penrose, it was realised that the provision of optimal care, though important, was not enough. There was important work to be done in clarifying the aetiology of the conditions causing mental handicap, in developing methods of therapy and in research.

Research activity was particularly important in view of the fact that there were important gaps in knowledge and understanding of the conditions, and that radical advances could only be made through research and development. It is interesting to note that the early pioneers in the care and treatment of the mentally handicapped were medical. The first concern in the care of the handicapped was directed towards training and socialisation, and in general educational measures; the clinical approach which might be considered to be the first concern of the medical profession was not seriously taken up until the end of the second half of the nineteenth century, by workers such as Ireland. It is unfortunate that a polarisation into one or other of these activities has been allowed to creep into the services for the mentally handicapped, whereas in fact they are complementary.

The services for the mentally handicapped have to contend for allocation of funds in rivalry with other services that are provided by local authorities and central government and, unfortunately, have not fared too well. In the past its neglect led to the description of the service for the mentally handicapped as the "Cinderella service", and only recently has recognition been given to the need for more financial support.

The arguments of the critics of the traditional methods of care are frequently subsumed by the term "normalisation" and can be outlined as follows.

(a) The care of patients in large institutions leads invariably to institutionalisation of the inmates, who, having their lives regulated by others, tend to lose initiative, to lead very restricted lives, to have their personalities impoverished through lack of stimulation in a monotonous and regimented environment, and are defenceless if abused and ill-treated. Some social theorists such as Goffman go further and maintain that ill-treatment of the subordinated and dependent inmates is inherent in the social structure of institutions (Goffman, 1961), and see no essential difference between psychiatric hospitals, prisons and Nazi concentration camps.

(b) In the context of the mental handicap hospital, it has been asserted that intelligence tends not to develop and that hospital care "teaches people to become defective".

(c) On a different level, it is claimed that institutional care is rooted in the desire to banish the handicapped from the midst of the social group, and that isolating the handicapped represents a flight from the inacceptable and harsh reality of physical and mental malformation. It follows that mature and responsible social groups accept their responsibilities and care for their handicapped in their midst and treat them as full members of society. In other words it treats the handicapped as normal members of the community — hence the term "normalisation" — and that under such a regime the handicapped develop faster and further, and lead happier and much more satisfactory lives. An important corollary of this approach is that the mentally handicapped should live in small groups in the community so as to be able to integrate with it.

(d) It is also pointed out that the fact that the nursing staff work in shifts and that junior nursing staff are moved from ward to ward in the course of training leads to lack of continuity, and failure to provide emotional security and a stable environment to the patients. This is particularly important in the case of children who need a stable, emotionally secure environment for their optimal social and intellectual development. It is also claimed that such an improved environment can be obtained much more easily in small units.

(e) Critics also point to the abuses which have occurred in the hospitals for the mentally handicapped in the past and have been the subject of official inquiries, and state that conditions that were revealed by these inquiries should not be tolerated in a civilised society.

The supporters of the more traditional methods of care make the following comments on the preceeding arguments.

(a) The above assertions are statements of belief unsupported by any convincing experimental evidence, and often contradicted by clinical experiences. The problems of the handicapped living alone or in small groups in the community have already been discussed, and the insistence of "normalisers" on small "family" units demonstrates their unawareness of the social needs of adults.

(b) The handicapped never become full members of the community in practice, and it is not sensible to expect people with the mental ages of children to be accepted as equals by normal adults. It is true that the public at large is much more sympathetic now to the mentally handicapped (and here the credit must be taken by the campaigners for community care) and there is much more kindness and tolerance to them than formerly, but normally the mentally handicapped remain separate from the community at large and form an inward-looking group of their own, which is much more restricted than the one found in hospitals. This is true even of married patients leading "normal lives" who cling to the old friendships formed in hospital and live in a self-imposed ghetto separate from the community at large.

(c) There is a false antithesis between hospital and community care, and modern hospital practice encourages patients to go into the community for recreation, shopping, holidays and other needs. Living in hospital does not preclude mobility or contacts with the community outside the hospital.

(d) Abuses have occurred in hospitals and these have been all too frequent, and completely inexcusable. One must not, however, lose sight that all systems of care, particularly of the helpless and inarticulate, are liable to abuse and that the frequency of these occurrences in the hospital service can be explained by the fact that the majority of those mentally handicapped not with their families were being cared for in hospitals. Now that community care has been established, one hears of similar abuse creeping into the hostels. Penrose used to say that when he became interested in the specialty in the 1920s, the scandals over ill-treatment of patients in the community were as common as the hospital scandals in the last decade, and that they were less easy to detect. It is considered that to abolish institutions where abuses have occurred rather than to reform them, ignores the problem of why they occur, and tends to throw the baby out with the bath water.

(e) It is unscientific and illogical to judge the service by its worst examples. There are a number of hospitals that are centres of excellence, and where in addition to concern for the patients' well-being and dignity as a human being, the quality of clinical work and the research and development of treatment constitutes an example and a model for less well-developed institutions. The assessment of the contribution that hospitals make should be made by considering their achievements rather than the faults of bad hospitals. Also the critics of the hospitals do not take into account the progress and development in hospital care, which has made enormous strides in the last twenty years.

(f) On the practical level it has been found that the social services have been unable to meet the obligations that have been laid upon them in recent years. It has also been found that the tolerance of hostels or of other places in the community for disturbed behaviour is much lower than had been expected, and it has been the practical experience that as soon as any disturbed behaviour or psychiatric disorder manifests itself that urgent admission to hospital is demanded by the social services. As the departments of social services have such wide-ranging, onerous duties laid upon them, the provision of care for the mentally handicapped is not always treated as a priority need, and problems of recruitment and training of social workers have been very severe in some local authorities. The turnover of staff has been very great indeed, and it was found in practice that hostels even for children could not ensure the continuity of care that was provided by sister and senior ward staff in hospitals. The public too, have demonstrated an ambivalance towards the mentally handicapped. Although in principle they are in favour of community care, in practice they object to community facilities being set up in their neighbourhood, and show little tolerance and understanding of deviant behaviour.

(g) The other point is that there has been no attempt to assess the cost effectiveness of community care. Although the protagonists claimed that community care was cheaper than hospitals, these assertions were not borne out by practice, and as long as ten years ago the Government was prepared to spend £200 millions on the shift to community care. At present the figure would need to be two or three times greater. It is irresponsible to spend such large sums without pilot schemes and experiments. It is contended that if such a sum were injected into the existing services, they would in all likelihood show better results for the money.

In the last ten years or so the Government has become converted to a more extreme form of community care. While accepting that there is a role for the smaller hospitals they had decided that the major part of care should be in the community, and that there should be no further building in large hospitals even when that meant that no further hospital based developments could take place.

Owing to the difficult economic situation, it was not found possible to inject the vast sums of money that had been planned. As a result the development of community services lagged far behind their planned extension. At the same time the run-down of hospitals continued as there was an urgent need to reduce the intolerable state of over-crowding, the extremely bad living conditions for patients and the working conditions of staff. The consequences have been increasing problems in providing residential services. In some areas the impossibility of making adequate provisions of services has led to a very serious situation. It is aggravated by problems of recruitment both of paramedical, nursing and medical staff. In the case of medical staff, the denigration of the medical role by a large number of bodies, the acceptance of diminished medical involvement and the planned run-down of hospitals made the specialty insecure and unattractive to members of the medical profession, and the lack of medical staff in some areas is rapidly reaching crisis point. Nothing short of a rethink about services policies, coupled with more intensive training in the medical schools of both undergraduates and post-graduates could remedy this situation which is alarming to those who believe in the importance of the medical contribution to the care of the mentally handicapped.

In this climate of discussion and argument it is impossible not to take a partisan view. It would seem to the authors, however, that the overriding consideration in the provision of all services for the mentally handicapped should be the consideration of the needs of the handicapped, and of the best way in which these could be met. From such a point of view it is obvious that very broad and integrated services are needed, and it must be admitted that we still know too little about the best way of dealing with the problems posed by the handicapped. Under the circumstances all types of services should be given an opportunity of development and their contribution given an impartial assessment. There is obviously a place in the community for the handicapped, and the needs of the handicapped, in a number of cases, can be best met by continuing life in small units where interpersonal relationships are easily established and manageable — this must, however, be combined with a wider social environment where there is a good opportunity to interact with one's peers. The idea of "village communities" which was the original rationale of the colonies is coming back into fashion, but it is essential that such organisations should be scientifically studied and scientifically developed. The authors see the provision of such a community as a possible role for the large hospital. The other role of the hospital would appear to the authors to be acting as the centre where all the skills and expertise can be concentrated and where training and research can be carried out, as well as providing clinical services. The link of the hospital with the community is most essential, and the hospital is seen as a centre from which clinical services can be deployed into the community.

Undoubtedly the best form of care for the mentally handicapped will be achieved by a close liaison between local authority and health services, thus assuring that the social support, educational facilities, training and treatment appropriate to the needs of the handicapped person and his family will be provided.

REFERENCES

Bobath, K. and Bobath, B. (1956): "Control of motor function in the treatment of cerebral palsy", *Australian J. of Physiotherapy*, 2, 75.

Burt, C. (1937): *The Backward Child*, London University Press, London.

Cravioto, J., Delicarie, E. R. and Birch, H. G. (1966): "Nutrition, growth and neuro-development: an experimental and ecologic study", *Paediatrics*, 38, 319-72.

Doll, Edgar A. (1941): "The essentials of an inclusive concept of mental deficiency", *American J. Mental Deficiency*, 46, 214-19.

Doll, Edgar A. (1953): *The Measurement of Social Competence: a Manual for the Vineland Social Maturity Scale*, Educational Test Bureau, Washington D.C.

Gesell, A. and Amatruda, C. (1947): *Developmental Diagnosis*, Paul B. Hoeber, New York.

Goffman, E. (1961): *Asylums*, Anchor Doubleday and Co. Ltd.

Griffiths, Ruth (1955): *The Abilities of Babies*, London University Press, London.

Gunsberg, H. C. (1965): *Progress Assessment Charts: Manual*, Sefa (Publications Ltd.), England.

Heaton-Ward, W. Alan (1975): *Mental Subnormality*, H. K. Lewis, London.

Hilliard, L. T. and Kirman, B. (1965): *Mental Deficiency*, 2nd edition, J. and A. Churchill Ltd. London.

Spearman, C. (1911): "Experimental test of higher mental processes", *J. Exp. Ped.*, 1, 101.

Tizard, J. and Grad. (1961): *The Mentally Handicapped and Their Families*, Maudsley Monographs No. 7, Oxford University Press, London.

Wechsler, D. (1958): *The Measurement and Appraisal of Adult Intelligence*, 4th edition, Williams and Wilkins, Baltimore.

FURTHER READING

Bobath, B., *Adult Hemiplegia: Evaluation and Treatment*, Heinemann (William) Medical Books Ltd., London, 1970.

Bobath, K., *Motor Disorders in Cerebral Palsy*, Heinemann (William) Medical Books Ltd., London, 1966.

Clark, A. D. B., *Recent Advances in Study of Subnormality*, National Association for Mental Health, London, 1972.

Gunsberg, H. C., (Ed.), *Advances in the Care of the Mentally Handicapped*, Baillière Tindall, London, 1973.

Heaton-Ward, W. Alan, *Left Behind: A Study of Mental Handicap*, Macdonald & Evans, Plymouth, 1977.

Kirman, B. and Bicknell, J., *Mental Handicap*, H. K. Lewis, London, 1975.

Penrose, L. S., *Biology of Mental Defect*, 4th edition, H. K. Lewis, London, 1972.

Tizard, J., *Community Services for the Mentally Handicapped*, Oxford University Press, London, 1964.

Tredgold, R. F. and Soddy, K., *Mental Retardation*, Baillière Tindall, London, 1970.

Childhood Emotional Problems in Medical Practice

Dr. Anthony G. Carroll,
M.B., B.Ch., M.R.C.Psych., D.P.M.
Clinical Director of Child Psychiatry to the Western Health Board and Clinical Teacher in Child Psychiatry, Medical School, University College, Galway, Ireland

Childhood Emotional Problems
in Medical Practice

In addressing himself to illness, any illness, in a child, the medical practitioner, for a number of reasons, has to make some immediate adjustments. First of all, it is almost always someone other than the patient who requests his help, who describes the symptoms and in many ways defines the problem. This brings a new dimension to the clinical situation. Next, children are smaller than adults. One only has to ask what is the dose of any drug for a child to see the sort of question this raises; size is a point that has wide implications and, for example, explains why it was not felt necessary to build mental hospitals for children. Another important point is that children are growing. In other words, the pace of biological and psychological change in a child is much more rapid than is that of an adult and this has important significance when one seeks to influence it. The age of the child is extremely important in itself, frequently determining whether a presenting problem is pathological or not, as, for example, in the difference between bed-wetting in a two-year-old and in a fifteen-year-old. There are many other, at first sight self-evident points, which have to be given some thought when determining one's approach. Another instance, for example, is the fact that, to a considerable extent at least, adults can be expected to use speech as a main communication medium whereas this is not at all the case with children. These differences with children in general when given some consideration, rather than being impediments may be put to therapeutic advantage.

Apart from any possible difficulties in communicating with physically ill children, some general practitioners feel uncertain with problems from the relatively new field of child psychiatry. This unfamiliarity may lead to the reaction of dismissing it as being irrelevant or alternatively to feeling so overwhelmed as to refer all childhood emotional problems for specialist attention. I hope to show that the child psychiatrist's closest professional colleague can be the general practitioner and that both fields have a lot to offer each other. Certainly, child psychiatry has been developing rapidly in recent years and a brief historical review should offer a useful framework.

HISTORICAL REVIEW OF CHILD PSYCHIATRY

Since the dawn of time man has observed his neighbours and himself reflecting on individual differences, in particular seeking explanations for idiosyncratic behaviour and unusual personalities. Indeed from classical times, both eminent thinkers and popular lore made perceptive associations between adult behaviour and childhood experiences, and offered many profound insights. However, while it has many roots in the past, child psychiatry is very much a twentieth-century creation and only in recent decades has it emerged as a specific scientific discipline. New ideas and scientific advances in quite a number of fields led to its development. While, within psychiatry itself, the nineteenth-century systematisation of knowledge and classification of mental diseases led to greater clarification, it was undoubtly the development of psychoanalysis which had the greatest significance for child psychiatry.

Although, apart from the well-known case of Little Hans, Sigmund Freud (1909) did not on the whole base his writings directly on the study of children's emotional development, nevertheless, his methodical enquiries into his adult patients' histories, tracing their current psychiatric problems to childhood experiences, directed enormous attention to the latter. It remained for his daughter Anna, amongst others, to focus attention directly on the children themselves. In the early years of the present century, educationalists addressed themselves to the question of devising specific curricula for particular children. In Paris, the psychologists Binet and Simon tested large groups of school children and devised intelligence tests, since when educational and clinical psychologists have contributed enormously to our knowledge and practice.

Changes also occurred within legal systems as lawyers and legislators recognised the specific needs of children. The writings of Dickens in particular, focused public attention on the many abuses. By the end of the nineteenth century, there were juvenile courts in some of the states of Australia and the United States and these spread to Europe. Throughout the twentieth century, as the social and environmental contribution to delinquency became recognised, enlightened attitudes spread and reformatories and industrial schools humanised their regimes. Research increased and policies of prevention and rehabilitation were adopted.

Paediatricians vary in the degree of emphasis they place on the emotional and sociological contribution to childhood illness and this is reflected in paediatric textbooks. Child neurology and mental retardation at first were the main areas shared with child psychiatrists, but since the 1930s and particularly in the United States, the two professions have interacted much more to mutual benefit with the result that now the child psychiatrist is probably closer to the paediatrician than to his adult psychiatric colleague.

The founder of what proved to be the first child guidance clinic was William Healy, who, in 1909, established his Juvenile Psychopathic Institute in Chicago, where he adopted a rational approach to the diagnosis and treatment of those delinquents coming before the children's courts. He recognised the significance of the developments in psychometry and recruited an educational psychologist to his team. It was in the Boston Psychopathic Hospital's children's clinic that the first psychiatric social worker was trained specifically for the job. By the 1920s what were called "Demonstration Child Guidance Clinics" were established in many cities and the movement had also spread to Europe. In Britain they started in London, Birmingham, Glasgow and Stoke-on-Trent and again were primarily concerned with the juvenile courts, and by 1927 a Child Guidance Council was in existence (Burt, 1944). The psychoanalytic movement had also gained in strength and within it the child analysts had shown that play was a natural investigative and therapeutic instrument with tremendous potential. In the 1930s, the upsurge of interest in social anthropology, sociology and the behavioural sciences in general, gave tremendous impetus to child psychiatry, with Leo Kanner's text book in 1935 representing an important milestone (Kanner, 1935). The Second World War brought large-scale population movements and evacuations. Residential homes, prisoner-of-war camps and later rehabilitation centres were opened and led to developments in social psychology in general and group dynamics in particular. Important observations were reported from the Hampstead Nurseries (Burlingham and Freud, 1942 and 1944) and the Tavistock Centre and, in 1950, W.H.O. asked John Bowlby to advise on the mental health of homeless children. This led to his important studies in infant-parent relationships and his development of attachment theory (Bowlby, J. 1951, 1965, 1969, 1973, 1977 (1), 1977 (2)).

In post-1945 Britain the political philosophy which led to the establishment of the welfare state and the National Health Service placed very great value on children's welfare in general and led to the development of a wide range of services catering for their needs. Child psychiatric practice was located in the child guidance clinics run by Local Authorities and in hospital based child psychiatric units. The establishment of a number of professorial child psychiatric departments within the teaching hospitals represented another major milestone.

CHILD PSYCHIATRY AND GENERAL PRACTICE

There has been a tremendous amount of research in all aspects of child development and the most recent contributions to child psychiatry have come from such diverse fields as psycholinguistics, ethology and systems theory. This has given it a vast literature. Whereas in the past, some individual authorities wrote from a highly subjective standpoint, in recent years more rigorous research, such as the valuable prospective epidemiological studies, have added a sound scientific base. There is an increasing number of professionals who are involved with children with problems. Apart from child psychiatrists and paediatricians there are educational and clinical psychologists, social workers, remedial teachers, speech therapists, child psychotherapists, educational welfare officers, probation officers, play-group leaders, art therapists and a host of others. Clearly the busy general practitioner cannot possibly keep himself informed of all these developments, nor indeed does he need so to do. What is required is some information and guidance on what practical implications these developments may have for his work. In seeking to encompass the task in a chapter, it is with regret that at times it seemed necessary that a didactic note be struck.

As in the rest of medicine the treatment adopted of course depends on the diagnosis. However, with childhood emotional problems this is not at all as straightforward a process as many parents expect. There seems to be a widely held belief, based in part on Hollywood's mispresentation of one of Freud's early observations, that the diagnostic task is to uncover a repressed, specific, emotionally-traumatic experience, which occurred earlier in the child's life. Hence, questions such as, "Have you found out what's behind it yet, doctor?" or even, "Has he told you what's worrying him yet?" The reality is that the problems are almost invariably multifactorial in origin and that frequently some of the causes will still be operating at the time the child is seen. Indeed with emotional problems in general, treatment and diagnosis are closely interrelated and both can be part of one continuing process which starts as soon as the patient enters the surgery. Therapeutic outcome is often dependent on the approach which is adopted from the start. How he conducts the clinical relationship depends on the doctor's personality of course, and the following points are made with the hope that each doctor will maintain his individual style. At medical school, we were taught that the first part of the clinical examination is keen observation and in child psychiatry particular attention is paid to this. Not only can it quickly indicate the line of enquiry but at times it suggests the diagnosis and even how and where therapy should be applied. The following might be the first observations in the case.

The patient was a 10-year-old boy with chronic encopresis. He and his two younger siblings clustered around their relaxed father while the tense, drawn mother sat some distance away looking at them.

In very many of these cases the doctor should be mindful of his role as family practitioner, putting an emphasis on the word "family". He maintains an open mind that silently questions the questions, as it were. Usually, it is the mother who brings the child. Who first enters the room? How are they dressed, what is their demeanour and gait and most importantly, how do they relate to one another? Body language, now very much in vogue, can reveal a lot. This is nothing new to medicine and we recall that the fictional character of Sherlock Holmes, that expert in understanding non-verbal communication, was based on a Scottish general practitioner. It is very worth while consciously to attend to body language and the time is never wasted. Is the mother protective or rejecting? Is the child sullen and hostile or does he proudly recite his symptoms? Why is it the father who has brought the child on this occasion? Or indeed why has the entire family come? Sometimes a mother will report a child's difficulties, frequently a behavioural problem, in his absence. Is she afraid of her child? Or is it that she is seeking help for herself?

This last is a very important point in child psychiatry, that of the location of the pathology. Balint has shown us how the adult patient and the doctor negotiate over the illness and introducing a child increases the scope for this (Balint, 1968). Winnicott emphasised the crucial interactional significance of the mother-child relationship by startling his students one day with the observation "there is no such thing as a child"; and Apley has reminded us that patients and doctors find it easier to believe in physical than in emotional causes for symptoms (Apley, 1975). In addition, family therapists view the entire system of family relationships as the clinical entity and network therapists go even further. I am sure that, in most of their cases, general practitioners, at least unconsciously, have been implementing these points in their practice. From a home visit, for example, through observing the family's values and attitudes as revealed in their furniture, photographs, sleeping arrangements, pets, and life style in general, and incorporating this in his history-taking and physical examination, the doctor may reach the appropriate diagnosis within minutes. Many sound clinical decisions, apparently intuitive, have been based on unconsciously recorded information of this sort. The more awareness one has the better, and this is particularly important with the puzzling, unusual or resistant case. The development of a habit of rapidly noting these relationship points and especially of reflecting on them in difficult or intractable cases, will frequently lead to insight, which then indicates the appropriate action. The doctor should ask himself such questions as: "What is this symptom doing for the family? What is it preventing the mother or the family from doing? What is it preventing the child from doing?" and he can also ask the patients these questions, in this way getting clues as to the function of the symptom or illness. The stomach pain which prevents the child from going to school is the obvious example, but the enquiry must go much further than that. What is the child's presence at home doing for the mother? What is it doing for the family in general?

The following case history illustrates the family factors which may be involved.

A 10-year-old girl was referred for persistent refusal to go to school. She came with both her parents and presented as a plump sullen girl who remained mute throughout most of the interview. It seemed that she had remained at home from school since her mother returned from a short spell in hospital a year previously, having had attention for her varicose veins. Presumably, the child was insecure and stayed at home to keep an eye on her mother. What was the appropriate treatment? During a general discussion about home-life and some aspects of the family history, points which the parents did not feel were relevant were pursued and proved highly significant. Apparently, the father was not working but it was unclear whether this had to do with some illness or difficulty in finding a suitable job. Indeed, he had not worked for many years and again the 17-year-old son, who had left school a year previously, likewise was unemployed and at home. Two older sisters who were married lived nearby but they too spent much of their time in the parental household and their husbands used frequently to joke about it. Indeed the only member of the house who seemed to be discharging role-responsibility appropriately was a 12-year-old sister who attended school happily and who was barely mentioned in the session. The family myth proved to have to do with a general anxiety that mother was very vulnerable and needed continual support lest she have a breakdown. The mother's own fear of this had stemmed from experiences within her family of origin and she had transmitted it unconsciously to her own family, nearly all of whom stayed at home to prop her up. The system could have remained unchanged except that the school authorities brought the focus onto their absent pupil. In a number of family therapy sessions the myth was challenged, revealing the underlying anxieties which were identified and worked through, and, *inter alia*, the little girl had taken herself back to school.

Children's physical and emotional welfare is linked intimately with the health and welfare of the community in general. It is salutary therefore for the medical profession to remind itself that children's health reflects general living standards and is probably more influenced by the decisions of politicians and economists than by any specific medical contribution. There are fashions in child rearing practice and each generation has had one or two immensely popular authorities. How much these experts are chosen by the public because they reflect its attitudes to such issues as authority and responsibility is a debatable question. It may be that these fashions represent sociological changes rather than resulting from any scientific research. However, the latter may be beginning to have some impact and certainly Bowlby's work has had a significant effect on professional practice within the United Kingdom. Child psychiatrists always have placed emphasis on their preventive role and this may also be the most important one for the general practitioner. We know that because of the intense feelings aroused, parents with otherwise sound judgment may over-react to children's problems and quite unnecessarily seek referrals for circumcision, cutting of tongue tie and residential schooling, or even summon police assistance in certain circumstances. Indeed professionals, too, at times, under intense pressure to do something, have given injudicious advice or taken inappropriate lines of action. Many children have been the victims of unnecessary procedures or, at tender years, have been despatched for specialised education or treatments because attention has been focused on a specific symptom, without consideration for the well-being of the child as a whole. Rather than pretend to expertise which he lacks, it is much better for the professional to confess to bewilderment and join the parents in seeking to understand a child's bizarre behaviour. It is essential that the doctor be ever mindful of the first principle of medical practice: *primum non nocere*. Doctors, like everyone else, have formed their views on child rearing on the basis of their own childhood experiences, modified by their training and clinical practice. A professional standpoint is necessary, however, to maintain objectivity and for this reason the following contributions from theory are offered.

THEORETICAL PERSPECTIVE

Many people now are familiar with some aspect of the research done on maternal deprivation and on the adverse effects on children of certain features of institutional care. John Bowlby is widely known through his popular writings and so are his colleagues, James and Joyce Robertson, through their excellent film series; *Young Children in Brief Separation* (Robertson and Robertson, 1976). Indeed since the 1930s there has been much research into the social behaviour of both children and young animals and, in recent years a great many studies on mother-child interaction from the moment of birth. It has been proposed that there is a primary drive amongst humans and most mammals to establish an emotional bond (an attachment) to another individual who is usually perceived as stronger or wiser. This is most clearly seen in the attachment between the infant and mother which occurs during the first nine months of life. When the mother is present, the child usually ceases to display attachment behaviour and is able to move away and explore the environment. Hence a crucial function of parents is to provide the child with a secure base and to encourage him to explore from it (Bowlby, 1977 (1)). It is also proposed that subsequent emotional relationships later in life, and indeed many other experiences, are strongly influenced by the way the first attachment developed and was experienced. This first attachment bond is an intensely emotional one and a threat of its loss results in anxiety and anger while the loss itself leads to sorrow and also anger. Where the attachment has been established on a reasonably secure basis, and is then disrupted, a pre-school child typically displays a sequence of behaviour which has been divided into three phases for descriptive purposes. He will display *(a)* protest, *(b)* despair and *(c)* detachment.

In the *protest* phase, the young child is obviously very distressed at having lost his mother, crying loudly, throwing himself about and usually angrily rejecting offers of comfort or distraction. The phase of *despair* is marked by a more hopeless crying and sobbing with the child no longer making demands but instead withdrawn and mournful. Following this is the phase of *detachment* where the child gradually begins to eat and play again and will relate to caring figures. This could be seen as indicative of recovery, but when the child meets the mother again it can be seen that the former intense attachment has gone. He may turn away, appearing uninterested and the renewal of the relationship is usually difficult and distressing to both mother and child. Where the mother is not reunited to to the child, he develops attachments to the main care-givers, e.g. nurses in the case of hospital wards, and where these are broken, in turn, will experience repetition of the earlier loss although with decreasing intensity. In the event of a prolonged stay in an institution, having lost several such figures, he ultimately appears to be unconcerned and new care-givers can come and go without his being distressed.

Some of the most valuable research work in child development is found in the prospective epidemiological surveys. Support for the effect of early hospital admission on subsequent development and behaviour has been reported by Douglas. His study comprised a large cohort of children born in the first week of March, 1946, which has been followed up regularly since. Data reported in 1975 revealed that "one admission to hospital of more than a week's duration or repeated admissions before the age of 5 years . . . are associated with an increased risk of behaviour disturbance and poor reading in adolescence". The children who had experienced these early admissions are more troublesome out of class, more likely to be delinquent and more likely to show unstable job patterns than those who were not admitted during the first five years. In a critical appraisal of his study, Douglas found that he was able to exclude the other variables which might have accounted for the result. In the five years after March, 1946, it was extremely unlikely that mothers would have been admitted to hospital with their young children as this was not then the practice (Douglas, 1975).

Relevant work on the emotional experiences following the disruption of attachment bonds has also been carried out at the other end of the human life span. Studies of bereavement in the cases of individual widows and widowers, and also following large scale natural disasters, described behaviour and experiences very similar to those seen in the young child. There was a phase of shock and numbness associated often with denial and frequently the sense that the dead person would return or somehow was around. At times this amounted to hallucinatory experience. This was followed by a gradual period of depression in which the loss was more deeply felt and during which time anger was sometimes felt and expressed. It was a period of gradually giving up and there followed a longer period of detachment. A recovery phase then ensued in which the bereaved person was able to get on with life and re-establish relationships, forming new bonds. Many cases have been described where this mourning was not experienced fully or was interrupted or blocked, with the result of many long-term adverse effects, such as depression, hypochondriasis, anxieties and the general failure to cope (Parkes, 1972; Pincus, 1976). Indeed it seemed that the capacity to have a successful mourning experience was associated with a good capacity for relationships in general and it has been linked with the quality of the first attachment experience in early childhood.

Of course there are many other influences that affect our relationship patterns, nevertheless, attachment theory and the work on bereavement and grief have wide-spread implications. A psychotherapeutic approach which has enabled patients to work through failed grief reactions, has been effective in removing symptoms and helping people to cope better. It has led to the recognition of the importance to health of a normal grief reaction and that measures taken to avoid it, such as the use of tranquillisers, may be ill advised. It has had implications for obstetric practice and maternity hospital routines as well as in rehabilitation following the loss of a limb, or a special sense. It can be seen to operate in society in general as in emigration, adherance to childish ways or to tradition, capacity to set up a new home, and in adjustments of many sorts. In child psychiatry it has relevance for the social structure of children's units and wards, adoption and fostering procedures, as well as in such clinical presentations as school refusal, separation anxiety, anorexia nervosa and many cases of childhood insecurity (Robertson and Robertson, 1974).

THE PREVENTIVE ROLE OF THE GENERAL PRACTITIONER

The potential of a preventive role for the general practitioner in cases of bereavement may be illustrated by the following cases.

Tim, aged nearly 14, was referred because of severe anti-social behaviour which had brought him before the courts. He was the second youngest of seven children, an eighth one had died some six years before he was born. Two years before the referral, the youngest one, Michael, had died tragically by drowning at the age of 4½ years. The older children had left home and established their own careers and at the time of referral there were three boys at home, Philip, aged 18, Peter, aged 15 and Tim. At the first appointment Tim and both his parents were quite depressed and unable to talk about Michael's tragic death. They were in a state of chronic bereavement reaction. Both parents had virtually stopped going out of the house as they did not want people to commiserate with them over the death. Whereas beforehand Tim had been well behaved and was getting on all right at school, since then he had been involved in anti-social behaviour and seemed to be a very unhappy boy. Prior to Michael's arrival he had been the youngest for ten years and one suspected that he had resented the newcomer. To some extent it could be said that his behaviour was very much that of a 4½-year-old and one wondered if he was unconsciously replacing Michael. Therapy consisted of a number of sessions in which the family, particularly the depressed father, was helped to discuss the bereavement and to experience some of the mourning. Tim made considerable progress, becoming more involved in social activities, joining a youth club, and became quite proficient in athletics. There had been no recurrence of his anti-social behaviour at a review two years later.

Another illustration was the case of Thomas.

Thomas, aged 8, was referred because of a developmental delay. He functioned at an immature level and was still sleeping in a cot. In the history it emerged that the much-longed-for first-born child in the family had a congenital cardiac defect and died at the age of 2 months. The mother was advised to banish the incident from her mind and to become pregnant again, which she did. She was full of anxieties throughout the pregnancy but Thomas was born a normal baby at term. From the start the mother was excessively solicitous for his welfare and became pathologically over-protective. At the time of referral, a school report on Thomas's level of functioning was at variance with the mother's report to some extent. Further enquiry revealed that Thomas behaved in a less immature way when away from home but still not age-appropriately. It was clear that his self-concept had been considerably moulded by his mother's anxieties. Treatment was at the Child Guidance Clinic and focused on some grief work with the parents, as well as giving them direct feed-back on Thomas's abilities through video-tape recordings of play group sessions.

Parents in similar circumstances or following stillbirths not uncommonly apply to adopt a child. While in the past such injudicious placements were made, social workers and adoption societies, recognising the implications, nowadays offer the appropriate counselling. Unfortunately it needs to be emphasised still that adoption or fosterage are no solutions to marital conflict or other parental problems, and in such cases usually only add to the stress.

In his preventive role the general practitioner, apart from intervening to protect the welfare of children, such as in cases of non-accidental injury or where institutions are insensitive to emotional needs, also has to guard lest unwittingly he contribute to the problem himself. A positive role towards childhood emotional development is called for and it is appropriate to discuss this, starting with pregnancy. In the vast majoirty of cases this is a normal physiological event and should be approached as such. It is essential that early antenatal care be established and any anxieties the mother may have, not only in the case of first pregnancies, should be discussed and resolved. Increasingly, nowadays, where the nuclear family has settled away from relations, it is important that such support be available. The preparation for childbirth often is best carried out in groups where mothers can support one another. Indeed increasingly, and particularly in preparation for natural childbirth, fathers are also welcomed at an early stage and the term "the pregnant family" has been coined. Nearly all babies now are born in hospitals and this has helped to reduce the infant mortality rate. Many maternity hospitals also give greater recognition to the individual needs and feelings of our pregnant families through seeking to establish a warm and homely atmosphere. Many mothers who have babies by natural childbirth do report experiencing it as a very special event which brings them close to their new babies. In those cases where various interventions, such as caesarean section, are clinically necessary and extra support and care has to be given to promote the mother-infant bond on these occasions. Most obstetricians now would agree that induction of childbirth should not be done just for convenience. There also is growing recognition that some anaesthetics affect the new-born infant so that it is drowsy and the establishment of a relationship with the mother is delayed. There are sound psychological reasons for the practice of rooming-in, where the mother keeps the newly-born infant with her. Likewise, apart from the nutritional and immunological reasons, there are sound psychological grounds for the promotion of breast feeding and the general practitioner has an important role in maintaining this. It is the mutual mother-infant, infant-mother relationship that is being fostered. Measurable differences lasting for as long as a year have been reported as occurring between the children of mothers who had early and extended contact with them in the early hours after birth, and those who were separated from them. One study reported a disproportionately high percentage of mothering disturbances, such as child abuse and deprivation-failure-to-thrive, occurring in those cases where the mother had been separated from a sick new-born infant.

In the case of the unmarried mother-to-be or where there are adverse environmental or social conditions, it is important for the family doctor to invoke the appropriate social support and ensure that these important relationship aspects are attended to. Doctors have always played an important role in advising on infant care and it is tremendously reassuring for a mother to learn that her baby is developing normally. It is all the more important that the doctor be careful not to add to any parental anxiety by such comments as, "he has a slight heart murmur, but it is of no significance", or even "he is looking pale", or, jokingly, "the poor fellow, don't you ever feed him?". One never knows which are the cases where such casual asides will resonate with conscious or unconscious anxieties in the mother, resulting in grossly obese children or cardiac cripples.

The general practitioner will not lightly refer a child for hospital admission, even though most paediatric units are now making arrangements whereby mothers can accompany their children to hospital. Care has also been taken to minimise the emotional damage where the separation is inevitable because the mother has to be admitted to hospital. Here it is best to leave the child in his own home with a familiar adult who can arrange frequent visits to the mother if possible and certainly keep the memory of the mother alive until she returns (*see* Table 1 on p. 381). Perhaps society will come to appreciate that the father is the person best suited to look after the young child in such circumstances. Children are capable of much greater understanding than is appreciated and can be prepared for such separations when they are imminent. Indeed there are simple play techniques which can be used to explain hospital procedures to children themselves and this has been shown to reduce the emotional stress otherwise caused (Harvey and Hales-Tooke, 1972; Vaughan, 1957). Play is essential to children as this is the way they acquire control over their emotions, grow in self-confidence, develop new skills, rehearse new roles, express anxieties, learn to co-operate with other children and in general widen their interests and knowledge of the world (Winnicott, 1964). The family doctor may have to enquire into this and suggest pre-school play groups where necessary. Similarly, some parents seem to wait for their children to start speaking and it has to be emphasised that language has to be put into a child before it emerges. This is particularly important in the cases where there are sensory impairments. The general practitioner's role in preventing emotional damage and in promoting positive attitudes and practices can be discharged in relation to children of all ages and can be the one that brings most professional satisfaction.

ASPECTS OF CHILD DEVELOPMENT

Apart from the mother-child relationship, children have also been studied in relation to their social, neurological, cognitive and emotional development and how these various functions interrelate. In child psychiatric practice different specialists will pursue their individual interests and this is reflected in their clinical practice. The child psychoanalysts have written extensively on the infant's and young child's emotional life with his developing concepts of self and of the world. From the perspective of the adult consensus on reality, some of these concepts seem bizarre and unfamiliar, but they are close to the psychotic phenomena of adult patients. Gradually, the growing child increases his capacity to tolerate frustration and to experience various emotions which become less intense. This increasing capacity in the child to contain himself and his feelings is partly what emotional maturation is about. When one considers the great pace with which the various processes change throughout infancy and young childhood, it is amazing that there can be sufficient stability for a consistent sense of self to develop. It is easy to understand why it is essential that basic trust has to be established and that the external environment be secure, for these interpsychic processes to come about in an integrated way.

Amongst the most interesting work of the child psychiatrist is that which occurs when he is able to reach an understanding of the symbolic concepts of the developing child and through using play, painting, and other means of expression, to enter into a therapeutic relationship. To help an inhibited child work through terrifying fantasies and become liberated is an exhilarating experience, as one has the privilege of observing creative forces in operation (Winnicott, 1977; Axline, 1971). In some cases the therapist's main function has been to provide the secure conditions within the safety of which the child is enabled to work through the problems with a minimum of intervention. Clearly the time schedule of the busy general practitioner will not permit him to undertake play therapy of this kind, but often he can help to bring about the conditions which will enable the working-through to proceed.

Children are born with temperamental differences and at the time of birth the new infant will already have acquired something of the mother's daily rhythms as for example her sleeping and waking pattern. Gradually, the new baby fits in more and more with the habits of the household and later on, other important lessons have to be learned such as the danger of fires, electric sockets, the fragility of crockery and so on. These and other lessons are learnt through direct experience and social relationships. At the same time the infant is exploring the potential of his body, manipulating objects and, through play, forming hypotheses and carrying out experiments, and thereby acquiring a vast amount of information. The infant starts off in total dependence on the mother or mother substitute, and has to develop ways of getting his needs met. He is helpless and yet very powerful and one has met parents who feel totally persecuted by the demands of a young infant. Much of what goes on in the interaction is negotiated over control and autonomy, with the child learning to become more self-reliant as he matures.

Indeed the act of creation on the parents' part does not end with the birth of the child, but the family, through its expectations, hopes, the behaviour it promotes and what it inhibits and so on, continues to mould the personality development and pattern of social interaction of the child. The family has its own growth and is subject to inward pressures coming from developmental changes in its members and to pressures to accommodate to the demands of the outside society. There is therefore constant transformation of the position of family members in relation to one another so that they can grow while the family system maintains continuity (Minuchin, 1974). From starting life within the mother, and then within the family, the child, gradually moving outside, encounters school and other social institutions and the community at large. Many of our social institutions are structured on the family model. This may be seen in the case of school, where the teachers would occupy the parental roles and the classmates that of siblings. However, there are differences and the school is not as sensitive to the child's individuality as is the family. It also embodies more of the general culture of society requiring conformity to social norms.

How the problems may present

Children therefore function in three main social arenas, i.e. the home, the school and the outside community. Their emotional problems which can manifest themselves in a very wide variety of ways, may present in any one, or all three, of these life situations. The diversity of presenting problems includes, for example, symptoms of anxiety, such as night terrors, insomnia, phobias, clinging behaviour and social isolation, or somatic symptoms such as headaches, stomach pains, loss of appetite, or a child may be depressed and withdrawn, isolated and inhibited and behind with school work. Children can present with developmental or habit disorders such as bed-wetting, soiling, speech impediments and tics, as well as such conduct problems as fighting, lying, shop-lifting, truancy and overactivity in general. As well as this, there are children with neuro-psychiatric disorders, including epilepsy, psychosomatic problems and psychotic disorders. Pinkerton has stated that, whereas organic pathology is disease specific, emotional pathology is case specific, and certainly this is true with many childhood emotional disorders (Pinkerton, 1974). The way the child manifests the problem including the choice of symptom, often can be best understood in the context of the child's experiences and life situation, as is illustrated by the following cases.

Two new referrals, both boys, attended a child guidance clinic on the same day with similar symptom patterns but of different origins: Adrian, aged 9, the eldest of six children and the only boy, had become quite timid, and had developed a hesitancy in his speech and a habit spasm, which was getting worse during the year prior to referral. He had been born in Manchester, of Irish parents. When Adrian was aged 7 the paternal grandfather became ill and the family returned to Ireland to look after him. The paternal grandmother very much indulged Adrian and there was considerable friction as a result of this. The father also had an adjustment problem as his parents continued to relate to him as a teenager and the grandfather (who had recovered) declined to sign the farm over although this was promised. Adrian was a bright boy and had been able to exploit the family tensions in many ways and so was able to run things much as he liked. This resulted in his becoming very insecure. Here was a case where it was important to reinforce the generation boundaries. Some work was done on introducing more social structure into Adrian's life by drawing up routines for meal times, bedtimes, etc. and recruiting the father to implement these. A psychiatric social worker, through home visits, facilitated communication between the adults which led to greater understanding and more appropriate role relationships. Following an initial testing-out period Adrian lost his symptoms and gained in self-confidence.

James, aged 10, the second of four children, had become overactive in the months prior to referral and had also developed a speech impediment and a tic. It emerged that he was experiencing increasing difficulties at school and psychological assessment revealed that his intellectual functioning was at the dull/normal level. He had been trying very hard to keep up with his classmates and to meet the demands made on him but the pace was too much. The therapeutic approach included an explanation of the situation to the teacher and a sensitive discussion with the parents who became more supportive. Remedial teaching was instituted and James became a happier boy and his symptoms gradually diminished.

Classification of childhood emotional problems

Many scientific disciplines have contributed to child psychiatry as a specialty, and, as childhood emotional disorders are invariably multifactorial in origin, together these have led to considerable difficulties in achieving a consensus on an acceptable classification system. Quite a number of proposals have been made; for example some have tried to fit the childhood syndromes into adult psychiatric diagnostic categories, but this has not been satisfactory. Other systems proved to contain a mixture of descriptive and aetiological categories and some cases would have to be listed under two or even three sections, while others had important features in the presenting picture which were not capable of being reflected in the diagnosis at all.

In 1967 a multi-axial system of child psychiatric disorders was proposed at a W.H.O. Seminar in Paris and this has been modified and further developed since (Rutter et al., 1975). To a large extent this system acknowledges the main variables which contribute to the presenting picture of the child's emotional problem and reflects the professional fields of the traditional child guidance team. In clinical practice this system has been proved to be reliable and valid and something along its lines is likely to meet with international acceptance. In essence the system has five axes: the first is the child psychiatric syndrome; next the level of intellectual functioning; thirdly are associated or aetiological biological influences; axis four is the medical diagnostic code from the I.C.D.; and the fifth one represents associated or aetiological psychosocial influences.

Agreement on a classification system will give tremendous impetus to scientific research in child psychiatry permitting properly controlled clinical trials to be compared and repeated in different settings.

It is well however, that the general practitioner need not concern himself with this debate and will develop his own method of formulating the cases he sees in his clinical practice. Something along the following lines may suit his purpose:

Is the main source of stress:

(a) from within the child?
(b) from within the family?
(c) from the outside community?

Having answered these questions in many cases it will emerge that the problem lies between two or more of the groups as in the case of James above, where there was dissonance between the environmental demands and the ability of the child. There treatment was at two levels, one aimed at diminishing the outside demands and the other at enhancing the child's ability and in this way removing the dissonance. The specific approaches adopted in practice will depend on their feasibility and it is a good principle to try the easiest one first.

THE DIAGNOSTIC PROCESS IN THE CONSULTING ROOM

As has been mentioned already, adults vary in their ability to establish a direct relationship with children and this is no less true of doctors. In most practices, the management of illness in children is carried out through the parents and frequently this is quite satisfactory. It does have limitations however, particularly where there are emotional difficulties and it is disappointing when one meets children at the child psychiatric clinic who have not seen the doctor, the referral having been made entirely on the mother's hearsay. In this chapter, emphasis is placed on a treatment approach that focuses mainly on working with parents or families. This is done partly because it is felt to be an appropriate and familiar role for the family practitioner, but also in recognition of the limitations on his time. It is not intended to suggest that the individual child does not have an important, sometimes a major, and occasionally the only, part to play in the treatment relationship. He certainly cannot and should not be excluded at the diagnostic stage, when a little time with the child may convey a lot, as well as ensuring his co-operation with treatment.

First of all, even where it is clear that the problem is entirely psychogenic, it is important to carry out a physical examination of the child. As Apley has pointed out, one may make an incidental finding such as carious teeth or a hernia (Apley, 1975). Probably more important, however, is the symbolic function the examination may subserve. A mother may feel inadequate and a failure when she has a sick child and the tremendous reassurance she gains through having him pronounced physically healthy may play a not insignificant part in modifying her feelings towards him. It is probably the same factor which prompts some mothers to present their young children frequently and with different complaints, when they have the negative relationship towards them, which sometimes proceeds to non-accidental injury.

It is a good idea to have a corner of the surgery set aside for children. There, one can place a couple of stools around a low table on which are a range of toys, jig-saws, Plasticine, books, drawing paper and crayons. Nearly all children are apprehensive when they come to the surgery, their experience being that doctors inflict pain rather than relieve it. The doctor can quickly settle the child in this corner and a useful technique is to suggest that he draw all the members of the family doing something together. Then the history may be taken from the accompanying parent and observations can be made on the child's behaviour, attention span, right-handedness or left-handedness, etc. Apart from what the drawing itself reveals about the family, it serves as a conversation piece from which to commence a discussion and may be used as part of the case record. Children like being asked questions to which they know the answer and, while they are intensely loyal to family members, are usually quite happy to provide the names and ages of siblings, their classes at school and such things as the sleeping arrangements at home. The mother's reactions and the child-mother interaction can be monitored while this is going on. Does she interject? Does she correct him? Does he look at her to answer the questions?

One should not talk down to children, who invariably view the doctor, a member of the adult world, as an agent of their parents. This is particularly true of adolescents but they will usually accept undertakings of confidentiality. With younger children the doctor may have to give the lead in play or in drawing and may find Winnicott's squiggle game useful, in which the child's squiggle is turned into a picture and then it is the child's turn to do likewise with the doctor's one (Winnicott, 1971). Children's ability to appreciate what is going on is almost universally underestimated and it is not sufficiently appreciated that they have the ability to understand a considerable amount about their anatomy and physiology. Where the doctor feels that it is appropriate that the child himself be viewed as the patient, it is important that he follow this through consistently. The confidence of even quite young children can be gained and a direct treatment relationship established, the parents having ancillary or facilitating roles. Such an approach is outlined below in the management of enuresis and encopresis and may also be used in many other cases.

General practice is both an art and a science, as indeed is child psychiatry, and how he approaches the case varies with the personality and style of the doctor and depends on his clinical judgment. Children's problems can present in a myriad of ways and so the treatment has to be tailor-made for each case. Indeed the presenting symptoms themselves are not indicative of the diagnosis, for example, one child reacting to the death of his father might develop school refusal, a sibling might commence shoplifting, another have a recrudescence of asthma, thereby illustrating Pinkerton's observation (*see* p. 357). One relies, therefore, on general principles, modifying these to suit the needs of the occasion. In the following account some of these principles stated baldly seem quite trite and yet they have proved very helpful as a guide for clinical practice.

GENERAL GUIDELINES FOR THE TREATMENT APPROACH

Parents who come to the doctor for help with their child's problem will already have tried a number of approaches; these will usually include a phase when they ignored the problem, a phase of leniency and a phase of attempted coercion. They will often feel guilty and occasionally angry and it is important that the therapist does not add to either emotion. It is supportive to make a comment which acknowledges these feelings, such as, "I am glad you brought Johnny here today, I have great respect for parents who bring problems like this to the doctor. Many parents are embarrassed and blame themselves for their children's difficulties, and I imagine you may have felt this way as well."

In practice, biology is a reliable guide and this reminds us of such simple but crucial facts that children have two parents, they are reared in families where there is a hierarchical age structure, the parents belong to a different generation to the children, and so on. If these biological facts had been adhered to many children's homes would not have developed the way they did. For example, it is of course not biologically possible for parents to have twenty children of the same age; nor could the instruction to staff not to get emotionally involved with the children have been given. Nowadays most adoption societies implement this principle and where parents applying for a child are beyond the biological age for childbirth themselves their application usually would not be successful.

It is important to remember the age of the child and a good principle is that a child should "be his age". It is sometimes helpful to think of four age dimensions for children: chronological age, intellectual age, emotional age and physical age. Where these ages are in accord all should go smoothly, while discrepancies lead to problems.

To illustrate this, an extreme example would be the case of an 8-year-old boy with the physical development of a 10-year-old, the intellectual level of a 6-year-old and the emotional level of a 4-year-old. Here the diagnostic task would require an investigation of how such a situation came about and the treatment approach would be to devise a method of redressing the imbalance. Not infrequently, in the case of an intelligent child with symptoms of insecurity, one finds oneself relating in a way appropriate to a much older child and the cues for this pattern have come from the patient himself. The parents may be doing likewise, which would mean that some of the child's emotional needs are going unmet. One would need to explore further to see why the child was rejecting his childhood so strongly. It may be that as a younger member of a grown-up family within which he has acquired verbal fluency, people related to him as an older child or it may have been that he was required to function as an adult before his years. One would seek to work through the cause when identified and certainly seek to have the parents relate to the child in a more age-appropriate way, perhaps quietly cuddling him a bit more, playing less advanced games and generally lowering the expectations for social functioning. It is true that children can function at an older level and frequently enjoy so doing. One often comes across young teenage girls successfully running a household and caring for younger siblings where the mother is chronically sick or perhaps deceased. For short periods of time, such "acting" can be a good thing and seen as role rehearsal but where the teenager's own emotional needs go unmet for a long time, emotional damage can occur. This could result in some limitations in personality development or later in life behaviour appropriate to a young teenager may emerge.

By and large, children are conservative and do not much care for change. As with everybody else, under stress they *regress*, functioning at a level appropriate to a younger child. A common example is the case of a family moving house due to the father getting promotion or changing jobs. Depending on the age and personality of the child many different symptoms may present, such as bed-wetting, temper tantrums, clinging behaviour, aggression towards younger siblings, etc. The treatment would be to increase the social structure, thereby introducing more predictability into the daily life of the child and also allowing for the regression and relating in a way appropriate to a younger child for a while. This might involve helping the child to keep a diary in which the week's events were planned, to have very definite meal times, play time, story-telling time, time with father and perhaps earlier bedtime. The symptoms often disappear quickly and this reminds us of another point, and that is that children's experience of the passage of time is different from adults, three or four days being a very long time in a young child's life.

Strategies for parental guidance

Society holds parents responsible for their children and by and large parents accept this. Therefore they do not find it easy to seek help for emotional or behavioural problems, which is one of the reasons why the problems are often framed in terms of physical symptoms. In a sense, the parents are testing the water, and the further description of the problem will depend on the therapist's response and line of enquiry. Michael Balint has brilliantly described this process as one of negotiation over the illness (Balint, 1968). It may have taken the parents a lot of courage to take this first step and, as has already been mentioned, it is extremely important for the therapist to adopt a supportive line from the beginning. It is therefore best that he accept what is offered and by an open approach seek to widen the frame of reference. Parents already will have received advice of all sorts from many quarters and will have discounted the glib reassurance of the "he'll grow out of it" kind. In order to understand how the family has got to its present position and to ensure the co-operation which is essential for treatment, it is crucial for the therapist of get onto the parents' wavelength. This is not to say that he should see himself as the parents' agent, as of course he does have a clinical responsibility for the child whose interest and welfare he must promote. Where significant disturbance in a parent is the cause of a child's emotional problem, the child psychiatrist has to decide on the line of treatment. Should he treat the child directly, should he adopt a family therapy approach, should he undertake treatment of the sick parent or should he refer the parent to an adult psychiatrist? Where he undertakes the treatment himself, the family doctor is faced with no such dilemma. However he does have to decide on where and how to focus the treatment and this will depend on his clinical assessment of what is needed and what is acceptable. It has been mentioned above that the main sources of stress on the child may come from within himself, within the family or from the community and that in many cases the problem stems from "poorness of fit" between any two of these. At times, the doctor will work primarily with the child, and frequently on behalf of the child and the family, will seek to bring about changes in the outside community, for instance through influencing the opinions of teachers or employers, or advocating the improvement of housing and social conditions. However, in general practice it is usually more feasible and more appropriate to involve the parents in a major way in the treatment transactions. In a sense, one is joining the parents as a co-therapist and the following are some of the ways in which this is done.

1. Provision of information

Supplying factual information is one of the doctor's main functions

and at times it may be the only one required. Frequently, one is reminded how little real knowledge of human biology there is in the
community and, in the face of difficulties, one can understand how
anxieties can soar, giving rise to all sorts of fears and fantasies. The
very fact that the doctor is familiar with the problem and may even
have a name for it is tremendously reassuring. Parents compare
children, but know little of the variation in developmental norms.
To have their doctor explain that a child may indeed stop using his
few words, while concentrating on walking, is very reassuring. Whilst
they read many of the books now available, many parents do not
appreciate that regressive behaviour can be quite normal and having
this spelt out by their doctor in the case of their own child, is often
sufficient to free them from their anxieties.

2. Moral and social evaluation

In a rapidly changing society, parents may feel unable to evaluate the significance of their children's behaviour or what attitude
they should adopt towards it. The general practitioner, as an important member of the community, may be used as a sounding board in
this regard although this is rarely done directly. A parent may describe
in shocked tones, such behaviour as truancy, shoplifting, masturbation or illegitimate pregnancy, with the aim of getting some guidance
on how to form a moral judgment. As doctors, we are increasingly
advised to be non-judgmental in our approach and not to let our
personal system of values impinge on our clinical practice. When called
on to evaluate behaviour however, there is an opportunity to function as therapist. The approach will vary according to what is felt to
be appropriate, e.g. a supportive and understanding one in the case
of a pregnant school girl. The following case gives an example.

Bill, a 14-year-old, was seen because of a series of anti-social
escapades. The family had moved from a poor quarter of the East
End of London to the rural West Country and it later emerged
that this was because of the father's anxieties lest his children
became delinquent. From the previous history and the way they
functioned in the session, it was clear that the father took very
little part in the running of the family whereas the mother was
over-intrusive. To get away from his mother, Bill used to slip out
at night and get into trouble. The father likewise avoided tension
and was frequently in the pub during these times. The doctor's
approach was to turn to the father and virtually hold him responsible for the boy's misbehaviour. An agreement was reached
whereby the father was not to let the boy out of his sight in the
evenings and this effectively imprisoned both of them in the
home. Seen at weekly intervals, at first they reported a high degree
of tension and then it was suggested that the father help Bill with

his reading, followed by some family games. It was recommended that Bill should tell his father when he felt ready to be trusted, e.g. to go out for half an hour and remain where he said he was going. This was tested out and over a six week period trust was re-established between father and son. The doctor played an important role here, that of lending superego and encouraging the parties to face the tensions that they had been avoiding.

3. Modelling

The doctor, through his unemotional approach, seeking to understand the child's behaviour, offers a role-model to the parents, as in the following case.

Gerard, a small wiry 9-year-old boy came with his mother who said she had twisted her ankle. While Gerard was looking at the toys, the mother whispered that the ankle was a pretence and in fact the problem was that Gerard would not go to school. The doctor immediately addressed Gerard directly enquiring about the home situation etc. He then broached the question of school and Gerard replied that there were no problems. On this occasion his mother said "Oh, but Gerard, you have not been to school for weeks" whereupon the boy threw himself at her kicking, screaming and pulling her hair. The amazing thing was that the mother did nothing to protect herself and so the doctor grasped the boy and held him firmly on his knee while discussing the background further with the mother. It seemed that there was a major disagreement in the home over child rearing, the father being quite punitive and the mother consequently concealing many of Gerard's misdemeanours. Gerard was in effective control of his mother which no doubt lay behind his high level of anxiety. Throughout the discussion Gerard at times struggled and shouted abuse, but it was quietly explained to him that he would be released if he promised not to attack his mother. As soon as he gave this undertaking he was let go and he kept his word. Not only was the mother protecting the boy from his father but she was somewhat frightened of Gerard herself. She was very impressed by the doctor's ability to confront Gerard with his school refusal and way of coping with the temper tantrum and this represented the beginning of treatment. Some time later a social worker was able to do some very useful work in helping to resolve some of the marital conflict.

4. Confirming the parental role

Sometimes parents have already worked out the appropriate course of action and are really seeking endorsement for it. One of the unfortunate consequences of the publication of many guides on child rearing and the frequent mentioning of child-related topics on the media by experts, is that some parents feel deskilled and even intimidated. Needless to say it is imperative that doctors (including child psychiatrists), do nothing to undermine parents in their role. It is in the child's best interest to promote better parental functioning and an attitude of criticism or fault-finding certainly will not achieve this. Some doctors feel that they have to adopt an omnipotent role and of course this is unrealistic. In those cases where the doctor is quite puzzled it can be helpful for him to say so and, as it were, join with the parents in seeking to understand the child's behaviour.

One example of a doctor reassuring a parent by reinforcing the parental role is shown in the case of the young mother who had been feeling inadequate. She was much reassured when an eminent child specialist handed her back her wailing infant to comfort. She had not noticed that he had given the baby a little pinch!

In very many instances the general practitioner, through his enquiries, will clarify the issues for the parents thereby enabling them to act more appropriately. A common example is in helping parents to see how they ignore a child who is behaving appropriately and attend to him, albeit to correct and punish him, when he misbehaves. Increasingly one encounters parents who declare they do not understand teenagers and who have, in effect, abdicated from their roles. Here a discussion of the issues often results in a demonstration that the parents have in fact a good understanding of their child who is often behaving just as they did at that age but in a different style and possibly on a different battle ground. It is usually possible for them to see the importance of limit-setting and of not reneging on their own standards. There are some youth club leaders, teachers and, no doubt, doctors and parents, who solve their problems in communicating with teenagers by seeking to join them. Needless to say, they lose the teenagers' respect in this and are not turned to in times of crisis or anxiety.

5. Outlining behavioural methods
A wide variety of modifications of the behavioural therapy approach can be devised for specific cases. It includes such well-tried methods as star charts, time-out procedures and enuresis alarms. Contract therapy, in which written and signed agreements are drawn up between one or both parents and children, are frequently very successful. Some parents at first find this idea distasteful as they see it as a very impersonal legalistic approach to what should be the normal give-and-take of family life. However, one can introduce it from the child's point of view showing how children are very good in thinking in terms of "rules of the game" and it can become acceptable when this game quality is emphasised. Contracts can be drawn up in virtually any situation and they are particularly useful in helping to bridge

the gap between parental expectations and children's behaviour, e.g. personal hygiene, table manners, household chores and homework, and the rewards could include pocket money, television viewing, time required to be in at night, film going, attending football matches, etc. It is very important to attend to the details of the modes of behaviour and the rewards and getting agreement on them. Time spent on this will increase the likelihood of success. The contract is reviewed at weekly or fortnightly sessions and may be modified in the light of experience. One of the most important things in all the behavioural approaches is to keep trying — parents and children may get discouraged easily and revert to the previous maladaptive pattern.

In cases where one is satisfied that an insecure child is limit-testing, it is often possible to demonstrate the rationale of relating to the child at the level his behaviour indicates.

An example was the case of Nigel, a 10-year-old who had been involved in petty pilfering. Both Nigel and his parents were able to see that whereas he had the privileges of a 10-year-old, he was really behaving like a toddler who did not know that one is not supposed to take things belonging to others. The treatment approach was that his parents should relate to Nigel as if he were a 3-year-old and the doctor spent some time eliciting from the family members as to what this would entail. Three-year-olds go to bed at about 7 p.m., they are not allowed out unaccompanied and have to hold the parent's hand crossing the street, they are allowed to watch only children's television programmes, and so on. While the doctor joined the family in seeing the amusing side of this, he also indicated that he was quite serious and that Nigel seemed to need the security of such parental attention. It was agreed that where Nigel felt he could behave at an older level he should say so and the parents would test it out, e.g. asking him if it were all right to leave sweets or money lying around. Where this was successful they were to test him at his request in going to the local shop and coming back at the time specified. It was emphasised that Nigel was to give the directions in this but that it was his behaviour that was to be the guide and that the method was to be applied without anger or rancour.

Where such a developmental approach is implemented consistently, one finds that children quickly get the point and that to earn the privileges of one's age one has to accept the responsibilities. Parents need a lot of support to help them in the early days, because usually the child will test their resolve with increased misbehaviour and it is as well to say that this is likely to happen. It is important to see both the child and the parents at weekly intervals, though not necessarily for very long, as these are usually the parents who have been tending to capitulate to the child in the interest of a quiet life.

The success of behavioural approaches lies in the attention to detail. It is important to remember that it is behaviour that is being focused on and it is useful to use charts and records to monitor this. Children quickly grasp the idea of this and enjoy it. One of the major reasons for the failure of this approach is that the behavioural goals are unrealistic and the child does not attempt them. It is essential that the therapist break down the goals to attainable steps and that these are clearly understood. It is also important that it is positive steps that are recorded and that the rewards are ones of the child's choice.

A fundamental principle is that none of the treatments should result in the child being deprived or in his emotional needs being unmet. They should all be recommended within a caring context and nothing done to inhibit the family's nurturing capacity.

6. Parent as play therapist

Children with a good capacity for creative play are unlikely to present with emotional problems. Those needing play therapy include timid, anxious, children with poor self-concept, who are inhibited in their play, and also the insecure overactive children who are unable to contain their feelings but discharge them in wild activity. In the case of younger children sometimes one can direct the parents to a suitable play group but, frequently, there is no such opportunity. There is no reason why the parents themselves cannot take on this role and indeed it is surprising, when one looks into it, how few parents make a point of setting aside time to play with their children. In the case of a child with an emotional problem, it is often best for the parent who is less involved with the child to take on the role of therapist. The main point is to set aside a regular time that is suitable for both parent and child. This need not be too long, fifteen to thirty minutes per day being ample. Essentially the parent's task is to set up the conditions within which the child can play out his fantasies. With inhibited children the parent may have to give the lead. When the child feels secure he may demonstrate aggressive or destructive behaviour; the parent should be warned of this and advised to facilitate it as long as the child does not become overwhelmed. The parent should also ensure where feasible that attempts be made to repair and reconstruct broken toys. Attention to this restitution and restoration will prevent the child from being overwhelmed with depressing feelings of destructiveness. However, neither the parent nor the general practitioner should make any attempt to interpret the transactions at a symbolic level, and where it is felt necessary the child should be referred for specialist opinion and treatment.

FAMILY THERAPY

Recently there has been an increased interest in the family both in the general population and amongst politicians. However, for many years general practitioners have prided themselves on the fact that they treated their patients as members of a family and in the context of a community, and have rejoiced in the title "family practitioners". As we have seen earlier there are some relatively new concepts which involve regarding the patient and the members of his family as a relationship system, and of treating this system as a clinical entity. These concepts derive from many sources and are brought together under the general title "family therapy". Deriving from General Systems Theory (*see below*) most of the concepts in family therapy are easy to understand and can have wide application in general practice. In order to appreciate the significance of the theory and to see it in context, it will be helpful to review the development of some ideas in psychiatry in general.

In the nineteenth century, the mechanical age, medicine as a whole was preoccupied with the discovery and description of individual diseases for the purposes of classification. Emil Kraepelin, was the principal worker in the field of psychopathology. Although revolutionary in many of his ideas, Sigmund Freud adopted much the same approach: that of the analysis and description of the workings of the psyche, involving a careful exploration of the patient's mental processes with a strong emphasis on their historical development. This can be seen in the structuring and procedure of psychoanalysis. These are very intense individual one-to-one experiences and the analyst not only does not interview the patient's relations, but frequently might view independent information about them as a hindrance to the therapy. It is how the patient views them and his fantasies about them that is important. Some of the child psychoanalysts maintained the individual tradition and indeed Melanie Klein, at one stage, even forbade the child's mother from staying in the waiting room, realising that the proximity would continue to exert an influence on the child in the treatment session. There are other schools of psychiatry whose adherents feel that greater emphasis should be placed on other factors influencing human feelings and behaviour. There are those who hold that neurophysiology and biochemistry are of fundamental importance and others, such as Alfred Adler and Wilhelm Reich, who believed that Freud's intra-psychic focus neglected to place sufficient value on those powerful social forces which mould behaviour. Since the 1930s social psychiatrists, psychologists and other social scientists have explored and developed ways of harnessing such social forces for therapeutic purposes. We have witnessed a world-wide expansion of group treatments of many kinds, e.g. therapeutic communities, psychotherapeutic groups, weight-watchers, Gamblers Anonymous. Some gestalt groups and encounter groups, by and large, discount the previous history of the group members and concentrate on here-and-now experiences. They place emphasis on open emotional communication and feedback amongst the members. Feedback is a term used in computer technology and some of the language and concepts of cybernetics has been found applicable and useful in studying human interaction.

Apart from group psychotherapists, other psychiatrists could see that the social and emotional environments of their patients were of great importance. It was recognised, for example, that some patients with schizophrenia relapsed when discharged home and that the outcome was more favourable when they remained in hostels and other less emotionally-intense settings (Brown *et al.*, 1972). Indeed the same is true for some psychosomatic disorders. Increasingly, psychiatrists began to interview and counsel the patient's relatives. It became recognised that other members of the family might be contributing in a more direct way to some of the relapses; the wives of some alcoholics became depressed when the husband remained off drink, and indeed not infrequently one saw the situation of a marriage breaking down, not when the drinking continued but when it stopped. Likewise in families where a delinquent child was placed in a special residential school, it often happened that another, previously apparently well-adjusted, child started misbehaving. It was as if such families needed a "black sheep". There were many such examples, such as a patient's husband saying, "You know, I like her more when she is depressed". Therapists, in such cases, came to appreciate that unless they effected changes in the relationships of these patients, including the way they were related to by others, that there was little likelihood of long-term change. The next logical step in this line of thinking was the idea of treating, not the individual with the symptoms but the entire family, the interest moving from the family *of* the psychiatric patient to the concept of the family *as* the psychiatric patient.

In this, there was no question of blaming anyone for the patient's symptoms but it was a case of recognising that frequently these emerged from a pattern of relationships that was maladaptive, and that it was this pattern itself that required changing. Social anthropologists and sociologists had been familiar with tribes and societies whose traditions and ways of life had not taken account of changing circumstances and which had failed to prosper. Likewise, management consultants and businessmen generally have been accustomed to studying factories, and working groups of all sorts, seeking to eliminate inefficiencies and have employed systems analysts for this purpose. Within the medical profession, social factors have long been recognised as exerting an important influence particularly in such specialties as public health, community medicine, occupational and industrial medicine and rehabilitation. Yet this family therapy concept is a new one to the profession: the idea that the site of the pathology is not within the individual but in the group and that the patient's symptoms could be seen as stemming from faulty group interaction rather than from anything within himself. The consequence of this results in the therapist's task being to seek to bring about such changes in the relationships that the symptoms become unnecessary. It is impossible to change one member of the group without effecting a readjustment all round and so it is the system itself that requires change and it is to the family system that the therapist relates.

In many other branches of science, this systems way of thinking is very familiar and General Systems Theory (G.S.T.) offers a unifying framework for the natural and social sciences (Bertalanffy, 1968). The family system can be seen as a system just like any other and G.S.T. applies to it too. We can see that the definition: "a system is an interdependent organisation in which the behaviour and expression of each component influences and is influenced by all the others", could be applied to the family (Walrond-Skinner, 1976). Needless to say systems theory has its own language and until recently there has been little, if anything, in medical training or literature to assist doctors to work with these concepts. Sometimes people become worried at the very mechanistic sound of the systems language when applied to human interactions, with talk of subsystems, boundaries, components, organisations and so on. In practice however, in family therapy, people's feelings are given great value and attention and are very sensitively approached. Indeed the aim of the process is to assist towards a resolution of problems, and there is no sense of adhering to theory for its own sake.

All behaviour is multi-determined and a child is exposed to a vast number of learning contexts all of which help to mould his development. However it is the family which has the strongest and most enduring influence on his attitudes, values, hopes, ambitions, ways of relating and so on. Therefore it can be much more efficient if the therapist can bring about better family functioning rather than attempting to promote change directly in the individual child, although there is place for that too. These ideas apply not only to families whose members have symptoms, but to all families. It is worth while reflecting on normal family structure and how it comes about. Most families have a distinctive style, various family rules and understandings about decision making, power, authority, responsibility and so on, both consciously and unconsciously felt. Many of the transactions of courtship and early marital life have to do with subtle negotiations on these questions, each partner bringing to the relationship, ideas, expectations and life styles from their families of origin. The new patterns that evolve are not set for all time because the family has to be a flexible unit adapting to the influences that act on it from without and within. As the children arrive and grow, the type of caring needed and the functions it has to subserve require adjustments within the family while the system itself maintains continuity. Just as in the case with individual children, the family as a whole grows and matures through facing and overcoming the stresses that impinge on it and each member contributes to this. There are families which are subjected to extreme stress and fail and other families who seem to be unable to cope with the ordinary stresses of life. However most families seem to function quite satisfactorily most of the time, evolving from one stage to the next and promoting the development and fulfilment of their members. Each family develops uniquely through incorporating something from each marital partner and from their families of origin, coupled with the growth that comes from joint experiences. The new pattern is created from the many negotiations amongst family members, often around small daily events and frequently at an unconscious level. What an outsider observes on looking at a family has been compared to characters interacting in a play, the script of which has been lost (Walrond-Skinner, 1976).

Families vary in their capacity to change when new demands are made and there are strong homeostatic mechanisms with which equilibrium is re-established (Ackerman, 1958). Sometimes these mechanisms are ineffective and a family crisis occurs which results in outsiders becoming involved. Indeed a crisis can be a good time for therapy as the system has become unstable and the members may be quite open to a readjustment in relationships. The sort of issues which can produce crises are, for example, when one or more children, perhaps unwittingly, challenge an unresolved or a patched-over parental conflict that has been buried in the past. The parents themselves may have forgotten about it but it would have continued to influence their behaviour. Such faulty resolutions frequently have to do with guilt-ridden events, such as infidelities, betrayals, illegitimate pregnancies and such skeletons in the family cupboard as mental illness in a family member whose name is never mentioned, and sometimes they have to do with failed bereavement reactions (*see* pp. 351-53). These and other ghosts from the past can return and, as it were, torment the present. They may have to be faced and named before they can be exorcised and the family freed from their influence. It is not uncommon for such issues to arise during the children's adolescence when they are seeking to establish their own identity and questions about dependence and independence surface. A case illustration may be timely here.

Patrick, aged 16, had been caught stealing both at home and in the neighbourhood on a number of occasions; he refused to study at school and was threatening to leave home. He was the third of a family of five, the siblings being Kathleen, aged 20, a student nurse, David, 18, just finished school, Dora, 14, at secondary school, and Natasha, aged 3, still at home. He was brought by both his parents and presented as a tall, well-dressed, well-built, obese boy. He related in a bland unaffected way, in contrast to his very worried parents. From the start the mother took a more dominant role in the proceedings, she stared intensely at Patrick with whom she was very closely involved. The therapist sat beside the father bringing him more into the picture and the story was that he had given up chastising Patrick, who made him extremely angry, because he feared that he would severely injure him.

It emerged that Patrick has always been regarded as a charming intelligent boy for whom everyone had a special affection, although he had been stealing and lying since the age of 4. The father in particular had had a soft spot for him, partly because of similarities he had with the more admirable features in his own father. He agreed that he had never exercised the same authority over him as he had over the other children and so he had become very much a special child. Up to shortly before the referral he had had nocturnal enuresis and to some extent was a compulsive over-eater which resulted in his obesity. He was something of a compulsive gambler as well, at which he was quite successful and his practice was to take his school mates to restaurants for meals.

The family were taken on for family therapy. One of the features in the sessions was that Natasha would turn to Patrick for mothering and indeed all agreed that Patrick was the best to look after her. Various other features emerged, but the turning point came when the mother felt able to state that she too had stolen in her childhood and had come from a very deprived background. That there was strong identification between Patrick and his mother had been clear and to a large extent he had taken over much of her role. She certainly seemed to need him desperately and bailed him out whenever he got into difficulties. It was only when the State, through the police, started to intervene that they had presented for therapy. The mother revealed this in an intensely emotional session and it led to very definite changes. Patrick started attending a weight-watchers group and lost over six kilograms in weight. His school work improved and while he continued to associate with his mates he no longer felt under a compulsion to commit anti-social offences. In a sense he became more differentiated as a person. One of the therapist's aims was to promote the father into adopting a more supportive role to his wife, and to some extent this was achieved. The family itself was surprised at the changes, particularly when it was possible to employ Patrick during the holiday period in the family business, whereas in the past he had been absolutely forbidden to go near the premises as he had stolen hundreds of pounds there over the years.

Indeed just as in the community at large, families may have not only ghosts but also myths. Family mythology represents a body of beliefs that the family has about itself or its members and frequently these beliefs have never been explicitly stated (Byng-Hall, 1973). Such a myth for example existed in the case already mentioned where it was thought the mother was very vulnerable and would break down if unsupported. In those families chosen for family therapy, the therapist openly confronts the family myth with his own view and much of the work of therapy has to do with sensitively supporting the family, while the feelings that are uncovered are explored and worked through. Many techniques have been evolved by family therapists to help them with their work; some of them have to do with looking at non-verbal communication and ways of providing feedback to the family members on how they view one another. The use of videotape, one-way screens, and techniques derived from psycho-drama are amongst the many methods implied. Clearly the general practitioner is unable to undertake work of this sort. Nevertheless the family therapy concept, when used with awareness, has a potential for enriching family practice and deserves thorough study.

A ready example of how a family myth may arise is through the establishment of the idea that a child is delicate, as in the case of Thomas already mentioned (p. 352). The family doctor has an important role in anticipating and preventing such myths from gaining currency, and in promoting healthy family functioning. Opportunities arise at the time of family crises but frequently these are lost when doctors apply administrative solutions, including hospitalisations, and the use of medication. If instead of providing such answers the doctor permits himself to join the family in seeking a resolution or invites a social worker to do this, he may be of much more value to the family. By finding the strength within it to cope with its problems, the family would grow and in the long run this will probably prove time saving to the general practitioner.

Throughout the ages, philosophers and poets have written of the power of the myth, the lure of fantasy, the unconscious transmission of influences and the necessity to confront the feared object before being released from its spell. These and similar concepts are conveyed in Confucian teachings and Zen writings, as well as in much Western literature. George Santayana's statement, "Those who cannot remember the past are condemned to repeat it", is a valid perception.

Yeats has written:

> Let the new faces play what tricks they will
> In the old rooms; night can outbalance day,
> Our shadows rove the garden gravel still,
> The living seem more shadowy than they.

T. S. Eliot illustrated the family interactional theme in his play *The Cocktail Party*, and also has reminded us in "Burnt Norton":

> . . . human kind
> Cannot bear very much reality.
> Time past and time future
> What might have been and what has been
> Point to one end, which is always present.

These ideas, therefore, are not new. What is new is the linking of them to systems theory, by those seeking to relieve human suffering and bring about change. Various psychotherapeutic methods and strategies from diverse sources have been employed and a certain amount of evaluative research carried out. One of the earlier family therapy practitioners, Theodore Lidz, clarified important points in relation to *generation boundaries*. He felt that it was important that the parents should have an effective coalition, appropriately sharing their roles and offering models for the children. He saw that it was important that the generation boundaries should be maintained so that the children would not be required to, and should not attempt to, meet the adults' unmet needs. He also made some points about sex-linked roles which probably require modification because of the recent societal changes. Despite the vulnerability of the nuclear family, he could see that it was much more flexible and adaptable than the traditionally extended family and was therefore better suited to prepare children for adulthood in Western society (Lidz, 1963).

The concept of generation boundary is a valuable one and is not to be confused with the "generation gap" of the journalists. Indeed reports of teenagers from the National Child Development Study cohort show that the generation gap is not at all as wide as the media would lead us to believe and that, by and large, the views, attitudes and aspirations of Britain's adolescents are very similar to those of their parents (Fogelman, 1976). In looking at the problems of families, one can very often make a diagnosis in generation boundary terms and thereby gain guidance for the treatment approach.

SPECIFIC PARENTAL SITUATIONS

Introduction
All children have two biological parents who normally rear them to adulthood and this is the basic model in most societies. In very simplified terms, one could say that adolescents engage in various pairing relationships, during which they increase in self-knowledge and mature. Ultimately the adult man and woman then enter, by marrying, what they hope will be a permanent relationship within which they may or may not intend to rear children. Courtship and early married life are times when a lot of reality-testing occurs with both partners having to shed fantasies. Consciously and unconsciously they establish a relationship pattern using their own parents as models and using society's norms as conveyed from their friends and through the media. Negotiation goes on in many subtle ways and while from time to time conflicts arise, they are usually resolved, although sometimes buried. By the time of the first pregnancy a considerable degree of mutuality has been achieved. The arrival of the first child has tremendous significance as it is at this point that "the family" is created, the triangle has come into existence, and we have two generations in the household. Peter de Vries in his work *Tunnel of Love* has said, "the value of marriage is not that adults produce children, but that children produce adults". Certainly the role of parent is very different from that of young husband or wife, bringing its own demands and satisfactions. It is a period which can call for rapid change in relationships and the role-flexibility and conflict-resolving capacity of the couple is tested. The task of the new-born may be a difficult one as many parents do not make the required adjustment without a struggle. This can carry some emotional risk to the child and it may be one of the reasons why many societies put a special value on the first born — hence the tradition of primogeniture. Of course why this applies only to boys is another question.

Winnicott has reminded us that many of our institutions derive their social structure from the family model. In the past this was more the extended family, as in the traditional hospital hierarchy with the matron running the household and the senior surgeon or physician in the male authoritative position, the other staff representing various relatives and household servants, and the patients, of course, as children, being seen but not heard. With the modifications required by their functions, one can perceive that a similar structure operated in many other social institutions and no doubt in this way met the psychological needs of the staff and clients of the Victorian generations. With time, relationships within the family itself and in our social institutions have been modified at varying rates but the strong parallels still apply. It is true that many alternative child rearing approaches have been adopted in different countries, some on quite a large scale, as for example in Soviet Russia, the kibbutzim in Israel and multiple-parent groups and communes in the United States and Western Europe. Nevertheless the biologically-based family social structure seems to be a dominating one which deeply imbues our culture. If our aim is to help children to function appropriately in society as we expect it to be when they are adults, we need to reflect on the psychological significance of this, particularly for those who do not experience such family life.

Reflection along these lines suggests the tremendous importance of both father and mother figures for the growing child without needing to invoke the concept of the Oedipal situation at all. We can see that the parents or the consistent parent-substitutes offer role-models, parts of which are incorporated into the developing identity of the child. Increasingly, as other adults enter the child's life, and especially school teachers, they too are used in this way. Nevertheless the main care-givers, those attending to the feeding, toiletting, washing and dressing of the child and playing with, comforting and, in general, sharing the many experiences of the developing child, exert the most powerful influence, whether they wish so or not. The following verses by Anthony Cronin describe the process of such identity formation.

FOR A FATHER

With the exact length and pace of his father's stride
The son walks,
Echoes and intonations of his father's speech
Are heard when he talks.

Once when the table was tall,
And the chair a wood,
He absorbed his father's smile and carefully copied
The way that he stood.

He grew into exile slowly,
With pride and remorse,
In some ways better than his begetters,
In others worse.

And now having chosen, with strangers,
Half glad of his choice,
He smiles with his father's hesitant smile
And speaks with his voice.

Paradoxically, young infants entertain omnipotent feelings and maturation requires the shedding of these as they encounter the realities of the world. Indeed many adults are unable to acknowledge the extent of their individual insignificance and are sustained by feelings of self-importance. The young child gradually extends the boundaries and perceives his family as all-important and the centre of the universe (which it is for him). Parents are seen as tremendously powerful and we have all heard young children comparing the strengths, skills and importance of their parents. Maturation involves the piecemeal discarding of such fantasies through a process of a growing insight acquired in many ways, some of them quite painful. The shedding of power, real or imagined, is experienced as a loss, and a depression and bereavement reaction ensues. Indeed the giving up of childhood itself likewise has to be mourned, and there is a considerable fluctuation in levels of functioning throughout childhood and adolescence. The achievement of full adulthood involves the capacity to recognise one's parents as ordinary human beings with limitations and failings and individual personality characteristics, albeit in a very special relationship with oneself. It is the consistent presence of the parents which enables the reality-testing to proceed. Trust in the stability of the family offers the support necessary for the ventilation and working-through of destructive fantasies, as well as depression, and permits reparation, so that feelings of gratitude and love can be experienced. Where the family system holds it offers a powerful milieu for personality integration.

On looking into it one finds that there are very many children who were not reared to adulthood by both their biological parents in this norm of family life (Fogelman, 1976). These include illegitimate children as well as those whose parents are dead, separated, divorced or missing and some who have particular sensory impairments or physical or mental handicaps. They may be reared in a variety of caring situations, including children's homes, special schools and hospitals, in short- or long-term foster care or with adoptive parents. They may also be reared by relatives, in one-parent families, in a household with one biological and one step-parent, move regularly or irregularly between the household of one natural parent to that of another, or live mainly in a one-parent family. Many children experience a number of these life situations, in some of which they meet and relate to full siblings, half-siblings, step-siblings and foster siblings. All of this can be very confusing indeed and even the adults involved can find it difficult to unravel the relationships. What guidance can we give?

It is most important that children know where they stand and one should follow the old counsel that honesty is the best policy. Children should know who their natural parents and siblings are and they should have regular contact with them, through which they may modify their views and attitudes and gain deeper understandings as they grow older. We relate to others as we perceive them and it is such perceptions that we incorporate into our identities. Children who continue to entertain fantasies of either overwhelmingly destructive or idealised parent figures will be governed by such in their adult relationships leading to many difficulties. Of course for a wide variety of reasons it is not always possible for such regular contact to be maintained. It is helpful to reflect on the experience of households where it is accepted that one parent has to be regularly and frequently absent for socially acceptable and "justifiable" reasons. These include the families of sailors, lighthouse keepers, servicemen, long-distance lorry drivers and, increasingly, of politicians, business executives and members of the professions. When the relationships are intact, the remaining parent transmits to the children a positive image of the absent parent in a myriad of ways and of course there is also mutual contact through correspondence, telephone calls and regular home leave. We must remember that "absence makes the heart grow fonder" and the image presented by the parent at home may be somewhat idealised, resulting in the children occasionally learning the truth somewhat harshly during actual confrontations. Indeed communication is of the essence, as everyone has the capacity to use such psychological mechanisms as projecting and splitting.

While every family is unique, there are those which can be grouped according to their life-situation or particular experiences or circumstances and which I shall mention. It is not possible to treat fully all their needs here and so attention is drawn to just a few points in each case, while the principles of parental counselling in general should be applied. I would emphasise again that in practice each case must be assessed on its merits and will make two further points. Firstly, social structures continuously change and the roles and role responsibilities appropriate to one generation are not necessarily those of another generation. The general practitioner, therefore, must remain sensitive to the changing dynamics both of the family and of society as a whole. Secondly, while every intervention we make in one sense is a social experiment, by and large we should adhere to social norms and it is rarely therapeutic, even if ethically acceptable, to try out novel life styles with our patients. Our obligation is to give our patients the best advice we can and they should not be used by us as society's trend-setters.

Working mothers

This is a subject surrounded by intense feelings of anger, resentment and guilt and one on which almost everyone has an opinion. In other words it touches on some very vital issues in our culture and within ourselves, having to do with the concepts of good and bad mothers and with sex-linked social roles. Caring for young children is very arduous work indeed and so the question really has to do with to what extent the biological mother should be the prime care-giver to her children. We have only to reflect on the number of children legally removed from their mothers' care by authorities concerned for their welfare, to realise that society fully accepts that children may be much better cared for by people other than the biological mother. Most general practitioners know of mothers who feel frustrated and resentful at having to remain at home with young children in the role of the dutiful mother. Yet it has been regarded as outrageous to suggest that such a mother could discharge her duty much more satisfactorily were she to work outside the house and employ someone who feels fulfilled in caring for young children. There is a popular belief that in previous generations children were reared in extended families and there was always a motherly relative standing by to help out when necessary. No doubt such situations did obtain in rural areas and at times in the settled working-class areas of our cities, but there was far more fragmentation of families than is realised and the popular belief may well be mythological. Nevertheless a number of social forces have brought about changes so that the nuclear family is now the social norm and a considerable percentage of Britain's working population now consists of married women. The question of the implications of this for children's emotional development has been somewhat bedevilled by a loose and inaccurate reading of Bowlby's work which is particularly inexcusable as his writings are so precise, unambiguous and scientifically documented.

There is no research evidence for the commonly advanced view that the children of working mothers are behind at school, uncared for and delinquent. As Rutter outlines in his popular book, *Maternal Deprivation Reassessed*, reliable research in this field is difficult to undertake because of the many variables affecting the emotional development of the child. However, it is becoming evident that it is the mother's attitude to her child, and the quality of the interaction between the care-giver and the child, that are the significant factors for his development. For the child to become well adjusted, it is important that the mother be contented and have role satisfaction and whether she goes out to work or not is incidental. The National Child Development Study showed that, at 7 years of age, children whose mothers started to go to work after the children had begun attending school, were slightly less well adjusted than children whose mothers started to go to work when they were of pre-school age. Indeed there is now a vast amount of research in this field and for the purposes of offering guidance, it is crucial to adhere to the data as presented and avoid speculation. In general practice, the following quotation from Rutter remains a reliable guide:

> When the mother goes out to work, there is good evidence that children do not suffer, provided stable relationships and good care are provided by the mother surrogates. If such mothering is of high quality and is provided by figures who remain the same during the child's early life, then multiple mothering (at least up to four or five mother

figures) need not have adverse effects. The only group of children of working mothers to suffer were those who went from pillar to post in a succession of unsatisfactory and unstable child minding arrangements.

(Rutter, 1972)

Of course, there can be no absolute blueprint and doctors will use their judgment in each clinical case. Certainly flexibility must be the keynote and where a child is displaying symptoms of stress, modifications including the giving-up of work, will have to be recommended. There are many factors which need consideration, not only in the question of working mothers, but in all situations where children experience change in their circumstances and environments. Sensitivity to their feelings is basic and they should be fully prepared in advance. In the cases of very young children, toy figures, houses, hospitals, cars etc. are most useful for this purpose. I am grateful to James and Joyce Robertson for permission to reproduce the table below which indicates these factors (Robertson, James and Robertson, Joyce, 1971).

TABLE 1. FACTORS WHICH COMBINE TO DETERMINE INDIVIDUAL DIFFERENCES IN YOUNG CHILDREN'S RESPONSES TO SEPARATION FROM THE MOTHER

A *Factors in addition to loss of the mother which are likely to cause stress*	B *Factors likely to reduce stress*	C *Child's psychological status which may increase or reduce overt distress during separation, may increase or decrease the overt upset after separation, may increase or decrease the long-term effects*
(1) Stage environment	(1) Familiar substitute caretaker	(1) Ego maturity, level of
(2) Inadequate substitute caretaker	(2) Known foods and routines	(2) Object constancy, level of
(3) Strange caretaker	(3) Toilet demands unaltered	(3) Quality of mother-child relationship, facets of
(4) Multiple caretakers	(4) Own belongings	(4) Defence organisation
(5) Cues/language not understood and responded to	(5) Unrestricted body movement	(5) Fantasies about illness, pain, physical interference, disappearance of mother etc.
(6) Unfamiliar food and routines	(6) Familiar environment	(6) Preseparation experience of illness/separation
(7) Unusual demands and disciplines	(7) Reassurance of eventual reunion	
(8) Illness, pain, body interference	(8) Keeping apart fantasy and fact ("My Mummy doesn't love me")	
(9) Bodily restriction	(9) Reminding the child of parental disciplines	
	(10) Support from father	
	(11) Willingness of caretakers to talk about parents and previous life	

(Robertson and Robertson, 1971)

Family conflict and broken homes

The general practitioner will often be asked directly whether it would not be in the children's interests for the parents to separate where there is chronic marital discord. Nobody can give a straight "yes" or "no" answer, although many are tempted to do so. The doctor's role surely is to seek to promote better mutual understanding and to help the parties to clarify the issues, see the options and consequences, so that they can reach a decision that is right for them and their children. While the interests of all members of a family are interrelated, frequently those of the parents are given more attention than those of the children and the doctor may find that he has to promote the interests of the latter. He should do this, not in any guilt-inducing way but through repeatedly introducing into the discussions points relating to their emotional and physical welfare. Even where children never see one parent, a father for example, they can have elaborate fantasies about them and so, psychologically speaking, a relationship continues in the child's mind, modified by what snippets of true or incorrect information he picks up as he matures.

It is important that parents should have their own adult life independent of their children and nowadays this is usually the case. It has been pointed out that in the case of women "instead of work being undertaken between school and motherhood, motherhood is taking place in the interval between school and work" (Finer Report, 1974). This is particularly important for two reasons: firstly, with the disappearance of the extended family there is much less call on grandparents to subserve their traditional roles; secondly, because of the greater life expectancy nowadays, parents have very many active years following the rearing of their families. There are parents who adopt the attitude that they should subordinate their own needs to those of their children and they practise great personal sacrifice. While no doubt many such are prompted by altruistic feelings, there are often other psychological reasons, having to do with feelings of personal inadequacy, behind such behaviour. Apart from the later identity problems that such parents may be faced with, they may also unwittingly have placed an enormous burden of guilt on their children which could prevent them achieving their potential.

The point is that there are sound psychological reasons for the generation boundary and parents should see to it that they have time for themselves. There is an independent parental private life which is not confined to sexuality, and to which children do not have access. However, having put this point, it is equally important that the generation boundary be permeable and that communication across it in both directions is free and easy. In other words a rigid policy of "pas devant les enfants" is as unwise as a full involvement of children in all parental transactions. Parents who never disagree in front of their children are rearing them in an unreal atmosphere and may be promoting a superego which is persecutory in its high standards. Such children may fear overt conflict and may have a limited capacity to sustain relationships within which conflict has arisen. On the other hand, young children are not able to cope with many of the anxieties of the adult world and, for example, they have little understanding of adult sexuality. While it is true that children's level of comprehension is usually underestimated, it is important to be aware that issues may have to be explained to them in terms which they can understand. Clearly a considerable amount of judgment has to be used and mistakes are often made. Usually, however, we err very much on the side of not involving them sufficiently in issues which importantly affect them. I would suggest that the doctor should make a particular point of recommending that children are given some information on all the important questions affecting the family and that their views are solicited. This does not mean that one is asking children to take the final decision in relation to house moves, changes of school, location of holidays etc., but it does mean that their views are given due weight. They should certainly be informed where there is a prospect of family breakdown and they need a lot of support during such time. They will be torn in their loyalties to both parents and usually a professional outsider is best placed to offer such support. Certainly their feelings in relation to their placement must be given serious consideration but the ultimate decision remains an adult one. The therapist should see to it that good arrangements are made or regular contact where separation does occur.

Throughout history most societies have regarded the family as central and there have always been strong taboos, traditions and legislation aimed at protecting it. Moves to enable the dissolution of marriage encountered strong resistance with fears of weakening family life and undermining society. There is an excellent short historical review of this in *The Tide of Divorce*, by William Latey. The Finer Report comments as follows.

> The institution of the family is buttressed, not weakened, by a divorce law which is well understood, respected and free from cant:
> It is a proper object of public policy to dispose of dead marriages in a manner that encourages and affords the spouses the best possible opportunity to make rational and conciliatory arrangements for their own and their children's future.

Single-parent families
In 1974 the Committee on One-Parent Families delivered its report (the Finer Report) to the Secretary of State for Social Services in

the United Kingdom. This report comprises two weighty well-documented volumes and I can do no better than offer a quotation of figures from it.

> We estimate that there were, in April 1971, 620,000 one-parent families with over one million children. Of these families 100,000 were motherless and the other 520,000 fatherless. Of the fatherless families 190,000 were separated, 120,000 divorced, 120,000 widowed and 90,000 single. One-parent families formed about one tenth of all families with children; and there are no figures available of the extent to which families move in and out of the one-parent category, but movement must be considerable and a significantly higher proportion must spend some time as one-parent families.

It was something of a surprise to learn that the children of the "typical" one-parent family, those of unmarried mothers, formed only 11 per cent of the total. Clearly the emotional needs of the children in these various sub-groups differ but the report emphasises one point common to all, which is frequently of over-riding importance: they found that one-parent families in general were financially much worse off than two-parent families and that there was widespread financial hardship; many of them relied on supplementary benefit and others struggled on maintenance payments and part-time earnings. Such economic circumstances obliged many lone mothers to enter full-time employment which added to the stress on her children and herself.

It is incumbent, therefore, on the general practitioner to make a specific point of enquiring into the financial situation of such families and to invoke the help of the social services. Advice which cannot be implemented because of economic circumstances is not only un-helpful but may be harmful through making the parent feel more inadequate or more guilty in relation to his or her children. These parents deserve a lot of understanding and support and this is best provided by those who have shared their experiences. They should be encouraged to make contact with such voluntary self-help groups as Cruse Clubs for widows, Mothers in Action, Gingerbread, Cherish, Adapt, AIM, and local clubs for the separated and divorced.

In many cases the parent may feel too inhibited to take the first step and the doctor should make a telephone call to arrange a personal contact. Apart from the important psychological support and social outlets offered by these groups, many offer such practical help as baby-sitting rotas, holiday schemes, home help etc. There are other voluntary and religious based organisations such as the National Children's Home, Dr. Barnardo's and the National Counsel for One-Parent Families which employ professional staff and provide a variety of services. The doctor should also ensure that the family has the support, where necessary, of home helps, relief mothers, nursery schools and play schools.

While concentrating on socioeconomic issues and legal formalities, the Finer Report contains a very useful review of the changing role of women in our society. It does not however attend to the social and psychologial factors which produce single-parent families, nor to their psychotherapeutic requirements. The general practitioner may well be the only source of advice acceptable to some parents who indeed may have approached him with an incidental medical complaint.

First of all the doctor needs to be aware of his own feelings in relation to the central issue at hand, be it illegitimate pregnancy, marital breakdown, adoption or whatever. Such feelings will have had their origins in his own childhood experiences and may well have led to very definite attitudes. Nearly all children strive to play one parent off against another and usually are skilled at ferreting out little cracks in parental relationships, seeking to enlarge them. Nevertheless, while fascinated by it, parental discord is the one thing they dread and parental separation is so terrifying as usually to be unthinkable. Where it happens, it is an abiding catastrophe although psychological defences enable partial readjustment to be achieved. The psychotherapist's task in relation to a parent or the child, first of all is to achieve empathic understanding and, through the support of such a relationship, to help the client face his or her own feelings and the emotional issues involved. The aim is to help the patient work through the traumatic experiences and, through growing awareness, gradually become able to leave such experiences safely in the past. The therapist's capacity to facilitate this work depends mainly on the degree to which he is at ease with such issues within himself. All therapists have their limitations and while they may seek to work through these, their responsibility to patients is to be aware of them and not to undertake work which they are unable to do. In other words the general practitioner should be honest with himself about his own attitudes and values and if he is unable to empathise with a patient he should admit as much to himself. Whether it is wise to admit it to the patient as well or not depends on the situation, but where necessary he should refer the patient to an alternative therapist for help. The principle is no different than that which obtains throughout medicine as for example in referring a patient with cholelithiasis to a surgeon. The doctor can continue to offer such support as he feels able to do and many general practitioners have the ability and skills themselves to help the patients achieve a satisfactory adjustment.

This work is by no means easy and can be very time consuming. People who have had painful emotional experiences feel very vulnerable and protect themselves with many defences and strategies. They are often rigid, evasive, angry, accusatory and resentful and have to project such feelings onto those who help them during the therapeutic process. Sometimes it is found that such intense emotions derive not only from the unhappy experience with the separated spouse but may have origins in childhood, the conflictual marital relationship to some extent representing a repetition. At times it may seem to the doctor that he should reunite the family or, in the case of a single mother, to encourage wedlock. Such solutions are appealing and society usually encourages them. However, they frequently have more to do with the therapist's and society's wishes and display insufficient appreciation of the realities or of the feelings of those directly involved. The approach should not be the seeking of solutions to problems but rather the helping of people who, amongst other things, have emotional problems. Following reflection, and with the agreement of the patient, it sometimes *is* appropriate to establish contact with a putative father, an estranged husband or a deserting mother if only to elicit their views and wishes on the situation. A short formal letter (marked personal and confidential), stating briefly the therapist's role, what information he is seeking and indicating respect for the recipient's position is probably best. Almost everyone likes to behave well and is relieved to be given an opportunity to do so, as long as they are not being manipulated, exposed to emotional blackmail or coerced in any way. It might be that the aim is to regularise contact between the children and the separated parent and, when he is sensitive to the feelings of all involved, frequently a doctor is able to achieve more satisfactory arrangements than a lawyer.

More often, however, the therapist's task first of all is to help the patient come to a realisation that the special relationship is over (if it ever in fact existed in reality) and a process of letting go has to be facilitated. Here again the therapeutic relationship offers supportive security and, in line with Bowlby's attachment theory, a grief reaction is promoted. Following the detachment phase, a rational approach to regular contact between the estranged parent and the children may be attempted. In any event the remaining parent will at least be able to communicate to the children a more balanced picture so that the estranged parent may be viewed in more realistic terms.

The approach outlined in the last paragraph is aimed at the adults and progress with them clearly is in the children's best interest. However, the children themselves need help to cope with what has been a shattering experience. Their psychological reactions will depend on their ages and levels of emotional maturity as well as their previous experience. But certainly their understanding will have a large fantasy component. While many psychological defences are called into play, blanket denial is a common one. The experience is thereby rendered inaccessible to consciousness and an emotional block occurs. This will result in a significant limitation in the subsequent range of behaviour and relationships. The repressed feelings will re-emerge within the context of a later relationship when it reaches a level of intensity and inappropriate hostility and resentment may be focused on an unfortunate boy-friend or girlfriend. The therapist's role is to provide the structure within which such feelings may be mobilised and worked through. While the pace at which this work is done has to be carefully monitored, children are able to use psychotherapy rapidly and effectively and the earlier such work commences the better. There are few general practitioners who have the time to undertake such work but an understanding of its importance should lead to the appropriate referrals, which will usually be to the local child guidance clinic. In the latter setting, the therapist is quite likely to use play material and little toy figures, as a communication medium particularly with younger children. Nevertheless the general practitioner through indicating his awareness of the emotions involved and through appropriate comments may have a significant supportive role to play. It is more likely, however, that he would prefer to take the issue up on a family basis and a therapeutic session carefully exploring the different feelings of the parent and siblings can be of great value.

ADOPTION AND FOSTERING

The psychological reasons for such human activities as choice of career or of spouse, decision to marry or to have children, size of family etc. are highly complex and usually unknown. One aspect of such questions has to do with personal identity. For instance, with many girls, there is often a growing identification with the mother and a shift from the position of being mothered to being a mother. The first pregnancy brings with it the requirement for this role change. The major anatomical and physiological changes of pregnancy cannot be prevented without terminating the pregnancy itself. However, the necessary psychological changes may not proceed in the normal way for reasons found in the earlier history of the pregnant mother and this can lead to considerable relationship and role problems. Sometimes such women are unable to assume the role of mother and they may have major personal identity crises in the puerperium including a psychotic breakdown. More often, negative and hostile feelings are focused on the child who may be completely rejected, occasionally physically harmed and sometimes the victim of infanticide. Emotionally deprived teenage girls who have become pregnant experience it as a time when they are valued and cared for and, while they may ultimately reject their babies, sometimes one finds that they become pregnant again and again. It can be seen that they are seeking mothering in their own right and so the help offered to them must include this in large measure. Such caring can often best be done in a group home where the mothers can care for and grow with their babies and reach the right decision in relation to them. Occasionally, one finds a family where the teenage girl is in effect bearing a baby as a present for her mother, who may have no social role other than that of caring for children. There are times when such a child has been reared in the belief that the grand-mother is the mother and the underlying tensions can lead to conflict and distress later on.

In cases of adoption there are usually four parties involved, viz. the parent or parents offering the child for placement, the child, the adopting parents seeking a child, and usually a facilitating agent or agency which undertakes the social work and relates to the legal authorities. It is usually the mothers of illegitimate and, to a lesser extent, extra-marital children who consider placing them for adop-tion. They usually seek the assistance of an adoption society or a social worker to whom they entrust the task of finding a suitable home. Most single girls, on finding themselves pregnant, react with shock and dismay and may be unable to accept the reality of the situation. With very many, the impulse is to reject the experience and to seek a termination of the pregnancy forthwith. Others remain ambivalent and, with varying degrees of dissociation, drift to term and childbirth. The social worker helps the unmarried mother to work through to the right decision for her child. All too often in the past the mother's tendency to reject has been colluded with, if not actually encouraged, through a misguided wish to help. New-born infants have been rapidly spirited away, frequently without the mother seeing them, and their subsequent fate shrouded in secrecy. Apart from the emotional damage caused to the mother, it also deprives her of an opportunity for growth and maturity. It has already been mentioned that there are some women who have re-peated pregnancies but reject them as negative experiences; it is important to help them to remain with their emotions and to get in touch with their deeper feelings thereby leading to personal growth. Such mothers can be helped to relate to their babies and care for them while discussing and thinking about the future. The decision to give up the baby to another family to rear, when emotionally experienced, is a painful one and mourning must occur. It goes without saying that the therapist must continue supporting these mothers after they have given up their babies. Such support may have to continue for quite a long time, at first through regular sessions and later on an "availability" basis.

The child
It used to be firmly held (and still is widely believed) that infants did not establish attachment bonds until 6 to 8 months of age when the

first "stranger response" was noted. It was therefore felt that there were no adverse emotional effects resulting from moving them from place to place as long as they were well cared for. Recent research has revealed the young infant's sensitivity to relationships in the very first hours and days of life and has shown, too, their rich repertoire of relationship skills. Careful attention, therefore, has to be directed at these relationships when a transition from one mother-figure to another is being contemplated.

Administratively, it would seem logical to do this by having the adopting or fostering mother meet the natural mother with the infant over a transitional period. Then, not only can the baby's routines of sleeping, eating, nappy changing etc. be exchanged but also his games, quirks and something of his individual style as well. Needless to say, such personal meetings have a tremendous emotional significance for both mother and foster mother and can be overwhelming or even explosive. Many skilled therapists find the prospect too daunting. However, they can be of great value to both women and to the infant's emotional welfare. Careful preparation is required and time has to be given to both the mother and the foster mother to voice their anxieties and reservations. Where both agree, it is probably best to decide on one meeting and the focus should be maintained on the baby. In the light of the experience, subsequent meetings may then be possible. This work is demanding and time consuming but it can be of such value to the parents and the child that it should always be considered.

A particularly valuable practice is for the infant to have his own folio. This might be a hard covered expanding file which contains, not only such official documents as birth and baptismal certificates and medical notes (including immunological dates) but also baby books compiled by the natural mother and foster mother including perhaps photographs of both and maybe letters to the child giving background family details etc. General practitioners, social workers and other professionals, too, might like to include notes and explanatory statements. All too frequently one encounters children in residential homes who know little of their past. The tragedy is that in very many cases it proves impossible to provide them with this type of information, their case files containing little more than brief notes on their legal and medical status. It would seem a basic human right that one should have access to one's own experience and background which is so intimately involved with personal identity. It is incumbent therefore on all the professionals involved to ensure that they do not deprive those in their care of this right.

Many natural children at times feel that they are adopted and certainly adopted children themselves have more intense questionings about their identities particularly during adolescence. Some, perhaps particularly those whose placements have been unhappy, do feel the need to seek out their natural mothers. Cases have been reported where this has happened and the experience has usually been described as empty and depressing. What seems to happen at such meetings is that long cherished fantasies are shattered and the adopted person has to face some realities which he had been avoiding. Such people with identity questions and other problems need to be, and should be, referred for skilled help and Dr. Barnardo's provides such a service. Most child guidance clinics report an over-representation of adopted children in their patient population. Apart from the likelihood of some increase in problems such as those just mentioned, there are other incidental reasons as to why this is the case. General practitioners and others presented with emotional or behavioural problems in a child, on hearing of adoption, tend to make an automatic referral which otherwise they would not have felt was necessary. In addition families who have an adopted child are more accustomed to dealing with social workers and helping agencies in general and they themselves may seek a referral where another family might not.

Those applying to be adoptive parents

At times doctors are approached by couples, with or without children, seeking advice as to whether they should adopt a child. Apart from some altruistic principles, often stated in vague terms, it is difficult to determine the right reason for such a decision. It proves much easier to outline inappropriate ones as, for example, to cement a threatened marriage, or to divert a lonely wife whose husband has to go overseas. While accepting that in human affairs, there are few if any absolutes, it has already been stated that biology usually offers good guidance in psychological matters. While accepting this in a general way it is important to remember that there are differences between the adoptive family and the natural or biological one. Such adoption relationships are being *socially,* rather than biologically, created and the consequences of this difference are often glossed over or denied. A sensitive and careful assessment of the couple has to be carried out and this usually includes an enquiry into physical health, financial circumstances and even police record. Fundamentally, however, it is the quality of their relationship to each other that is important, and this involves an exploration of the social and psychological history as well as an appraisal of the current life situation. Ultimately it comes down to the personal subjective judgment of the assessor, which is why it is a difficult and at times contentious task.

When a couple approach the general practitioner requesting advice on whether or not to adopt, he should, in a supportive way, seek to understand the motivation. In cases of infertility, it is particularly important to clarify the reasons for having no children. There may be a morbid fear of pregnancy or a psychosexual problem, and treatment should be offered for these problems while discussing the adoption application. It is widely known that the adoption of a child is frequently followed by pregnancy in the adopting mother, but should it be undertaken for that very purpose? Most people are unaware of the very real difficulties that can present in rearing handicapped or institutionalised children and the lack of discrimination in some aspiring adoptors may indicate this. The doctor has to provide such information in a sensitive and understanding way, both while discussing the question and while assessing the parents' suitability. To be adopted means to be somewhat different, and therefore there is much to be said for placing such children in ordinary "normal" families. The aim is to find a home where the child will get a good upbringing and the task of assessment is very much easier where there already are children. While recognising the possibility of sibling rivalry, it is usually much better for the child to be placed where there are other children. It is sometimes forgotten, particularly by applicants, that it is the emotional needs of the child that have primacy and some childless couples feel aggrieved when they see children being placed with parents who already have natural children. Similarly, when a family is succeeding with one child frequently a second and a third child is placed with them. The general practitioner may need to spend quite some time with an infertile couple, discussing their feelings so that they can have an informed understanding and a good adjustment to it. When they are at ease with this question and secure in their roles and their relationship, they are much better placed to cope with some of the problems which adopting a child will raise. They will be able to discuss what they know of the child's background with him, adopt a common-sense attitude to his fantasies and accept his rejection at angry moments for what it is. Once they have reached this stage, the doctor makes the recommendation to the adoption agency or social worker and continues to support the parents throughout the application process and subsequent developments.

The social worker

In all developed countries arrangements for the adopting process are governed by legislation which lays down very definite procedures which have to be attended to. These have to do with consent, confidentiality, qualifications for adopting parents, essential documentation and legal processes. As well as attending scrupulously to such details, social workers must be sensitive to the emotional issues involved and it is gratifying that the standard of work in this area has improved in recent years. The disapproving regimes of the Magdalen Homes are very much in the past and more unmarried mothers now elect to keep their children. The social worker's tasks

include helping the mother to understand what the various alternatives will mean both for herself and for her child. In most cases
there will be two social workers employed, one with the mother
and her baby and the other with the adopting couple and it is
important for both to understand their roles and their professional
tasks.

PLANNING FAMILIES: GENETIC COUNSELLING

In the welter of human relationships there is continual re-negotiation
over such issues as authority, dependence, responsibility and control
and a wide variety of strategies are used. Laing, Berne and others
have written on the politics and the games of the family. As we know
from stories and dramas from earlier times, such relationship questions have always been intriguing and have their tragic and comic
dimensions. In some societies relationships became highly formalised
and books on etiquette indicate that there were rules and conventions
governing a very wide range of social activities. Scientific and tech-
nological developments led to enormous changes in society in the
nineteenth century and these and other social and political developments have had great implications for interpersonal relationships in
this century. For example, divorce law reform, the suffragist movement and the women's liberation movement have required and
reflected changes within as well as outside the family. The advent of
more reliable contraceptive methods, too, has both enabled and
resulted in change.

No doubt general practitioners as well as child psychiatrists are
approached by parents wanting answers to such questions as what age
the first child should be before the second one should arrive. It will
now be clear that the guidance takes the form, not of providing direct
answers to such questions, but of exploring the issue with the parents.
One seeks to deepen their understanding of what is involved, thereby
enabling them to reach the right decision for themselves. Children,
likewise, where there is a new baby expected, should be told
of the mother's pregnancy and well prepared for the new arrival.
They should participate in family discussions about names and be
involved with the purchase and preparation of the baby clothes etc.
The parents need to understand that, despite all such preparation, the
children are still likely to experience the actual arrival as threatening
and they need continual support with their anxieties and regressive
behaviour. In other words, as far as a child is concerned, there is no
right time for the coming of a new sibling, although having a sibling
in many ways will prove a real advantage later on.

"Is he all right, doctor?", is one of the first questions mothers
ask about their newly-delivered babies and this indicates an important apprehension. Increasingly parents approach the family

doctor for information on the chances of transmitting a wide variety of conditions to their children. While many of the old wives' tales have now been discarded, there is a widespread misunderstanding of inheritance in the general population. Adoption societies are familiar with requests from prospective adopting parents for children with specific backgrounds, e.g. working-class or farming, indicating a belief that social attributes and skills are inherited. Likewise, it is thought that acquired illnessess, and in particular brain diseases or traumata, may be genetically transmitted. While the family practitioner will be able to reassure such parents, he should probe a little further to see whether the question does not indicate a significant ambivalence towards having another child, which may need to be worked through. When there is a genetic condition or a family history which may be significant, it is best to refer the parents to a specialist who can carry out the necessary chromosomal and other studies. In some cases the actual risk involved can be calculated and at times is no greater than that in the general population. Whatever the actual risk factor may be, genetic counsellors increasingly are aware of the important psychological element so that apart from providing the factual information, they find that their work includes a considerable amount of psychotherapy.

MANAGEMENT OF SOME SPECIFIC DISORDERS AND PROBLEMS

This section will cover some of the more common disorders and problems to be met in practice when treating children.

Habit disorders
In relation to the causes of symptoms, all too frequently within the medical profession one encounters an attitude which views the organic and the psychogenic as alternatives and almost mutually exclusive. Both dimensions operate in all our patients and this reality is recognised in the clinical approach of general practitioners more so than that of most specialists. Differences in the treatment approaches to some children's complaints have stemmed from such differences in the formulation of the presenting problem and *bed-wetting* (enuresis) is a good example.

Enuresis
Everyone starts life without bladder sphincter control and in part, therefore, one is talking about the age at which this is normally acquired. The wetting of the nappy is not viewed as a symptom in a one-year-old child and it is only at a later age that a not otherwise obvious anatomical defect would be recognised. Likewise, in an

infant it is other symptoms which would lead to the discovery of a urinary tract infection. When therefore does bed-wetting become a symptom? One immediately has to define the term bed-wetting, i.e. one wet bed per week, per month or whatever. Research reveals that, at one level, bladder sphincter control must be viewed as a biological variable which is linked with the psychosocial environment. At the age of 4 years, the percentages of boys and girls dry at night has been found to vary as follows (Oppel *et al.*, 1973):

Country of study	% of Boys	% of Girls
Australia	62	60
U.S.A. (Caucasian)	69	66
U.K.	86	89
Sweden	90	94

The Isle of Wight study (Rutter *et al.*, 1970) shows comparative figures which also indicate that in England girls are quicker to acquire urinary continence at night than boys. In the U.S. study above, which was carried out in Baltimore, between the ages of 2 and 3 years 45 per cent of girls and only 32 per cent of boys were dry at night, between 4 and 6 years the differences were still marked and, after the age of 7, the ratio of boy to girl wetters increases until by the mid-teens boys are twice as likely to be wet as girls. There seems to be a relatively sensitive period of aquiring night-time bladder control between the ages of 1 and 4 years. Much of the research in this field has been summarised and clearly presented in the book *Bladder Control and Enuresis* (Kolvin *et al.*, 1973) which those interested should consult. There, research is presented which indicates that in the third year of life, 40 per cent or more of children still wet become dry and after that the chances of nocturnal dryness emerging are approximately 15 per cent per year. Night-time dryness is also shown to be associated with such variables as social class, family size, presence or absence of maternal depression, and whether or not the child is in an institution or living with his family. These and differences in operational definitions very much limit the validity of comparing different studies. The figures tabled above illustrate this point and direct reference should be made to the studies themselves before any further significance is drawn from them.

Parents of enuretic children often report that they sleep deeply and are difficult to arouse, but in fact studies do not confirm that they sleep more deeply than others. Of course parents have less cause to awaken their non-enuretic children and therefore their judgment on comparisons is questionable. Wetting does not usually take place during R.E.M. (i.e. dreaming) sleep. Dosing with imipramine reduces enuresis, but the reason for this is not certain. Phenobarbitone has more effect on inhibiting the deeper stages of sleep, yet has no anti-enuretic action (Shaffer *et al.*, 1977).

Some have suggested that enuresis is an epileptic equivalent but further studies have not confirmed this. There is also the widely held view that bed-wetting is a sign of nervousness. Research in fact has confirmed that there is a greater prevalence of psychiatric disturbance in bed-wetters, although no characteristic psychiatric syndrome was found. The Isle of Wight studies show this also. They examined at the age of 14, those children who were both wet and disturbed at the age of 10. Of those who had stopped wetting, 59 per cent were no longer psychiatrically disturbed, whereas only 29 per cent of those who had continued to wet had lost their psychiatric symptoms. As a group, enuretics tend to have lower self-esteem and to be more passive than non-enuretics.

Much of the research into these questions must appear highly academic to the doctor confronted with a mother and her shame-faced child. For those who seek a fuller understanding of the psychological principles, I would recommend Anna Freud's clear exposition of these in her book *Normality and Pathology in Childhood* (1969). Before outlining a management approach I will draw attention to one further point. As most mothers know, bed-wetting may be a symptom resulting from the stress of such life events as house moving, commencing at school, change of teacher etc. It is a regression to an earlier level of functioning and following a period of increased attention and understanding, sphincter control is usually achieved again. In some cases, however, it maybe that bed-wetting continues while the source of stress has been removed and in these cases the bed-wetting can be seen more as a habit than as a symptom. In line, therefore, with the approach outlined ealier, it is important for the general practitioner to ask himself what is the source of stress on this child or in other words what is the bed-wetting a symptom of. The reason for emphasising this is that it is usually not difficult to help the child acquire dry nights, but one may not be doing him a service if one has not helped remove the source of stress. Alternatively where the bed-wetting is a habit the direct task is to help overcome it.

Nocturnal enuresis is best managed by the family practitioner who is usually the first one consulted on it. As each treatment approach fails, the patient and relatives become discouraged and the chances of success diminish. As a working definition, one could accept as a problem, night wetting at least once a month after the commencement of school and this should probably be linked with overt concern in the parents. There are two groups of bed-wetters, those with primary nocturnal enuresis who have never acquired bladder sphincter control, and the group of secondary or "onset" enuretics who have become dry and then resumed bed-wetting. In the latter group it is much more likely that there is no anatomical neurological or physiological abnormality.

First of all it is important to establish what is the problem. It is nearly always the mother who complains, the child being embarrassed and awkward and frequently not wishing to be present at all. However, in the case of an older child such denial is sometimes absent and overt distress is experienced occasionally focused on inability to go on holidays to summer camps etc. It is essential to achieve agreement on the aim of treatment. It is not just a matter of avoiding laundry difficulties by any means to hand; the doctor in particular aims to help the child achieve bladder sphincter control at night. In order to achieve this direct doctor/child relationship, one adopts the approach outlined earlier in the chapter. It is now generally agreed that the most important single therapeutic factor is a sympathetic and enthusiastic approach by the doctor. Why is the patient being brought at this time? It may be that the mother has come under extra stress, perhaps she is pregnant and wishes to have one child out of nappies before a new one arrives. How often does the wetting occur? Was the bed wet this morning? Does the boy tell his parents in the morning if he is wet and what happens then? Who washes the sheets, pyjamas etc.? Has he his own bed? Who else sleeps in his bedroom? What time does he go to bed? Do they lift him at night? Where is the toilet? Is there a potty? Has he a torch? In some houses the problem is self-reinforcing, for example the child is brought into the parent's bed after he has wet. A general enquiry should be made into the toilet training of the patient and of his siblings.

A full history including a family history is taken. Enuresis commonly runs in families and approximately 70 per cent of all enuretics have a first degree relative who is or has been afflicted with the same condition. The child usually derives support from such information and it helps him acknowledge the problem. A history of his general health is taken, enquiring into the possibility of other developmental delays. The rare neurological causes of enuresis are likely also to disturb bowel function and usually interfere with such normal activities as running and playing. Where such social and environmental aspects as poverty, inadequate nutrition and clothing, parental delinquency, repeated disruptions of maternal care and large overcrowded households are found, it is essential to share the treatment with a social worker. A sensitive appraisal of the parental response is important for as with such other functions as eating, sleeping, school attendance and social behaviour, bed-wetting can become an issue over which the battle for control is fought. If such proves to be the case, it should be recognised, as it is a very different question from that of helping the child acquire night-time sphincter control.

Following the history taking, a general physical examination should be done. Careful abdominal palpation may reveal large kidneys, or severe constipation and the examination of the lower spine for dimples may suggest *spina bifida occulta*. This in itself is not evidence of neurological involvement and ankle jerks and gait should be observed routinely, with testing of saddle-area sensation if it is thought that neurological cause is likely. The only obligatory investigation is examination of the urine. A Diastix test for glucose will exclude diabetes and a freshly-collected clear urine specimen should be sent for culture. Of children with severe enuresis 10 per cent have a urinary tract infection which should be treated. Spinal X-ray is not indicated unless there are neurological symptoms or signs and I think most urologists would agree that I.V.P.s and cystography are not indicated unless there is strong suggestion of a major anatomical fault or proven urinary tract infections. About 15 per cent of children with urinary infections present as enuretics and a girl aged over 5, who wets the bed, has a 15 per cent chance of having such an infection. It may be that the wet perineum may predispose to such infections; successful treatment cures the enuresis in about one-third of the cases.

Practitioners who treat many enuretics continue to be surprised by the frequency with which parents do not seem to think of such common-sense measures as giving the child a flash-lamp or a potty, or removing his nappy and arranging his own bed etc. The enthusiastic advocacy of such practical procedures often meets with success. Frequently parents already have a practice of lifting the child at night and in such cases it is probably as well not to advise that it be discontinued. However, in the course of treatment a test week every month without lifting, should be tried to see how the regime is going. Apart from a common-sense attitude, fluid restriction should not be recommended as there is no evidence that it helps and it may be introducing another anxiety.

As has been mentioned, the child should be directly recruited into the management of the problem. This is done by having him record his dry nights (not the negative wet ones) and through this relating directly with the doctor about his own physiological performance. In the first instance, this offers a good base-line record and indeed in itself is sometimes sufficient to lead to complete dryness. A simple star chart is used and constructing this with the child helps to individualise it and turn the procedure into something of a game. The child should be seen after a fortnight and a behavioural approach to treatment adopted. Depending on the current performance, rewards may be added for two dry nights or three dry nights in a row, and all the siblings should be rewarded as well, as sometimes there is a danger that one of them may resume wetting.

The child should be seen at weekly or at most fortnightly intervals and these visits may be quite brief. Where the regime is being implemented, if progress is slow it is occasionally appropriate to introduce drugs. One of the main values of these is to raise confidence through demonstrating that dryness can be achieved. There is a wide variety of drugs which have been used and the tricyclic antidepressants are the only ones which have been shown to be superior to placebos. It should be said that, with increased recognition of the cardiotoxic effects of these, the justification for their use in cases of enuresis is being questioned. Imipramine is the drug of choice in a dose of 25 mg to young children and 50 mg for those over 10 years of age. Where it is known that the child wets before midnight, drugs should be given at 5.00 p.m., otherwise at bedtime. The dosage may be increased in 25 mg stages at one or two week intervals according to response up to 100 mg daily. It is essential that the general management features continue to be implemented and the response, of course, can be monitored on the star charts. Where a sustained improvement occurs, a gradual reduction of the drug dosage should be tried while continuing to reinforce the star chart approach with rewards for the appropriate number of dry nights.

Enuresis alarms are quite popular and result in a higher proportion of cures than other forms of treatment. While they have a sound basis in learning theory, it is likely that the social factors are as important as the conditioning ones. The main reasons for their failure is either because the full details surrounding the enuresis have not been uncovered or because the alarm is not used correctly. One usually asks the mother to become co-therapist and it is essential to prepare both her and the child in the surgery. The details outlined in the instruction sheet have to be rehearsed carefully and some points require emphasis. First of all, one wants the buzzer to sound as the aim is to achieve the conditioning. This must be explained to the parents and they must be cautioned not to lift the child in the hopes of having an undisturbed night. The child should not wear the trousers of his pyjamas and the alarm must be placed so that he has to get out of bed to switch it off. He must then go the the toilet, micturate and on return help the mother to change the sheets. The older child can do this for himself, switching on the buzzer again before returning to bed. The child is asked to record on the chart both the number of times the alarm calls him each night and the nights when he has been completely dry. On the whole, children of 7 years and older can successfully use such an alarm and so can a number of 5-year-olds who understand its purpose. The parents and child should be instructed not to try to discontinue using the alarm but should adhere rigidly to the doctor's instructions. In most cases improvement occurs and in one reported series the success rate was 92 per cent. Two techniques help reduce the relapse rate: firstly intermittent reinforcement which involves switching off the alarm three or four nights a week once dry nights have been achieved, and secondly, that of over-learning. For this after dryness has been achieved, the child can be given a fluid load of one or two pints at night.

In the vast majority of cases the above approach will meet with success and the steps again are as follows.

(a) *Primum non nocere*. Rather than embark on a series of unnecessary investigations, each with their own risks, or add to a child's stress with unwanted treatment regimes, it would be better to make a statement such as "he is not ready to be dry yet" or even to use such traditional remedies as feeding the child on raisins or concoctions of magnolia blossoms, while redressing other problems.

(b) Careful history taking, focusing on the details of the circumstances of the enuresis.

(c) An enthusiastic, sympathetic and common-sense approach, with the doctor recruiting the child directly into the management of the problem.

(d) Very frequent if brief follow-up appointments, approximately every two weeks for two to three months.

Some patients such as those with intractable urinary tract infections and those showing evidence of anatomical or neurological disorders will need to be referred to specialist clinics. Where the above management approach does not achieve success, a referral should be made to the local clinic specialising in this problem. The child psychiatric clinic is appropriate for those who show emotional disturbance which is commoner in combined day and night wetters. Frequently, it is just the change of therapist which brings about the desired effect and so referral should be made sooner rather than later.

Encopresis

Faecal soiling seems to be the most unmentionable of childhood practices — even more so than masturbation. Parents feel embarrassment and disgust, while these children are full of shame, resentment and anger. Indeed, by the time they come to the doctor for treatment, anger and mutual recrimination are usually the order of the day. Bellman's definition (1966) is a useful one: "encopresis is the repeated involuntary defecation into clothing, occurring in children over 4 years of age and of at least one month's duration". There are some cases where the faeces are deposited at inappropriate places around the house rather than in the pants, and at times this behaviour represents an almost conscious act of aggression. Three different groups of cases have been described.

(a) Cases where there has been failure ever to gain bowel control, reminiscent of the primary enuretic.

(b) Cases where control, having been achieved, breaks down temporarily.

(c) Cases of constipation with over-flow soiling.

When one reflects how proud children are of mastery of their physiological functions and the contempt they have for those whom they view as babies, it is unlikely that the problem is due to laziness. This is frequently, however, the parental view and one needs to discuss it. Most mothers acknowledge their fury at seeing their sons wandering around apparently blissfully unaware of the putrid smell. This denial on the part of the child is defensive and seems to be the only way he can cope with his feelings of hopelessness and helplessness. Such children frequently do look miserable and the illustrations showing such misery in popular advertisements for laxatives may have some validity. As in enuresis, the role of the therapist is to help the child acknowledge the reality of the problem, and the same confident approach is adopted, thereby cutting across the intense child/parent focus on this symptom.

I shall concentrate on boys since the problem is three to four times more common with them than with girls. In the constipated group, they are usually highly controlled, frequently have high standards in relation to school work and their drawings are precise and definite. Indeed they cannot stand a mess and are frequently described as being very good. In particular, feelings of aggression rarely emerge and may be completely repressed. Not infrequently one finds that the entire family is controlled and maintains a rigid boundary with the outside world. Metaphorically, things are "held inside". It is of course impossible to defecate when one is tense and the pity is that some treatment regimes lead to an increase in this tension.

Adopting the interview approach already outlined, one identifies background contributory problems and deals with those that one can. A physical examination may reveal that the child is constipated and, in severe cases of faecal impaction, manual removal may have to be done. However, it is usually best to use enemata. The child is brought directly into the management of the question and helped to acknowledge the fact of the soiling so that it can be overcome. One should emphasise that one is not going to coerce the child into using the toilet but instead must request that he take over its management. One checks with the mother where she wants him to deposit his soiled pants and the routine then is that the child will make some attempt to clean himself and change his pants. A star is given by his mother when he carries out this management procedure correctly. A point to emphasise is that unfortunately star charts for clean pants frequently lead to more constipation. While this is going on one is seeking to relax the child and the mother and defuse the issue. It is often noticeable that the soiling occurs on the way home from school or when the child is playing, i.e. when he is least tense. Having achieved this step the next one is to ask the child if he wishes the doctor to help him to use the toilet in the normal way. He is also asked which parent he would like to assist him. Sometimes the bowel habit can be regained by outlining a specific toilet schedule, for example going a half-hour after meals, and it is often best to start at weekends. Laxatives such as Senokot and stool-softeners are of value but, where acceptable, a regime using a suppository may be more effective. The point is to ensure that the child achieves a bowel movement thereby giving him confidence. The regime with this is to have the chosen parent insert the suppository (bisacodyl) once daily for three days, explaining to the child that a successful movement will occur into the toilet within half an hour. The programme requires three days with suppository, then three days without and should faecal retention recur the suppository is tried for another three days. The atmosphere in which this is carried out has to be supportive to the child and to the parents. In particular the family may need to be helped to permit of a more open discussion on emotional issues and the acceptance of more assertive behaviour on behalf of the child. Some psychotherapists recommend helping the child express aggressive feelings.

Sometimes a short period of hospital stay is necessary for the establishment of a proper bowel habit and where the above approach has been unsuccessful it is usually best to refer the case to a child guidance clinic.

Autism, mental handicap and language problems

There is no need for the general practitioner to get caught up in the controversies as to who should treat children with the above problems. In many cases there are a number of specialists involved, and even different services, throughout a patient's childhood. The primary role of the general practitioner will be supportive to the family and to this may be added the important role of co-ordinator of services as well. He therefore needs to be in a position to provide clear information to the family in relation to diagnosis and not infrequently to explain what specialists may have meant by various comments. On seeking information to help him with this task however the doctor very often finds himself confronted with confusion.

The reasons for this are partly that specialists are slow to attach diagnostic labels to young children, partly because such diagnosis cannot be made with much confidence without a prolonged period of observation and also because of the fear of the self-fulfilling prophecy. The other main cause for the confusion has been disagreement over classification of childhood psychoses and the criteria for their diagnosis. The following observations are made with the hope of clarifying the situation somewhat.

There has been a wide debate on the nature of intelligence at least since the middle of the last century and psychologists have put forward various concepts from time to time. The value of the intelligence quotient (I.Q.) has been questioned and the belief that it is in fact intelligence that "intelligence tests" measure has also been fiercely debated. Over the years a large number of other psychological tests have been devised to assess children's cognitive functions, skills, aptitudes, language and motor development and social skills etc., and the predictive value of many of them has been established. Increasingly it is becoming clear that what is of most value is a range of tests that discriminates between these different functions giving a much broader picture than heretofore. These enable more appropriate prescriptions to be made in such areas as language development, speech development, remedial education, word recognition, numeracy, behavioural modification, and so on. Similarly, amongst the treatments can be added individual psychotherapy focusing on areas of definite conflict or on specific relationship problems within the family. This is true of children both of normal intelligence and those within the different groupings of mental retardation. When we look at children in an ordinary school we can see that just as they differ in physique, hair colouring etc. so have they different abilities in their level of cognitive functioning and to some extent the examination system is a crude measure of this. The same situation is equally true in a group of children who have been assessed as moderately mentally handicapped.

Rutter has pointed out that *autism* was a misleading term for Kanner to have used for the syndrome he reported in 1943 (Rutter, 1978). Bleuler had used this term for the active withdrawal into fantasy of some schizophrenics and this is not at all the sense in which the term is used with autistic children. Other workers confirmed that the syndrome did seem to exist but confusions arose — some of them to do with genuine misunderstandings and over-enthusiastic hopes in relation to therapy. The idea became current that autistic children were somehow locked within themselves and that if one could find the key they would quickly function like the normal, intelligent children many of them appeared to be. It was also thought that autism was an alternative diagnosis to mental handicap. Many voluntary groups were established, research was funded, assessment and treatment centres were set up and books and journals dealing with autism published. Lists of clinical criteria for the diagnosis were issued by various workers but the position remained confused. In the U.K., the working party under Mildred Creak was established to study the schizophrenia syndrome in childhood (Creak, 1961). One of the difficulties was that some of the features which were associated with autism were also seen in other conditions. It was then felt that some of the disorders were primary and led on to other secondary ones. Although the debate continues the following points are beginning to gain general acceptance.

(a) Childhood schizophrenia is a clinical condition different to autism and is characterised by the presence of thought disorder.

(b) It may yet be found that there is a number of syndromes covered by the term autism.

(c) Autism can occur in children at all levels of intelligence and it seems to be more handicapping in the more retarded children.

(d) While evidence (immunological, biochemical and other) is accumulating to suggest that there may be damage to some area of the developing foetal brain, so far the cause is unknown.

(e) While there can be considerable variation between autistic children, the following four features are essential for a diagnosis of childhood autism.

(i) The disorder begins before the age of thirty months.

(ii) There is impaired development in the capacity to relate to people socially.

(iii) There is impaired language development which is out of keeping with the child's general intellectual level. This language impairment is linked with a general impairment in symbolic thinking. These children display little imagination and seem to fail to make the association between toys and the objects they represent. Likewise they seem limited in making general observations about the identity of things of one order, for example that tables of different shapes belong to the same group. This results not only in a delay in the acquisition of speech but also major impairments in the understanding of gesture and in learning in general.

(iv) Insistence on sameness: Kanner observed this characteristic which describes a rigidity in play and behaviour patterns and an intense attachment to specific objects which they insist on carrying with them. They frequently have definite rituals and compulsions which have to be adhered to and later on they can become preoccupied with learning and repeating long lists of timetables, sports results etc.

(f) Neurological disorder is sometimes present but more usually in those autistic children who are also mentally handicapped. The incidence of E.E.G. abnormalities increases with age and, in a considerable number of cases, fits commence after puberty.

(g) The prevalence is something between 2.5 and 4 per 10,000 children.

(h) The syndrome is severely incapacitating and special education facilities are always required, frequently on a residential basis. Specific behaviourally-oriented programmes have to be developed for each individual child and require very high staff/child ratios. The families require much supportive psychotherapy and family members must be viewed as co-therapists.

(i) In general the prognosis is poor, with many of these children remaining functionally handicapped into adult life, although surprising improvements in social functioning have occurred in some cases. Those who have acquired some speech by the age of 5 have the least unfavourable prognosis.

(j) The syndrome is world-wide and the male to female ratio is approximately four to one.

From the above it can be recognised that the general practitioner's role, by and large, is to ensure that the child is seen by the appropriate specialist and, following diagnosis, the major task is a supportive one to the family. As has already been mentioned parents have to be helped to work through the mourning of the normal healthy child they consciously or unconsciously expected and it is important that this process be started as soon as they begin to suspect that their child is handicapped. This work requires courage and sensitivity and cannot be hurried. Again and again as the child grows older the parents are confronted with his limitations and they need more intensive support at such times. The introduction to parents of children with similar problems and the involvement in voluntary societies is very helpful and may have to be initiated by the family doctor.

It is very understandable that parents of infants and young children are frequently concerned about their development and wonder at the significance of apparent delays. In very many cases the family doctor will be able to reassure them but it needs mentioning that mothers in particular are very sensitive to their individual children and it is essential to check whether there is any basis to their concern. Frequently the doctor will be approached by a mother asking the significance of her child's speech delay. Of course there is great variation in the age at which the first words appear and in some children it may well be not until shortly after their second birthday. Children understand speech before they are able to use it and it is important that this be assessed. Of course language includes not only speech but also gesture: children will point and wave bye-bye, etc., before they have speech. The clinical assessment of speech and language is a highly specialised one but the general practitioner can make a good assessment through a careful history taking and a simple examination in the surgery. Table 2 below (reproduced by kind permission of Professor Rutter) includes the differential diagnosis as well as the points that need attention (Rutter and Hersov, 1977). On the basis of this the general practitioner would be able to be of help to the parents, and where there is doubt-the appropriate referral must be made.

TABLE 2. COMPREHENSION IN DIFFERENTIAL DIAGNOSES

	"Inner language"	*Hearing*	*Attention to sounds*	*Watching face*	*Under-standing spoken language*	*Under-standing gesture*
Severe deafness	+	—	—	+	—	+
High frequency loss	+	low. freq. only	+	+	limited	+
Mental retarda-tion	limited	+	±	+	limited	±
Autism	—	+	—	No	poor	±
Elective mutism	+	+	+	+	+	+
Psychosocial retardation of language	+	+	+	+	+	+

KEY: Present: +; Absent: —; May or may not be present: ±

(From Table 29.2 of
Child Psychiatry: Modern Approaches,
Rutter and Hersov)

Psychosomatic disorders

Despite much current talk about treating the patient as a whole, there still is the tendency to think of organic and emotional causes for pathology as separate alternatives. The truth is that just as the physical and emotional constantly interact in everyone in ordinary day life, so do they in illness. There are emotional dimensions to even the most physical of illnesses, such as a fractured leg, as each person experiences such an injury in an individual way. In many medical schools the teaching still is that all likely organic causes have to be thoroughly investigated and ruled out before one should start thinking of emotional ones. The patient, however, is a person, a physical and emotional entity, and how these aspects interact must be borne in mind throughout the investigation of his or her illness. In some cases the physical aspect will predominate and in others the emotional. While it is true that both dimensions contribute in all illness, this is more generally accepted in cases of what are called psychosomatic illnesses. In children these would include asthma, peptic ulcer, eczema, failure to thrive, some psychogenic eating disorders (including obesity and anorexia nervosa) and some cases of epilepsy and diabetes mellitus.

As the medical profession finds it difficult to accept a psychological cause for symptoms, it is not surprising that many patients find it even more so. Indeed their feeling that their integrity and even honesty is being questioned is sometimes partly justified by the attitude of some clinicians. One finds that arguments occur, with the patient strongly resisting his doctor's explanations and all too frequently changing doctors. However, in order to treat such conditions, it is not necessary to convert the patient to the belief that their illness has an emotional origin. Indeed, in the case of children it is frequently unwise to adopt such a line with parents, certainly in the early sessions. A more advisable approach is to say that while any investigation into an organic cause will be carried out where it seems appropriate, the emotional factors need attention and treatment will be continued along those lines.

Minuchin (1974) and his co-workers have identified certain patterns of family organisation and functioning associated with psychosomatic illness in children, and they have shown convincing results from family therapy with some severe psychosomatic conditions. The following are some of the characteristics which they have described in these psychosomatogenic families.

1. *Enmeshment*
These family members are much too intrusive with one another and there is very little privacy or individuality amongst them. The generation boundaries are weak and there is much role confusion, each member being very involved with all the others.

2. *Over-protectiveness*
In the case of the sick child, one finds the whole family is showing great care and concern, and, indeed, there is a high level of protectiveness by all the members of the family towards one another.

3. *Rigidity*
These families are fairly inflexible and have well defined routines. They are quite resistant to the idea that any change within the family system is necessary, and maintain that everything is fine except for the patient's illness.

4. *Lack of conflict resolution*

There is very little overt conflict in these families. One finds that emotionally important subjects are rarely, if ever, discussed and indeed frequently the family members will volunteer that they never have rows. One finds that the ill child is an important focus and indeed that there may be reasons why the family needs one of its members to be a patient. Glimpses of submerged parental conflict may be seen as the patient gets better.

In some of these cases it is helpful to think of the patient as therapist to the family. In other words, one asks what is this ill child doing for the family, in what way is he helping it? The answer to that question may give clues as to how treatment should be taken up. Certainly, any work that can be used to open up communication and to help the family members face unresolved conflicts with less anxiety would be of help. However, because of the rigidity, this work is often unsuccessful and other treatment strategies may have to be tailor-made for a particular family (Haley, 1963). Family myths may have to be challenged and a lot of support given while the uncovered anxieties are worked through (Byng-Hall, 1973). The strengthening of the generation boundaries and the promotion of individuality within the family are also important aims. A keen understanding of the society in which he works is necessary for the practitioner adopting a family therapy approach and the experiences of general practice provide this. How much socio-cultural factors affect illness can be seen not only from the changing prevalence of smoking related diseases but also in the increased prevalence in recent years of anorexia nervosa. Ogden Nash expressed social emphasis on slimness and its consequences neatly in his couplet:

So I think it is very nice for ladies to look lithe and lissome,
But not so much that you cut yourself, if you happen to embrace and kissome.

A case history will serve at this point to illustrate some of the problems of psychosomatic disorders.

Thomas, aged 15, is the eldest of four children of a professional man and his wife. The other children are Lara, aged 12, Michael, aged 10, and Adam, aged 9. When Thomas was 9-years-old he went off his food and complained of tummy pains. At times he also vomited. In the background history his mother had hospital treatment for a lung infection twelve years previously and his father had hospital treatment for a liver viral infection three years before Thomas' symptoms started. Thomas had been a normal delivery at term and the parents were delighted at his arrival. His early developmental history was rapid — at ten months he was walking and was already saying a few words.

Apart from the normal childhood illnesses there were no difficulties. When he was 2½, his father went abroad on business for a prolonged period and Lara was born shortly afterwards. When Lara was 6-months-old the mother joined the father for a couple of weeks, but then returned and things proceeded normally. The father returned from business eight months later and the two younger boys were born. The family lived a few miles outside the city where their social and business life was focused and did not integrate with the local people in their area very much. When Thomas was old enough he proceeded to the local school and in due course was joined by his sister and young brother. They were all regarded to some extent as outsiders, partly on account of the way they dressed and partly because there were no family contacts.

When Thomas was seen by the doctor, he examined him and carefully took a history, with various investigations (including a barium meal, and a cholecystogram). These revealed that he had a duodenal ulcer, which was treated in the usual way by diet and antacids and it cleared up. The symptoms recurred a few months later and he was readmitted to hospital but they cleared up and he went home. Two years later when he was eleven the symptoms emerged again and he was so sick that he could not go to school. The whole family were invited to a family therapy session and the following is an assessment of the situation. The mother, an attractive looking woman, took the lead and presented as a matter-of-fact person, who was good at coping with practical matters. Her husband presented more as an intellectual, quiet-spoken and casually dressed. He acknowledged that he kept his feelings in, except occasionally when he "flared up". Thomas was a pale, timid, immature boy who was very attached to his mother and irked his father by continuing to play childish games. The father had quite high aspirations for him in fact and was annoyed that he had been falling behind at school. However, it was a close family and they focused very much initially on school problems which were quite real. Psychological investigation revealed that Thomas indeed had above average intelligence but he was more than three years behind at reading and numbers. He was something of a loner and was afraid of his classmates at school who used to bully him. When one looked at the other children one found that Lara, aged 9, was an intense, serious girl who was obsessionally thorough about her school work and very upset if she missed even a day. Michael, aged 7, had a nickname — Jerky — because he jumped about so much. In fact he proved in the session to be tense, agitated and over-active and had limited capacity to contain his feelings. Adam, aged 6, seemed well adjusted.

It was fairly clear that Thomas was under considerable stress at school but also there were stresses in the family which were manifested in the three older children. Treatment involved focusing on the interfamilial relationship, as well as helping Thomas on an individual basis to express and work through his repressed feelings. Culturally and educationally it seemed appropriate to move him to a city school which was more sensitive to his individual needs. He had remedial teaching there and rapidly caught up with his peer-group and he became particularly good at athletics. His symptoms cleared and there was no recurrence at follow-up three years later.

THE USE OF DRUGS

While the over all thrust of child psychiatric treatment is psychotherapeutic, there is certainly a place for the judicious use of medication. It hardly needs to be emphasised that children should be prescribed psychotropic drugs only in the context of a full treatment programme which is under continual review. Few doctors would condone the casual administration to children of minor tranquillisers and pain-killers, yet this seems to be a practice which is increasing and frequently without a diagnosis being reached. While condemning this practice, it has been difficult to insist that all such prescribing be done only on the basis of properly controlled clinical trials, as up to recently there were so few reliable studies carried out in the field of childhood psychopharmacology. However, with increasing agreement on diagnostic classification, the position already has improved and it is likely that there will soon be a vast increase in the necessary research.

In general medicine, drugs may be used to control and contain symptoms, as well as to treat disease processes, and the same is true in psychopharmacology. Drugs may be used to contain, to bring under control, the behavioural excesses of a patient, as in the case of manic excitement or bizarre psychotic behaviour in an adult. They can be used also to treat and terminate a disease process itself as in the case of antidepressant drugs. Sometimes, it seems, that both functions are subserved simultaneously by one drug, e.g. the exhibition of chlorpromazine in acute schizophrenia. Clinically, and perhaps ethically, it is important that we appreciate which functions our drugs are performing.

For centuries, infants and young children have been given teething powders, gripe waters, herbal and chemical elixirs, as well of course as alcohol. While mostly harmless, some, such as those containing mercury, were quite toxic. Clinical psychopharmacology as a scientific discipline derived from the nineteenth-century interest in the natural hypnosedatives, opium and cocaine, and could be said to have been christened, if not born, on the Feast-Day of Saint Barbara, 1862, when Bayer synthesised barbiturates. Childhood psychopharmacology did not emerge until the 1930s and indeed all drugs for the treatment of behavioural and emotional problems in children were first studied in adults. In 1936 a series of studies showed that benzedrine (a combination of dextro- and laevo-forms of amphetamine) was a central nervous system stimulant which affected mood and behaviour and possibly speeded up behaviour. In the following year, Bradley reported the effects of benzedrine on children with behavioural problems in a residential setting and this marked the beginning of scientific clinical childhood psychopharmacology. Further studies showed that the improved intellectual performance stemmed from a better attitude by the child towards the intellectual task. Controlled studies following the introduction of dexedrine showed that it was equally effective to benzedrine, in half the dose and there was a lower incidence of excessive stimulation.

This "paradoxical" effect of some drugs on children has been much studied but remains unresolved. The psychostimulants seem to relax some overactive children and to increase their attention-span. On the other hand, barbiturates frequently bring about overactivity, irritability and behavioural difficulties in some children, whereas with adults they usually function as sedatives. Unfortunately, one still encounters too many children where phenobarbitone, prescribed to treat these problems, has only increased them.

Methylphenidate (Ritalin) was first synthesised in 1954, and it was hoped that it would be free from the abuse-potential of the amphetamines, but with adults, this has not proved to be so. In the United States, it has been widely used for the treatment of children with "minimal brain-dysfunction" (see below).

In 1950, Charpentier in France, synthesised chlorpromazine, thereby initiating a new era in psychopharmacology. At first, because of its hypothermic and sedative effects, it was used in anaesthesia particularly for open-heart surgery. Delay and Deniker in 1952, were the first to report on its value in psychiatric practice (Delay and Deniker, 1952), and in child psychiatry the first report of its use was for psychomotor excitement in 1973. The anti-histamines also, were introduced around this time and are of value as hypnotics and mild sedatives in children as well as adults. Mepro-bamate, at first, was thought to be of particular value in childhood behavioural and emotional problems as well as for nocturnal enuresis. However, further studies have been disappointing and it is now prescribed much less frequently.

In the 1960s two further phenothiazine compounds were intro-

duced into child psychiatry: the piperazines (example, trifluoperazine) and the piperidine compound, thioridazine. As a tranquilliser,
this latter drug is probably the most suitable for children being
prescribed as a syrup. It is unwise, in the case of children, to try to
memorise a drug-dosage, as the compromise over the age-span leads
to giving too much to a young child and too little to the young teenager. It is safest to develop the habit of prescribing for the individual
child, weighing him, consulting the pharmacopoeia or formulary
and monitoring the response.

Various drugs have been investigated for their value as anti-
psychotic agents in children. The phenothiazines now are the most
widely used. In the mid-1950s, reserpine was reported to be of
limited value in the treatment of some autistic children, but has not
been adopted in clinical practice. In 1962 and 1963, Bender and her
co-workers in Bellevue Hospital, New York reported favourably on
the value of L.S.D.-25 in hospitalised, severely-disturbed children
with schizophrenia and autism (Bender *et al.*, 1962 and 1963).
These findings were confirmed by Simmons in 1966, but there have
been no follow-up studies since. Compounds from two additional
categories of major tranquillising drugs have also been found of
value in psychotic children; they are thiothixene from the thioxan-
thine group and haloperidol from the butyrophenone group, the
latter in doses very much greater than are usually prescribed.

In the 1960s lithium was used in some children with emotional
difficulties, especially those given to explosiveness and aggression,
and the results were equivocal. It must therefore continue to be
viewed as at the investigational level, at present.

Apart from the anticonvulsants, which will not be reviewed
here, the two most widely used groups of drugs in child psychiatric
practice are the antidepressants and the psychostimulants. Despite
many clinical trials, the value of antidepressants must continue to
be viewed as unproven, apart from their use in nocturnal enuresis.
The conflicting reports reflect methodological as well as classification difficulties. Pearce, in a review of depressive disorder in childhood, stated, "clear diagnostic criteria are necessary, before it is
possible to talk of incidence, aetiology and prognosis" (Pearce,
1977). Frommer, after some years of studying antidepressants in
children, in a report in 1972 stated, "without a general basis of
classification, it is not possible to know where to begin with a
systematic study of treatment and prognosis" (Frommer, 1972).

Where he considers using antidepressants in a child, it is probably
wiser for the general practitioner to seek a specialist opinion. Much
helpful guidance can be gained from consulting *Pharmacology in
Childhood and Adolescence* (Wiener, 1977) on which some of the
material here is based. Most child psychiatrists will be prepared to
use them in carefully selected cases, usually with older children.

In the United States, the commonest condition for which children are prescribed medication is the hyperkinetic syndrome. It is a diagnosis extensively employed there and the symptoms are attributed to a syndrome said to result from minimal brain dysfunction. The term, hyperkinesis, is applied to an overactive child with aggressive behaviour, frequently experiencing failure at school associated with low attention span. Wender in a book, *Minimal Brain Dysfunction in Children* (Wender, 1971) stated that it is "probably the most common single diagnostic entity seen in child guidance clinics", and that "many minimal brain dysfunction children are neurologically intact. There is no doubt that the syndrome can appear with total absence of neurological signs or symptoms or E.E.G. abnormality." The treatment usually includes one of the psychostimulant drugs, methylphenidate or dextro-amphetamine. Winsberg and his colleagues in Brooklyn reported a series of studies of the drug treatment of children with this disorder (Winsberg *et al.*, 1974). These are well conducted double-blind clinical trials where, through randomly assigning the subjects to all possible sequences of drugs and placebo, they functioned as their own controls. They employed a number of rating scales of established sensitivity to the effects of psychostimulant therapy, behavioural change was measured through parent and teacher ratings, and drug-effects on attention, short-term memory and impulsivity were evaluated on laboratory tasks. In a recent study, they report that amitriptyline and methylphenidate were largely comparable in attenuating hyperactivity and aggression. Previously, they had found that dextroamphetamine and methylphenidate were similarly comparable in effectiveness, while in another study imipramine was found to be effective when compared with dextro-amphetamine.

Another authority on this subject, Connors from Harvard, refers to the many myths about the hyperkinetic child (Connors, 1972). He, too, found that dextroamphetamine and methylphenidate were equivalent in action except that the latter produced better results on W.I.S.C., arithmetic and similarities sub-test, and in another study found that magnesium pemoline and dextroamphetamine were similar in effectiveness after eight weeks.

These authors and others refer to the many side-effects from these drugs. Apart from the obvious ones of insomnia, anorexia, weight loss and irritability with the psychostimulants, they also included the more serious ones of hallucinosis and suppressed height. With the tricyclics most authors recommend caution because of the possibility of cardiac abnormalities.

A most valuable contribution to the consideration of the drug treatment of hyperkinesis was Barkley's review of all the published work available (Barkley, 1977). He looked in detail at more than 110 studies and concluded that the results of follow-up studies suggest that stimulant drug therapy is not a panacea for treating hyperkinesis. While the drugs seem to facilitate the short-term management of hyperactive children, they have little impact in the long-term social, academic or psychological adjustment of these children. He calls into question the practice of prescribing these drugs to most hyperactive children without due consideration for the modes of intervention that might be used in conjunction with or as alternatives to them.

Rutter has demonstrated that the relationship between hyperkinesis and minimal brain dysfunction does not hold (Rutter, 1977). While brain damage is a factor contributing in a substantial way to the genesis of child psychiatric disorder there is no behavioural stereotype. In other words conduct disorder or hyperactivity is not specific to brain-damaged children, who are as likely to display the whole range of psychiatric symptoms as non-brain-damaged patients.

Again, in view of these controversial opinions and conflicting research findings, it is probably better that the general practitioner refrain from prescribing psychostimulants. Certainly, they should be introduced later rather than earlier in a treatment programme and always with regular monitoring of height and weight, and psychological evaluation of educational progress.

There is little evidence to suggest that sedatives and minor tranquillisers have any role to play in the treatment of minor behavioural or emotional disorders. However, the doctor will use his judgment here. Where a young child has so intimidated his parents by screaming, and demanding throughout the night, that they have acquired the bad habits of taking him into their bed, or even playing with him, a hypnotic may well have a part to play in helping a regular normal sleep-pattern be re-established. In such a case, chloral or an antihistamine elixir in a sufficient dose, may be effective. They should be used only for a short period, remembering that a week is a long time in the life of a child as well as of a politician.

The butyrophenone, haloperidol, has been shown to be effective in the treatment of some children with tics, habit spasms and stammering and may well be worth considering, especially where other treatments have been ineffective. One has to warn the parents and teachers of the possibility of the child developing parkinsonian side-effects.

By and large, at present, it would seem that the role of drugs is with major and seriously-disabling child psychiatric disorders, but they may have a limited role to play in general practice. One is always conscious of the negative educational dimension, when one prescribes for children. Much further research is needed and it is gratifying to see this now proceeding. I conclude with a quotation from Eisenberg: psychoactive drugs in children:

> . . . should be used only when a condition exists that requires treatment, when the agent prescribed is likely to be effective in treating that condition, where the likelihood of benefit outweighs the risk of toxicity and then only for the shortest period possible. Indeed it is an error of equal magnitude to overprescribing to deny a patient an agent which can help relieve his symptoms and hasten his recovery.

(Eisenberg, 1971)

REFERENCES AND FURTHER READING

Ackerman, N. W. (1958): *The Psychodynamics of Family Life*, Basic Books, New York.

Apley, J. (1975): *The Child with Abdominal Pains*, 2nd edition, Blackwell Scientific Publications, London.

Arnold, L. Eugene (ed.): *Helping Parents Help Their Children*, Brunner/Mazel, New York.

Axline, V. M. (1971): *Dibs in Search of Self*, Penguin Books Ltd., Harmondsworth.

Balint, M. (1968): *The Doctor, His Patient and the Illness*, Pitman Medical Publications, London.

Balint, Enid and Norrell, J. S. (1973): *Six Minutes for the Patient: Interactions in General Practice Consultation*, Tavistock Publications, London.

Bellman, M. (1966): "Studies on encopresis", *Acta Paediat. Scand.*, Suppl. 170.

Bender, L., Goldschmidt, L. and Siva Shanka, D. V. (1962): "Treatment of Autistic Schizophrenic children with LSD-25 and 4ML-491", *Recent Advances Biol. Psych.*, 4, 170-177.

Bender, L., Faretra, F., and Cobrinik, L. (1963): "LSD & UML. Treatment of hospitalised disturbed children", *Recent Advances Biol. Psych.*, 5, 84-92.

Bertalanffy, L. von. (1968): *General Systems Theory*, Allen Lane, Penguin, Harmondsworth. (First published by Braziller, New York, 1948).

Barkley, R. A. (1977): "A review of stimulant drug research with hyperactive children", *J. Child. Psychol. Psychiat.*, 18, 137-165.

Bowlby, J. (1951): *Maternal Care and Mental Health*, Geneva, World Health Organisation.

Bowlby, J. (1965): *Child Care and the Growth of Love*, Penguin Books, Harmondsworth.

Bowlby, J. (1969): *Attachment and Loss Vol. 1: Attachment*, Hogarth Press, London.

Bowlby, J. (1973): *Attachment and Loss Vol. 2: Separation, Anxiety and Anger*, Hogarth Press, London.

Bowlby, J. (1977 (a)): "The Making and Breaking of Affectional Bonds", I. *Brit. J. Psychiat.,* **130**, 201-210.

Bowlby, J. (1977 (b)): "The Making and Breaking of Affectional Bonds II", Ibid. 421-430.

Bradley, C. (1937): "The Behavioural of Children receiving Benzedrine", *Am. J. Psychiat.,* **94**, 577-585.

Brown, G. W., Birley, J. L. T. and Wing, J. K. (1972): "Influence of family life on the course of schizophrenic disorders: A replication", *Brit. J. Psychiat.,* **121**, 241-258.

Burlingham, D. and Freud, Anna (1942): *Young Children in Wartime,* Allen & Unwin, London.

Burlingham, D. and Freud, Anna (1944): *Infants Without Families,* Allen & Unwin, London.

Burt, C. (1944): *The Young Delinquent,* 4th Ed. University of London Press, London.

Byng-Hall, J. (1973): "Family myths used as defence in conjoint family therapy", *Brit. J. Med. Psychol.,* **46**, 239-250.

Connell, P. M., Corbett, J. A., Horne, D. J. and Matthews, A. M. (1967): "Drug treatment of adolescent tiqueurs", *Brit. J. Psychiat.,* **113**, 375-383.

Connors, C. K. (1972): Symposium on Behaviour Modification by Drugs II: "Psychological effects of stimulant drugs in children with minimal brain dysfunction", *Pediatrics,* **49**, 702-708, 1972.

Creak, M. (1961): "Schizophrenia syndrome in childhood. Progress Report of a working party", *Cerebral Palsy Bulletin,* **3**, 501-504.

Delay, J. and Deniker, P. (1952): "Réactions Biologiques observées au cours du traitement par le chlorhydrate de dimethylamino-propyl-N-chorophenothiazine (4560 r.p.)", *Congrès des psychiatres de langue française,* Luxembourg, July 22-26.

Douglas, J. W. B. (1975): "Early hospital admissions and later disturbances of behaviour and learning", *Develop. Med. Child Neurol.,* **17**, 456-480.

Eisenberg, L. (1971): quoted in *Psychopharmacology in Childhood and Adolescence,* ed. Wiener, J. M., Basic Books, New York, 1977.

Finer, M. (1974): *Report of the Committee on One-Parent Families,* H.M.S.O. Cmnd. 5629, London.

Fogelman, K. R. (Ed.) (1976): *Britain's Sixteen-Year-Olds: Preliminary findings from the third follow-up of the National Child Development Study* (1958 Cohort), National Children's Bureau, London.

Freud, S. (1909): *Analysis of a phobia in a five-year old boy,* Standard Edition, *Collected Works,* Vol. **10**, Hogarth Press.

Freud, Anna (1969). *Normality and Pathology in Childhood,* Hogarth, London.

Frommer, Eva, Mendelson, W. B. and Reid, M. A. (1972): "Differential diagnosis of psychiatric disturbance in pre-school children", *Brit. J. Psychiat.*, **121**, 71-74.

Guerin, P. (1976): *Family Therapy, Theory and Practice*, Gardner Press, New York.

Haley, J. (1963): *Strategies of Psychotherapy*, Grune & Stratton, New York.

Hardgrieve, Carol and Dawson, Rosemary (1972): *Parents and Children in Hospital*, Little Brown & Co., Boston.

Harvey, Susan and Hales-Tooke, Ann (Eds.) (1972): *Play in Hospital*, Faber and Faber, London.

Heuyer, G., Gerard, G. and Galibert, J. (1953): "Traitement de l'excitation psychometrics chez l'enfant paré (le 456rp)", *Arch. Franç. Pediat.*, **9**, 961.

Kanner, L. (1935): *Child Psychiatry*, Charles C. Thomas, Springfield, Ill.

Kolvin, I., MacKeith, R. and Meadow, R. (1973): *Bladder Control and Enuresis*, Spastics International Medical Publications, Heinemann, London.

Latey, W. (1970): *The Tide of Divorce*, Longman, London.

Lidz, T. (1974): *Marital and Family Therapy*, Grune & Stratton, New York.

Lucas, A. R. and Weiss, M. (1971): "Methylphenidate hallucinosis", *J. Amer. Med. Ass.*, **217**, 1079-1081.

Minuchin, S. (1974): *Families and Family Therapy*, Tavistock Publications, London.

Oppel, W. C., Harper, P. A., Rider, R. V. (1968): "The Age of Attaining Bladder Control", *Pediatrics*, **42**, 614.

Parkes, C. M. (1972): *Bereavements: Studies of Grief in Adult Life*, Tavistock Publications, London.

Pearce, J. (1977): "Depressive disorder in childhood", *J. Psychol. Psychiat.*, **18**, 79-83.

Petrillo, Madeline and Sanger, S. (1972): *Emotional Care of Hospitalized Children*, Lippincott, Philadelphia.

Pincus, Lily (1976): *Death and the Family*, Faber and Faber, London.

Pinkerton, P. (1974). *Childhood Disorder. A Psychosomatic Approach*, Crosby, Lockwood and Staples, London.

Robertson, James and Robertson, Joyce (1976): *Guide to Five Films: Young Children in Brief Separation from their Mother*, Robertson Centre, London.

Robertson, James and Robertson, Joyce (1971): *Young Children in Brief Separation*, Quadrangle Books, New York.

Robertson, James and Robertson, Joyce (1974): "The Importance of Substitute Mothering for the Long-Stay Child", *Health and Social Service Journal*, April 20th, 1974.

Rutter, M. (1972): *Maternal Deprivation Reassessed*, Penguin, Hardmondsworth.

Rutter, M., Tizard, J. and Whitmore, K. (1970): *Education, Health and Behaviour*, Longman, London.

Rutter, M., Shaffer, D. and Shepherd, M. (1975): *A Multi-Axial Classification of Child Psychiatric Disorders*, W.H.O., Geneva.

Rutter, M. (1977): "Brain damage syndromes in childhood: Concepts and findings", *J. Child Psychol. Psychiat.*, **18**, 1-21.

Rutter, M. and Hersov, L. (1977): *Child Psychiatry: Modern Approaches*, Blackwell Scientific Publications, London.

Rutter, M. (1978): "Diagnosis and definition of childhood autism", *Journal of Autism and Childhood Schizophrenia*, **8**, (2), 139 -162.

Sargant, W. and Blackburn, J. M. (1936): "The effect of Benzedrine on intelligence scores", *Lancet*, December 12, pp. 1385-7.

Shaffer, D. (1977): "Enuresis" in Rutter, M. and Hersov, L. (Eds.) *Child Psychiatry: Modern Approaches*, Blackwell Scientific Publications, London.

Shapiro, A. K. and Shapiro, Elaine (1968): "Treatment of Gilles de la Tourette syndrome with Haloperidol", *Brit. J. Psychiat.*, **114**, 345-351.

Simmons, J. Q. III, Leiken, S. J., Lovaas, O. I., Schaeffer, B. and Perloff, B. (1966): "Modification of autistic behaviour with LSD-25", *Am. J. Psych.*, **122**, 1201-1211.

Vaughan, G. F. (1957): "Children in hospital", *Lancet*, i, 1117.

Walrond-Skinner, Sue (1976): *Family Therapy, the Treatment of Natural Systems*, Routledge and Kegan Paul, London.

Wender, P. H. (1971): *Minimal Brain Dysfunction in Children*, Wiley, New York.

Weinberg, W. A., Rutman, J., Sullivan, L., Penick, E. C. and Dietz, S. G. (1973): "Depression in children referred to an educational diagnostic centre: Diagnosis and treatment", *J. Pediatrics*, 1065-1072.

Wiener, J. M. (1977): *Psychopharmacology in Childhood and Adolescence*. Basic Books, New York.

Winnicott, D. W. (1964): *The Child, the Family and the Outside World*, 83, Penguin Books, Harmondsworth.

Winnicott, D. W. (1971): *Therapeutic Consultations in Child Psychiatry*, Hogarth Press, London.

Winnicott, D. W. (1977): *The Piggle*, Hogarth Press, London.

Winsberg, B. G., Press, M., Bialer, I. and Kupietz, S. (1974): "Dextroamphetamine and methylphenidate in the treatment of hyperactive/aggressive children", *Pediatrics*, **53**, 236-241.

Yepes, L. E., Balka, Elinor B., Winsberg, G. B. and Bialer, I. (1977): "Amitriptyline and methylphenidate treatment of behaviourally disordered children", *J. Child Psychol. Psychiat.*, **18**, 39-52.

CHAPTER TEN

Therapeutic Management of the Elderly

Dr. J. K. Binns,

M.B., Ch.B., F.R.C.P.E., F.R.C.Psych., D.P.M.

Consultant Psychiatrist and Physician Superintendent, Leverndale Hospital, Glasgow and Honorary Lecturer in Psychological Medicine, University of Glasgow, Scotland.

Therapeutic Management of the Elderly

INTRODUCTION

Projections made in 1976 as to the future size and age distribution of the U.K. population up to the end of this century show that people of retirement age and over will continue to increase in number until at least 1991. This will be accounted for particularly by those aged over 74, who will increase by 24 per cent from 2.9 million in 1976 to 3.6 million in 1991 (Office of Population Censuses and Surveys, 1977). Inevitably this means that there will be a further shift in emphasis towards the care of the elderly for all Health Service and community workers. This chapter covers the management of the elderly with psychiatric illness by consideration of the following:

(a) administrative considerations;

(b) present variability in patterns of care and general principles of management;

(c) psychological, physical and social characteristics of the elderly;

(d) interviewing;

(e) prescribing;

(f) psychiatric illnesses;

(g) emergency situations;

(h) legal aspects:
   (i) compulsory admission to hospital;
   (ii) appointment of receiver (or Curator Bonis);
   (iii) testamentary capacity;
   (iv) divorce;

(i) care of the dying;

(j) prophylaxis.

ADMINISTRATIVE CONSIDERATIONS

A doctor's time is most effectively spent if he works within a sound administrative framework. Planning for those with psychiatric disorders should not take place in isolation, but should be an integral part of the plan for the development of services for the elderly, for which advisory committees should exist at every level of Health Service administration. It is important to ensure that all those concerned in meeting the service needs are represented. As well as psychiatrists, membership of such committees should include geriatricians, community medicine specialists, general practitioners, nurses and paramedical workers. Having addressed themselves initially to assessing current needs and deficiencies, and having decided to what extent existing resources can be deployed more effectively, they should subsequently consider what future developments are required and establish priorities, since finances are inevitably limited. A continuing function will be to monitor the effectiveness of the service provided, and for this purpose the early establishment of an effective procedure for providing meaningful statistical information about patients will prove invaluable.

PRESENT VARIABILITY IN PATTERNS OF CARE

A comprehensive account of the emerging services for the elderly with mental disorder was published in 1970 (Scottish Health Service Council, 1970). At the present time, however, the pattern of care for the elderly mentally ill differs considerably between one part of the country and another depending on the facilities and professional personnel available. Where considerable expansion has occurred within recent years this is usually the consequence of local authority interest and activity in financing such developments as day centres, sheltered housing, group homes or hostels. This is in keeping with Government policy which aims to replace, to an increasing extent, the service based on the large mental hospitals by community-based services (D.H.S.S., 1975). In many parts of the country, however, such developments are still in their infancy and in these areas organically mentally ill patients have come to occupy beds within the mental hospitals to an increasing extent and also beds in general hospital medical, surgical, orthopaedic and other wards. In some areas the geriatricians accept some responsibility for the non-behaviourally-disturbed patient with dementia, but in others their policy is to regard such cases as the responsibility of the psychiatric service. It is the experience of most clinical psychiatrists that the mental disabilities of an ever-increasing number of patients in general hospital units are of the same quality and degree as many of the patients in their own psychiatric wards, although, in the non-psychiatric wards of a general hospital, the psychiatric diagnosis is likely to be omitted in the diagnostic formulation in case records. It is fundamental for those involved in planning services for the elderly to appreciate that such variability in the placement and recording of the elderly mentally ill exists and that it makes for difficulty in assessing the exact size of the problem in any one locality.

To an increasing extent during the past two decades the organically mentally ill have come to occupy beds which have become available as the chronic schizophrenic population of the mental hospitals has been reduced with modern methods of treatment. However, it is unlikely that any significant additional number of beds will become available in this way in the future, except perhaps by the provision of additional facilities for schizophrenic patients such as day hospitals, hostels and sheltered housing. Even with such developments it would seem unwise, for the future effectiveness of mental hospitals, to expect them to take a greater load of elderly patients than at present. Many psychiatric nurses who have acquired special skills in their training become discontented on finding that they are required to concern themselves predominantly in the nursing of elderly confused patients where few of these skills are applicable. The long-term nursing care required by the organically mentally ill with handicaps of helplessness, confusion, incontinence and dysphasia, for whom the most optimistic prospects are for a better quality of life, has a limited attraction, particularly for young people considering nursing as a career. To increase the load of elderly patients, the majority of whom will have dementia, in mental hospitals thus runs the risk of depriving these hospitals of beds and appropriately trained staff for younger non-organic psychiatric patients. Since the number of demented patients requiring some form of in-patient care will continue to increase in the years ahead, it would seem that the best quality of care for them is likely to be obtained by providing accommodation in small units, each situated in the community it serves, rather than in large centralised institutions.

A *multidisciplinary team approach* has many advantages and also general approval, yet up to the present time most hospitals have experienced difficulties in recruiting staff. Any of the professions which should form part of a comprehensive and integrated hospital and community psychiatric service may be deficient in numbers and because of this a considerable overlap in the role of the various professional groups has been necessary. The role of the major supporting professional groups is considered below.

Nurses

In recent years the nursing staff of most mental hospitals have extended their traditional role and developed a community nursing service. Whilst this is essentially to provide an after-care service for chronic schizophrenic patients on maintenance doses of antipsychotic drugs, by using their knowledge of the patient's background and illness the staff concerned play an important part by helping patients resolve their social and psychological problems.

Health visitors

With access to a general practice age-and-sex register health visitors can select persons who are likely to benefit from their care. It is beneficial in the preventive sense to visit in particular those who are living alone and without visitors, to encourage them to keep fit, active and independent and to discourage social isolation. Regular visits also enable changes in a person's general condition to be noted and appropriate action taken.

Occupational therapists

The important part that occupational therapists can play in promoting the well-being and sometimes the recovery of both the long- and short-term elderly psychiatric patient, either with or without intellectual impairment, is not always appreciated. In most hospitals a programme of activities will be provided within an occupational therapy department and at ward level for less ambulant patients. For those not requiring hospital care, a domiciliary occupational therapy service can be useful, although group activities are usually preferable. A day hospital should have as its basis a well-staffed occupational therapy department.

As normal ageing proceeds help can be given in mastering complexities of everyday living, e.g. heating and lighting equipment, labour-saving devices and the telephone. In the absence of a domiciliary dietetic service, instruction can be given in preparing an adequately nutritious diet. Through the hospital or local authority multidisciplinary team the occupational therapist (O.T.) can liaise with other relevant professionals, e.g. social workers, community nursing service or with neighbours and voluntary organisations, as is appropriate. A good service will have a basic principle of making every effort to prevent the isolation which so easily befalls the elderly.

In many areas there is a shortage of trained occupational therapists, however, and their lack has to some extent been overcome by the recruitment of untrained staff (O.T. helpers). Many of these, chosen on the basis of their personality and interest, are doing excellent work, but it should be appreciated that they lack professional training and thus a full appreciation of the subtle limitations often imposed by psychiatric illness.

Within the O.T. department or day hospital, the occupational therapy-programme is tailored to the individual patient's needs and may include physical activites such as exercises, ball games, dancing, mental activities such as games, quizzes, pottery and handicrafts, or social activities such as whist drives, bingo, sight-seeing trips. Particular emphasis is likely to be given to interaction with other patients and the maintenance of links with the community. Where symptoms are indicative of functional rather than organic psychiatric illness, the therapist will be able to assess the patient's ability to manage outside hospital in the various domestic situations and to provide training where necessary. The limitations caused by a patient's organic impairment can be defined and from there a programme devised for the individual which may decelerate further impairment. Encouraging the discussion of familiar people, places and events, and participation in everyday activities such as cooking, simple house-keeping and dressing may help to prolong the deteriorating patient's ability to cope at home without additional support.

Social work department

These departments have responsibilities towards the mentally disordered for their social welfare and their after-care. General practitioners, health visitors or hospital staff may become aware of the patient's social needs in the course of attending to their physical and psychiatric needs, and close collaboration and co-operation between the social and health services is necessary.

There is no doubt that active social work with the elderly can avoid or delay the need for the removal of many of them from their own home. Social assessment and, as appropriate, assistance in making appropriate claims for pension and other social security benefits, attention to financial difficulties which have already arisen, arrangements for the provision of a home help, laundry service, meals on wheels and attendance at a day centre or lunch club, are some of the very practical ways in which help can be given. Arrangements for a sitter-in service, or holiday admission to hospital, can often be arranged to give supporting relatives an occasional rest.

Finding suitable accommodation for patients, with their agreement, can be of crucial importance, preventing psychiatric illness in some, and in others in preventing relapse when psychiatric illness has already occurred and responded to treatment. If relatives are no longer willing or able to cope, it may be beneficial for the patient to move away. Homes which have been designed specifically for this age group, which allow easy access to neighbours, the local community and shops, to which the necessary support services are provided on a continuing basis and where social activities are encouraged, will be ideal.

Case work with the patient and family can also have a significant impact, not only by reducing the need for additional support or hospitalisation, but also by improving the well-being of all members of the group. Those living with an elderly patient may develop their own psychological problems, and a social worker's intervention involving all members of the family can be a useful insight-producing and therapeutic procedure.

Psychologists

The clinical psychologist contributes to the care of the elderly mentally ill by the assessment of psychological functioning and the provision of behaviour modification programmes.

Other professionals

Other professionals who have a signficant part to play include physiotherapists, chiropodists, dentists and opticians.

General principles of management

The successful management of elderly patients with psychiatric problems extends to other aspects of their care beyond the mere prescription of tranquillisers, and the initial role of the doctor, as always, must be to establish an accurate diagnosis upon which a rational approach to the patient's problems can be made. This is especially important in utilising most effectively and economically the services of other professionals who are likely to be able to make a useful contribution, e.g. social workers and health visitors.

CHARACTERISTICS OF ELDERLY PEOPLE

The psychological, social and physical factors to which any individual is likely to be subjected because of age must always be taken into account.

Psychological characteristics

As age advances, various abilities may become impaired, although to an unequal extent. The older person tends to be less energetic and to have less need for achievement. Decreased energy reserves necessitate some withdrawal from a full life, which increases as frailty becomes more pronounced. The elderly person tends to become more rigid, with a narrowing of interests and outlook, and tends to be generally more concerned with himself.

Significant impairment of memory and forgetfulness are not handicaps invariably associated with the elderly, although the capacity for learning, and recollecting contemporaneous events, gradually lessens. Except for those with gross organic impairment, however, given sufficient time and adequate motivation some capacity to learn new concepts and initiate new ideas will be retained. Reaction time becomes slower with increasing age and there is a decreased effectiveness in solving problems which involve dealing with new situations and making decisions. Adaptation to new life circumstances is slower, particularly if the change, whether physical or environmental, is of a major kind and of sudden onset. Much of the forgetfulness in the elderly can be accounted for by increasing self-preoccupation, and a less easy arousal and maintenance of the person's interests by external events. Emotional control sometimes lessens as age advances so that, for example, the individual is moved to tears by less than their normal degree of provocation. Sometimes the control over anti-social tendencies within the individual's personality is lost, possibly with legal consequences.

Physical characteristics

As age advances, physical frailty becomes more evident and the risk increases of more specific pathologies being added. Physical illness may be a direct cause of the psychiatric illness (e.g. cerebral arteriosclerosis; cardiac decompensation; respiratory infection). Sometimes the physical signs and symptoms are so obvious and demanding that the associated psychological problems may be overlooked (e.g. the patient with a hemiplegia may have some impairment of intellectual abilities and emotional control although these are much less obvious).

Physical illness may act indirectly as a non-specific precipitant of mental disorder and in the elderly illnesses restricting movement or impaired function (e.g. arthritis, "dizzy turns", or painful corns) are frequently detrimental psychologically because of the resultant increasing withdrawal and isolation.

Impaired hearing

The distress caused by impaired hearing itself is intensified by the embarrassment such people experience as a result of the misunderstandings which occur, and by their sensitivity to the awkwardness which friends and acquaintances experience in endeavouring to communicate with them. The hard of hearing adapt to the voices and associated mannerisms of those with whom they are familiar, and this often lessens the sympathy that they might otherwise justly receive from others. Especially when long-standing and severe, deafness has been shown to be an important causative factor in the onset of paranoid psychosis (Cooper et al., 1974) and in the development of feelings of isolation, insecurity and depression (Denmark, 1969).

Impaired vision

People with failing vision similarly may adapt and cope effectively in surroundings with which they are familiar, especially if these are brightly lit. However, if in surroundings to which they are unaccustomed, and particularly if there is also a low intensity of illumination, they may, deceptively, appear incapable of functioning independently.

Appetite

The food requirements of the elderly are normally reduced as a result of the diminished level of general activity, and a voracious appetite will often be indicative of organic cerebral disease. Decreased mobility, relative social isolation, a reluctance to make the effort of shopping or preparing food, the possibility of additional physical illness and financial anxieties, are all relevant factors which may increase the likelihood of sub- or malnutrition. Malnutrition was evident in 3 per cent of the elderly population in a study sponsored by D.H.S.S., although in the majority this was associated with an underlying medical condition (D.H.S.S., 1972). Dementia of several months' duration which showed complete resolution after treatment with folic acid has been described (Strachan and Henderson, 1967).

Bowel function
Preoccupation with bowel habit is a common feature in the elderly. Lack of exercise and increased weakness of the abdominal and other muscles leads to constipation. This often leads in desperation to self-medication with large doses of laxatives and consequent diarrhoea and abdominal pain.

Disturbances of sphincter control may discourage social contacts. Occasional soiling associated with the passage of flatus, with or without occasional difficulty in control of micturition, and possibly in association with a mild prolapse, may make an individual fearful of social situations lest she disgrace herself. The shame associated with any "accidents" may be so intense that disclosure to the doctor is avoided unless he makes a specific enquiry.

Sleep
The elderly often show changes in their sleeping habits. Often they take to retiring earlier and wakening earlier, sometimes coping with this latter in their own homes by rising to make tea or fill hot water bottles. A tendency to have an afternoon nap also becomes part of the daily routine. The majority adapt to this altered rhythm quite happily, but it can become a problem if they move to relatives or elsewhere, where such altered habits are not appreciated. It is important to realise that this sleeping pattern of the elderly is not readily controlled by medication, which may in fact simply confuse them and thus add to their difficulties.

Social characteristics
The demands of present-day society that an elderly person must retire from employment on reaching a specified age can have disastrous consequences. This one incident combines a reduction of income, a loss of self-esteem and, more significantly, a loss of daily contact and friendship with former colleagues. This imposed withdrawal can have particularly serious consequences for those with few interests initially, and it is such individuals who are the least likely to have attended

the preparatory courses for retirement which are now often available. Other factors of common occurrence in this age group combine to heighten the sense of social isolation and insecurity — increasing frailty, physical or psychiatric illness, the loss of relatives and friends and the preoccupation of their children with their own families. Decreasing financial security associated with a reduced income and, nowadays, the ravages of inflation on savings also leads to social isolation.

Feelings of insecurity and loneliness may be combated by the elderly person constantly seeking the company of friends or neighbours. Some will attempt to attract continuing attention by talking of their isolation and unhappiness whenever an opportunity presents itself. Some will become extremely possessive of their belongings, with resultant abnormal attachment to objects for which they no longer have any use, e.g., articles of furniture; others will become embarrassingly generous in an endeavour to ensure the continuing friendship of the recipient; others may become more self-reliant by intensifying their previous spiritual or emotional interests, although sometimes this may occur to a degree which is contrary to the best interests of their health.

Various studies have shown an inverse relationship between the amount of company a person keeps and the tendency to become mentally ill in old age. A study of the case notes of all admissions to the Bethlem Royal and Maudsley Hospitals over a three-year period showed that the number of patients whose illness followed the loss of a spouse was six times greater than expected, suggesting that bereavement had been a precipitating factor in their psychiatric illness (Parkes, 1964).

INTERVIEWING THE PATIENT

It is common for elderly people to feel that they should accept some degree of illness because they are getting older. On this basis they are often reluctant to seek medical attention and when they do they are reluctant to consume much of their doctor's time. It is necessary therefore for the doctor to convey a positive interest in elderly patients and their problems by what he says and by his attitude, and to show that he has time to listen. As age progresses, cerebration slows, so that the time needed in dealing with the elderly requires to be proportionately greater. Unless one has previous knowledge of the patient, it will not often be possible to make a full psychiatric appraisal in less than one hour.

All patients need to be put at ease and provided with an atmosphere which encourages them to tell their problems as spontaneously as possible. This is especially true of the elderly psychiatric patient.

The history should be allowed to emerge with a minimum of prompting, although the information should be organised in the interviewer's mind into a scheme of history-taking. In this way, no information will be lacking when making a full appraisal prior to planning a realistic treatment programme. An unhurried, uncritical and accepting attitude by the interviewer is required if the patient is to reveal thoughts of self-injury, self-destruction, guilt feelings about past misdemeanours, problems concerning anti-social behaviour and sexual behaviour or abnormalities.

Need to see relatives
With the organic patient much of the history of the illness, and the problems it has created and is causing in management, will only emerge if someone who has been living in close contact with him is also interviewed.

Physical examination
Physical examination, including a chest radiograph and examination of the urine, should always be carried out to ascertain whether there are any organic conditions present which could be contributory to, or causative of, the patient's psychiatric illness.

Catastrophic reaction
If, in the course of an interview, the elderly patient unexpectedly reacts to questions by bursting into tears or becoming irritable, agitated, and childishly aggressive in his behaviour, one should suspect that the patient may have been taxed beyond his current capabilities. Such symptoms may be indicative of the intellectual impairment and emotional lability characteristic of organic cerebral disease. Further enquiry may then reveal that over the past few months, whilst the illness has been developing, the individual has progressively reduced his interaction with his environment in such a way as to prevent exposure to situations which would have been likely to precipitate "catastrophic reactions". Such a reaction is extremely distressing for the patient and should not be provoked unnecessarily, even though it may be of diagnostic significance.

PRESCRIBING

A recent survey showed that psychotropic drugs were prescribed by general practitioners more often than any other group of drugs and accounted for almost one-fifth of all prescriptions (Skegg et al., 1977). The proportion of people receiving such drugs, i.e. sedatives, hypnotics, anti-psychotic drugs, tranquillisers or anti-depressants, increases progressively with age, the highest proportion for both men and women being in those aged 75 and over. In association with this trend, the findings of Learoyd are relevant. On reviewing the admissions of elderly patients to a medical and psychogeriatric unit he found that at least 20 per cent had been precipitated by the adverse effects of such drugs (Learoyd, 1972).

Special considerations are necessary when prescribing for the elderly because of the increasing likelihood of a significant decrease in mental and physical fitness as age advances. Various surveys have shown that, for all age groups, a high percentage of patients fail to take their medication as instructed and this must be especially true of the elderly since many, because of their age, show an impaired ability to grasp instructions and memorise these. This is particularly true if the instructions are of any complexity, e.g. if several drugs each with differing frequencies of administration have been prescribed. If the patient has an awareness of his own difficulty in comprehending the instructions anxiety may be added to his problems, and if not, the risk of accidental overdosage is increased. With their increasing rigidity in outlook, the elderly usually prefer, wherever possible, to take drugs with which they are familiar, especially any that they have found effective in the past.

Physically, impairment of renal excretion or liver metabolism may result in drugs having a more potent or prolonged effect and may increase the likelihood of unwanted side-effects, e.g. hypotension, dizzy spells and falls with some phenothiazines; confusion with tricyclic drugs.

The prescriber should be satisfied that there are clear indications of a need for ongoing medication and that there is every reason to believe that the objectives of medication can successfully be attained without undue risk of toxic effects. Often the elderly patient will have multiple diseases requiring treatment and where this is so it is best to make any necessary adjustments, e.g. alteration of dosage or prescription of additional drugs, one at a time and on a generous time-scale. With such a scheme, if there are any developments which may be attributable to drugs, the relevance of any particular medication will be more easily established.

Drugs should be prescribed in low doses and the dosage gradually increased, as tolerance permits, until the desired effect is achieved. Progress should be frequently assessed as to the benefits obtained, or the development of side-effects, so that treatment can be discontinued promptly if it is not proving beneficial, or is harmful.

The number of drugs prescribed should be kept to a minimum and a particular effort should be made to give clear instructions about their administration to the patient. Drugs introduced in recent years are the safest and most specific, and barbiturates in particular should no longer be prescribed as sedatives or hypnotics because of their tendency to cause depression, confusion and dependency. The form of medication, e.g. pills, syrup, and its palatibility should be considered.

Patient compliance with the prescriber's instructions will be improved if the patient feels that the prescriber is keen to help, has listened and understood the nature of his symptoms, and if doctor and patient each know of the other's expectations from treatment (Ley, 1977).

It is essential that unambiguous instructions are given to patients in simple everyday language. Most patients expect immediate results from treatment and on this basis discontinue medications which appear ineffective. In prescribing anti-depressants, therefore, it is important to explain that although side-effects may be experienced at once the anti-depressant effect is not likely to be apparent for at least another ten to twenty-one days. The verbal instructions given to the patient should be reinforced by the instructions on the label, which should be equally simple and unambiguous. Many patients will be more contented if actual times are stated, rather than "three times daily", and instructions such as "as directed" will often be found very unhelpful.

Many patients will fail to take their medication as prescribed, but careful records and a note of the medication left when the prescription is renewed will be useful in measuring the extent of "non-compliance". Hospital studies have shown that if a designated member of staff can spend time, as a matter of deliberate policy, with each individual elderly patient, to ensure that the discharge drug regime is fully understood and remembered, the number of errors in medication subsequently made by such patients will be substantially reduced (Macdonald *et al.*, 1977).

The significant breakthrough in providing safe and more specific psychotropic medication came in the late 1950s and early 1960s with the introduction of chlorpromazine, imipramine, iproniazid and chlordiazepoxide. The subsequent activity of the pharmaceutical industry in the psychiatric field has been mainly to introduce chemical relatives or derivatives of these substances, marketed for refinements such as quicker onset of activity. Some of these claims have been difficult to substantiate in clinical practice, and it would seem wisest to limit one's experience to two or three drugs of each group and to be fully conversant with advantages and disadvantages of each, so that they can be confidently prescribed for use and in a rational manner. In particular, each drug should be given in adequate dosage and for an adequate period of time before it is decided that its replacement is justified on the grounds of its unsatisfactory therapeutic effect.

The drugs referred to in the rest of this chapter indicate the author's own preferences.

PSYCHIATRIC ILLNESSES

The spectrum of psychiatric disorders to which a person may be subject is broadest in the chronologically old and includes the schizophrenic reactions, disorders of mood and neurotic reactions to which the person may have been subject for a large part of their life. Some psychiatric disorders, however, arise for the first time with ageing and these include the depressions of late onset, late paraphrenias and organic mental syndromes. These latter may be acute, and potentially reversible, or chronic, in association with widespread cortical neurone loss, and either may be complicated by the presence of paranoid or affective symptoms.

A study of 297 subjects, sampled at random, aged 65 and over and living at home revealed a remarkably high prevalence of psychiatric disorder (Kay *et al.*, 1964). Ten per cent showed evidence of an organic brain syndrome, due in the majority either to senile or arteriosclerotic dementia. In about half of this group the mental deterioration was of a similar degree to that found in demented patients in psychiatric hospitals; in the other half the diagnosis of dementia indicated less severe deterioration but of a greater degree than expected in someone of the subject's chronological age. A further ten per cent suffered from severe or moderately severe affective disorders or neuroses, the commonest being depression. Two per cent suffered from schizophrenia, and three per cent from other functional disorders, e.g. mental subnormality or marked personality deviation. Of the subjects studied and regarded as psychiatrically ill seventy-five per cent had sought medical advice within the previous three months for one reason or another, indicating the importance of psychiatric awareness for general practitioners.

Organic mental syndromes

The term "organic" is applied to those psychiatric syndromes which can be attributed to organic pathology demonstrable by post mortem and often during life by physical and laboratory investigations. This is in contrast to the term "functional" which is used in reference to those psychiatric disorders when no such pathology is demonstrable. In some of these latter, however, it is anticipated that biochemical abnormalities will at some future date be found to be aetiologically relevant.

Three types of organic mental reaction are generally described, common features to all of which are disturbances of consciousness and intellectual functioning, especially in the fields of attention, grasp, memory and orientation. These are:

1. acute confusional state;
2. dementia;
3. the dysmnestic syndrome.

The dividing lines between confusion, delirium and dementia are indistinct. The patient with an acute confusional state has difficulty in sustaining attention and concentration. He is easily distracted and there is considerable fluctuation in the extent to which the examiner can establish rapport and in the patient's level of awareness of what is going on around him. The condition may be described as delirium when transient hallucinations, illusions and delusions are prominent, often in association with obvious restlessness and a mood of fear. Dementia refers to an irreversible decline of functioning and is thus the term used when intellectual impairment and disturbed consciousness have been present for some time. In association with its duration there tends to be an impoverishment of the patient's thought content.

1. Acute confusional state

The following aetiological factors are those which are most frequently encountered in the elderly.

(a) Iatrogenic. Assessment of the patient should include deliberate enquiry as to self-administered or other medication that the patient may have been taking recently. Anti-depressants, hypnotics, tranquillisers and sedatives are common causes of confusion in the older age groups. The possibility of secret drinking should be considered, particularly when delirium develops within the first few days of the person going into a situation where he is likely to have been deprived of his usual sources, e.g. into hospital care or into prison.

(b) Systemic disease. Confusional states can be caused by any of the following systemic diseases. Cardiac failure, whatever its aetiology, as a result of a reduction in cerebral blood flow and the oxygen supply to the brain, e.g. in myocardial infarction. Respiratory disease, e.g. pneumonia, bronchopneumonia or chronic bronchitis, may be responsible for confusion also by causing hypoxia. The possibility of otherwise asymptomatic respiratory disease should always be considered whenever confusion is of sudden onset in this age group. Relatively minor infections, e.g. of the urinary tract, as well as acute generalised infections, may be associated with confusion in the elderly.

Other systemic diseases include the following. Neoplasms: carcinoma of the bronchus may be associated with confusion in the absence of cerebral metastases and the mental symptoms may precede clinical evidence of pulmonary disease by several months (McGovern et al., 1959; Charatan and Brierly, 1956). Thyroid disease: confusion may occur in association with hypothyroidism or hyperthyroidism. Diabetes: hyperglycaemia or hypoglycaemia can cause confusion.

(c) Cerebral disease or injury. Very transient confusion may be a feature of a developing sub-arachnoid haemorrhage, cerebral *embolism* or *cerebral haemorrhage.* Confusion is likely to be more prolonged in association with cerebral thrombosis and whilst there will usually be associated neurological signs these may be absent when the thrombosis occurs in the so-called "silent areas" of the brain.

Episodes of more marked confusion are frequently seen in the course of *arteriosclerotic* or *senile dementia.* Whilst relatives or close associates may have accommodated themselves to the progressive intellectual impairment, the development of more marked confusion and perhaps resulting anti-social or unacceptable behaviour is often the point at which medical attention is sought for the first time.

With all *head injuries* there is usually some alteration in consciousness but impressions of the presence and extent of this are dependent upon the thoroughness of examination. Some considerable time may elapse after an injured person is able to act in an apparently normal manner, but before his "ongoing" memory is regained. Patients with confusion following upon a head injury should be admitted for observation, in particular so that the question of developing complications, e.g. intracerebral haemorrhage, can be assessed. To facilitate such assessment these patients should not be given any drugs that may interfere with the level of consciousness in the following forty-eight hours.

In cases of *epilepsy*, some epileptics either following, prior to, or in place of a convulsion, may develop a "twilight state" in which they remain confused, disorientated and with impaired grasp and concentration. In some, consciousness is only slightly disturbed but in other cases the patient is delirious. Marked retardation of thinking and movements is often present and there may be vivid hallucinations often of a religious nature.

Cerebral neoplasms or infections may first manifest themselves as a confusional state, with or without focal neurological signs. *Subdural haematoma* is an uncommon cause of confusion which, if untreated, may result in dementia. It may result from quite a trivial head injury sometime previously, the significance of which is only appreciated in retrospect.

(d) Other causes. These include the following: *disturbances of fluid and electrolyte balance*, especially in association with severe sodium or potassium depletion. *Vitamin deficiency:* in thiamine deficiency confusion, general weakness, depression and irritability occur as early symptoms, usually long before other manifestations of beri-beri. Such a deficiency may arise from an impoverished diet, chronic alcoholism, repeated vomiting, or gastro-intestinal disease and associated malabsorption. *Anaemia:* delirium may occur in the fairly advanced stages of pernicious anaemia but it is not a significant feature of severe iron deficiency or anaemia arising from haemorrhage. *Hypothermia:* mental confusion, retardation of movement

and speech increasing over several days may be important presenting features. Decreased activity, poor nutrition, inadequate clothing and treatment with neuroleptic drugs are common contributory factors.

Management of the acute confusional state. Treatment is essentially directed to that of the underlying cause, e.g. infection, hypoxia or any of the causes already mentioned. When alcoholism or a vitamin B deficiency is considered contributory, large doses of Parentrovite (containing vitamins of the B group and vitamin C) should be given. Two pairs of Intravenous High Potency ampoules should be given twice daily for two days followed by one pair of either Intramuscular High Potency (7 ml) or Intramuscular Maintenance ampoules (4 ml) daily for seven days, as indicated clinically.

Restlessness and withdrawal symptoms may be controlled by one of the benzodiazepines – e.g. diazepam (Valium) 5 mg intramuscularly, repeated after an interval of not less than four hours, or 2 mg t.d.s. orally in less severe cases. For extreme restlessness haloperidol (Serenace) may be given starting with 5 mg intramuscularly and repeating this six-hourly until control is achieved, when oral dosage may be substituted in diminishing doses although haloperidol has no anti-epileptic function. Patients with arteriosclerosis or basal ganglial disease are particularly prone to develop dystonic reactions and the risk of such developing will be lessened if an anti-parkinsonian agent is given, especially when the haloperidol is first given, e.g. orphenadrine hydrochloride (Disipal), 50 mg t.d.s.

Most of the confused patient's behaviour is a result of the fear produced secondarily to his symptoms. This can be minimised by constant reassurance from his attendants. Well-lit and simply-furnished surroundings with minimal changes of staff and constant attendance by a small group of nurses will all prove helpful. Visitors should stay for only short periods and should be warned not to increase the patient's distress by overtaxing his comprehension and grasp of current affairs.

2. *Dementia*

Not all confusional states, even those of acute onset, are reversible. If the aetiological factor is severe in degree or prolonged in duration, irreversible damage to brain structure may occur and the clinical picture is then described as dementia. Often the causative agent will result in increasing brain damage which will be exhibited in a continuing decline of mental faculties and progressive deterioration. Disturbances of memory and orientation are particularly evident, but other symptoms may also be present, e.g. difficulties in comprehension and learning, emotional lability and deterioration in social behaviour.

Dementia may be primary or secondary. Senile dementia is by far the commonest form of the primary type and is associated with an underlying diffuse atrophy of brain tissue with neuroglial proliferation and characteristic senile plaques and neurofibrillary tangles. The condition rarely occurs before the age of 70. It affects both sexes and twin studies suggest that heredity is an important aetiological factor. Less common primary dementias include those associated with the names of Pick (1892) and Alzheimer (1907) and referred to as the presenile dementias because of their earlier age of onset. The neuropathological features of Alzheimer's disease are similar to those found in senile dementia.

Secondary dementia. Commoner causes are as follows.

(a) Trauma — head injury; subdural haematoma.
(b) Inflammatory — e.g. neurosyphilis; following encephalitis.
(c) Neoplastic — may be primary or metastatic, intra- or extra-cerebral.
(d) Toxic — alcohol; lead or mercury poisoning.
(e) Anoxic — asphyxia; carbon-monoxide poisoning.
(f) Vascular — arteriosclerosis; hypertension.
(g) Metabolic — B_{12} deficiency; chronic hepatic disease, hypocalcaemia.
(h) Endocrine — hypothyroidism.

Cerebral arteriosclerosis accounts for the majority of cases of secondary dementia. Its onset is usually in the sixth decade. Generalised arteriosclerotic changes are present in the cerebral blood vessels with consequent areas of ischaemia and cerebral softening. There is often associated hypertension. Various clinical features may be present which make this diagnosis more likely than that of senile dementia, but in many cases the distinction, clinically, between the two is impossible and as age advances pathological evidence of both conditions becomes more likely. Clinical features favouring arteriosclerotic dementia diagnostically are: earlier onset; associated hypertension; evidence of previous strokes; symptomatic epilepsy; better personality preservation and a more fluctuant and less steadily progressive course.

Methods of investigation. These may include:
Psychological assessment. A psychologist may be able to make a useful contribution by assessing objectively the extent and degree of any intellectual deterioration and by monitoring further developments.
Laboratory investigations of possible relevance include a full blood count together with B_{12} and folate levels, liver function tests, urea,

electrolyte and blood sugar levels, tests of thyroid function and serological tests for syphilis.

X-Rays such as a skull X-ray may be helpful by revealing calcification, local bone erosion, evidence of increased intracranial pressure or displacement of a calcified pineal gland. Chest X-ray for evidence of any primary lung pathology is routine hospital practice.

An electro-encephalogram can give useful information regarding a cerebral tumour or subdural haematoma, but a normal E.E.G. can occur despite widespread cerebral atrophy if this is developing slowly. The investigation involves the recording of changes in electrical potential from electrodes placed on the patient's head and involves no discomfort.

A pneumo-encephalogram involves lumbar puncture and the introduction of air into the subarachnoid space. From there it is directed into the ventricular system assisted by changes in the position of the head. Dilation of the ventricles may be seen, as may local or generalised cerebral atrophy. Distortion of the ventricular system or cerebrospinal fluid pathways may be evident when these are encroached upon by space-occupying lesions.

Computerised axial tomography (The E.M.I. Scan) has revolutionised the approach to the investigation of suspected space-occupying lesions, although scanning facilities are limited to major centres. It is a non-invasive investigation which can be used to differentiate between cerebral haemorrhage, infarction and tumour, and to demonstrate subdural haematoma or cerebral atrophy.

A brain biopsy, when brain tissue is obtained through a burr hole via a biopsy needle or at craniotomy prior to possible immediate neuro-surgical intervention. This is a rarely used procedure.

Management of patients with dementia. Either senile dementia or arteriosclerosis accounts for the vast majority of patients presenting with clinical features of dementia. There is no method of reversing or halting the progression of either of these, but this should not lead to complacency once a diagnosis of dementia is made, for a number of treatable conditions may be responsible for the same clinical picture, notably neurosyphilis, alcoholism, B_{12} deficiency, and hypothyroidism. Some gliomas, meningiomas, colloid cysts, benign tumours, subdural haematomas and giant aneurysms may be treatable space-occupying lesions which present as dementia.

Adequate history-taking, which must include an account of the development of the illness and its features and problems from the relatives, is as essential as is physical examination to elicit features which may lead to the diagnosis of a treatable causative condition. Correction of deficiencies or disease processes, or otherwise effective treatment of the various possible causes, will at least prevent further progression of the intellectual impairment and in some cases will result in dramatic improvement. It has to be accepted, however, that it is not always possible to obtain a useful history either from relatives or from the patient. The evaluation of any neurological signs may be difficult, and the question may arise as to what extent further investigation should be undertaken. This will depend on such factors as the duration of the illness, the degree of dementia, the extent to which there is doubt about the illness being other than senile or arteriosclerotic dementia and, in general terms, the extent to which the patient is likely to benefit if the investigation yields positive results and the discomfort to which the patient will be subjected by further procedures.

The majority of elderly people with dementia continue to live in the community and most old people want to go on living independently in their own homes for as long as possible. The extent to which an individual can continue to do so is dependent, not only on the extent of the organic brain disease, but also on the patient's physical health, the physical features of his environment and the support provided by relatives and neighbours.

All organic psychiatric illness in the elderly clearly requires *medical screening* as soon as it is detected, in accordance with the principles already outlined. Once the diagnosis has been established, then a scheme of management can be worked out. This is likely to be complex, involving far more than the mere prescription of drugs, and even these should be avoided unless there is a clear indication for their use. Regular medical contact is an essential part of the patient's further care. Demented patients often have difficulty in communicating their symptoms adequately, but a sudden change in the patient's well-being, e.g. sudden impairment of appetite, alteration in the level of activity, a tendency to fall, clumsiness, the appearance of incontinence, or an unaccountable accentuation of the degree of confusion, will call for reappraisal of the patient's physical state. Many easily treatable conditions will be uncovered in this way, e.g. intestinal obstruction, urinary retention, silent myocardial infarction, respiratory infection and gastro-intestinal bleeding. Changes in the general well-being will also call for a review of the patient's medication, for side-effects may be responsible for the patient's deterioration, e.g. postural hypotension, extrapyramidal symptoms, or hyponatremia associated with diuretic therapy. Sometimes the appearance of additional symptoms or other atypical developments in the progress of the illness will cast doubts on the initial diagnosis and thus call for further investigation.

Living in the community: patients with dementia can place a considerable burden on their relatives, friends and neighbours, and the personality of the patient can be crucial in determining to what extent and for how long, their co-operation will continue. Social workers and health visitors should be an integral part of the caring team. A full appraisal of the patient and his problems in the home setting with regular visiting will ensure that all necessary agencies are mobilised, such as home helps, meals on wheels, laundry, and day centres. It will be helpful for relatives and neighbours to be given some understanding of the personality changes commonly associated with ageing, as well as the nature of the patient's illness and the sort of difficulties to which it is giving rise, e.g. the tendency of a patient to become paranoid on the basis of forgetfulness and to misplace articles in his own home; the tendency to disintegrate into a state of tearful helplessness when faced with what would previously have been a trivial problem, like a fused light bulb, a broken window, a leaking tap, which now proves too much because of his failing faculties. It should be possible to assure relatives that should a crisis arise admission will be available within a very short period, if not immediately.

Sheltered accommodation, with some supervision by a warden or guardian, may be appropriate for mildly demented patients who are no longer able or willing to live in their own homes with support from the community and yet who do not require the full caring facilities provided by hospitalisation.

Assessment centres with their own multidisciplinary teams have been established in many parts of the country. The aims and organisation of these have been described in detail elsewhere (Robinson, 1975). Such centres have facilities for specialised investigation and have a close working relationship with geriatricians. The aim is to ensure not only full appraisal of patients, but also that they are maintained in the community as long as their physical and mental health permit and that, when this is no longer possible, appropriate placement in continuing care in a supportive environment will be arranged. Assessment centres originated from reports which showed many elderly people to be misplaced, i.e. in the wrong type of hospital (Kidd, 1962), but this is probably not a significant problem nowadays.

Many *day hospitals* are currently fulfilling many of the functions of assessment centres and thus have readily available access to laboratory services, radiologists, neurologists, audiologists, opticians, dentists, chiropodists, occupational therapists and speech therapists. A multidisciplinary approach is made and behaviour rating scales (e.g. the Crichton Royal Geriatric Behavioural Rating Scale) are often used to help involve all members of the team in diagnosis and assessment. Weekly conferences incorporating all the personnel involved are an essential feature for continuous appraisal of the patient and his progress, as well as for formulating plans for new entrants and for the subsequent care of those about to be discharged. Such conferences also play an invaluable part in maintaining staff morale at a high level, which in turn is reflected in a high quality of patient care. These units have a programme of activities, run by occupational therapists, designed to maintain or widen the interests, sociability and self-esteem of those attending. It has been shown to be advantageous for one member of staff to be assigned to reporting on a particular patient, thereby giving each patient the benefit of having a stable figure to whom he can relate.

Appropriate placement and support should be available on discharge as a result of assessment, whether in the assessment centre or in the day hospital. Some patients will return home with additional support from the social services; others will benefit from continuing attendance at the day hospital with or without sheltered housing; those requiring general nursing care will be appropriately placed in geriatric long-term care, whilst psychiatric hospital care will be appropriate for those behaviourally disturbed or requiring some security. It must be emphasised, however, that the efficiency of such centres is dependent upon the adequacy of the supporting services. If these are deficient, the day hospital or assessment centre cannot move people on and by default has to provide long-term care itself, thus becoming increasingly ineffective for assessment purposes, no matter how industrious, enthusiastic or knowledgeable its staff.

Within the institution, be it a local authority home, geriatric or mental hospital, much can be done to maintain the relative well-being of such patients at its highest level. Staff on long-term wards should be in a relatively permanent placement there, so that under-standing, tolerance and sympathy towards the individual patient and his progressively increasing disabilities can be developed to a maximum. Attention should be paid to the safety of the patients by ensuring, for example, appropriate footwear, floor-coverings, handrails, bed heights and the absence of fire risks. The individuality of patients should be respected by encouraging each to have his own personal possessions and clothes and by encouraging visiting. Regular toileting will avoid unnecessary daytime incontinence. A simple ward routine should be the aim, with short periods of stimulation, e.g. singing, simple games and handicrafts.

Whether the patient is living in the community or in hospital, undue anxiety or distress during the day, or in association with insomnia, is best treated by a small dose of one of the short acting benzodiazepines e.g. lorazepam (Ativan) 1 mg b-t.d.s. Alternatively oxazepam (Serenid-D) 10 mgm t-q.d.s. may be prescribed (see also p. 113).

From time to time, drugs have been introduced with claims that,

by increasing the supply of oxygen or other essential nutrients to the
cerebral neurones, they improve intellectual functioning. Unfortunately none of these has been impressive clinically.

3. *The dysmnestic syndrome*
The dysmnestic syndrome is a discrete entity characterised by impairment of recent memory, often with a tendency to confabulate and
a relatively intact memory for events earlier in life. The condition is
usually associated with thiamine deficiency occurring on the basis
of alcoholism, persistent vomiting or malnutrition. The distinctive
pathology of the syndrome involves congested blood vessels and
petechial haemorrhages in the dorso-medial nucleus of the thalamus
and mamillary bodies. Treatment is by large doses of the B-group of
vitamins. Vascular or neoplastic lesions in the same areas may produce
a similar clinical picture.

Depressive illnesses
The marked increase which occurs in the suicide rate for both sexes
beginning in the fifth decade (Stengel, 1965), serves as a reminder
not only that depressive illnesses are particularly common in the elderly, but also of the possible tragic consequences of failing to recognise
and treat these. Such illnesses frequently present themselves as minor
physical complaints, characteristic depressive symptoms also being
present but often elicited only on specific enquiry. Caution must be
exercised in diagnosing the occurrence of phobic anxiety, obsessional
or hypochondriacal symptoms as neurosis in this age group and a
search for symptoms indicative of an underlying depressive illness
must be the rule. Similarly, paranoid symptoms should not lead to
the assumption of a basic paraphrenic or dementing illness. It is well
recognised that the memory difficulties, inability to cope and general
disorganisation suggestive of an organic illness, such as cerebral
arteriosclerosis, may in fact be part of an agitated depressive illness.
It must also be said that psychiatrists for a long time have recognised
that many elderly patients who develop neurotic symptoms, without
clear evidence of a depressive illness, respond well to anti-depressant
drugs — suggesting the "masked" depressions described by Post
(1965).

Management
Depressive spells characterised by feelings of hopelessness and anxiety
are extremely common in the elderly and by no means confined to
those in poor physical health and socially isolated. These are often
associated with some precipitating event and may be of a few hours'
or days' duration and thus in the nature of a transient, reactive
depression. The brevity of such disturbances of mood means that

they often escape medical attention and are rarely seen by psychiatrists. If such people are encouraged to ventilate their feelings with discussion and reassurance this is often all that will be necessary. Follow-up should be carried out, however, to ensure that a depressive illness of greater intensity or duration is not developing.

General management of a depressive illness should be directed towards supporting the patient, at the same time as providing speedy relief of symptoms by the appropriate physical treatment. It is particularly important to protect the patient against the risk of suicide. Symptomatic and specific anti-depressant medication will be appropriate in a majority of cases.

Whenever a diagnosis of depression is made, the risk of suicide must be considered and if no indication of this is given spontaneously, specific enquiry should be tactfully made. Previous knowledge or assessment of the reliability of the patient will be important in deciding upon the validity of answers given and a history of previous suicidal attempts or impulsive tendencies will arouse particular concern. Suicidal talk should always be taken seriously and whilst suicidal intentions may not be disclosed at interview, those living with the patient may know of recently expressed tendencies in this direction. It is important to explain to the patient and to his associates the nature of his illness, giving every encouragement to expect a favourable outcome.

With less serious depressive illnesses, where the doctor is confident that there is no suicidal risk and where there is a good relationship between the patient and doctor, treatment may be given without hospitalisation. In a reactive type of depression the patient may feel most content continuing to work, if this is of fairly routine nature, but his ability to work effectively should be repeatedly assessed, otherwise he may incur the displeasure of his employers, thereby adding to his problems. Some reactive depressions will be helped by changing the current environment because of its unhappy associations and moving to somewhere more stimulating. When there is any evidence that the illness is of an endogenous nature, however, the patient should be firmly discouraged from exposing himself to more stimulation, as this will only draw his attention to his difficulty in concentrating and his social disinclinations, thereby accentuating his general state of unhappiness. Such patients should be encouraged to lead a quiet life, and well-meaning visitors and friends should be discouraged from visiting too frequently, or for too long a period.

When there is any risk of suicide the patient should be encouraged to seek hospital care, in order that adequate supervision can be provided. Sometimes, because of the nature of the illness — for example, delusions of unworthiness or guilt — the patient cannot be persuaded to seek hospital admission and in these cases compulsory admission may be necessary to safeguard the patient's interests. There is no doubt that psychiatric nurses are able to provide a more understanding and supportive environment for such patients, so that whilst the patient and his relatives may prefer to hide his mental illness by seeking admission to a general hospital or nursing home, this is unlikely to be the most appropriate form of in-patient care.

In more severe depressive illnesses particular attention should be paid to the patient's state of nutrition, hydration and general physical health, since these matters may have been neglected prior to coming into care. Persistent refusal of food is usually no longer a problem, once electro-convulsive therapy has been given. Patients with severe agitation and determined suicidal tendencies are also best treated with E.C.T. because of the rapid and dramatic improvement which results (*see* p. 446). Occupational therapy and some form of recreation will often be encouraged to stimulate the patient's interest and the return of his self-confidence. With some improvement, the patient and his relatives often plead for his discharge but this is discouraged until improvement has been maintained for two or three weeks, because of the risk of relapse. Relatives should be invited to help the patient to follow the doctor's advice. It is common policy to suggest that patients go home for short periods at first, as this gives them and the medical staff an opportunity to assess the extent of recovery in the patient's home environment. Psychotherapy will involve a discussion of the patient as an individual, his background and the precipitating factors. A social worker may be involved to help the patient with current social problems and any other problems of daily living.

The diagnosis of a depressive illness requires the prompt institution of appropriate therapy. Most of these patients will have some sleep disturbance and appropriate medication may be dichloralphenazone (Welldorm), 2 tabs (of 650 mg) nocte, or Welldorm Elixir, 10 to 20 ml (225 mg in 5 ml) nocte; or chlormethiazole (Heminevrin), 1 to 2 tabs (of 500 mg) nocte, or Heminevrin Syrup, 5 to 10 ml (250 mg in 5 ml) nocte.

The majority of depressed patients will respond to antidepressant drugs although E.C.T. may be indicated for the severely depressed, very agitated, stuporose or suicidal patient, because it takes effect more rapidly. A large number of antidepressant drugs are available, most of which are chemically related to imipramine or amitriptyline with both of which there has been long experience since their introduction is the late 1950s. Some of these are less troublesome in the extent to which they cause side-effects, but none of them has shown to be consistently better in terms of the proportion of patients responding or the quality of improvement (Morris and Beck, 1974). In healthy patients normal therapeutic doses of these drugs are free from clinically important adverse cardiovascular effects apart from postural hypotension, but in patients with pre-existing bundle branch block this can be increased. These drugs are therefore best avoided for elderly patients and particularly for those with a history of cardiac disease (Glassman and Bigger, 1981).

Nomifensine hydrogen maleate (Merital) is a safer alternative to the tricyclics as an antidepressant in that it has no significant cardiotoxic effects. It has minimal anticholinergic effects and no epileptogenic effect in therapeutic doses, and is well tolerated even in very high doses. There are no contraindications as to its use although it may antagonise the hypotensive effects of adrenergic neurone blocking drugs which the patient may be taking as anti-hypertensive therapy. In the elderly treatment should be commenced with 25 mg once or twice daily and gradually increased to a maximum of 100 mg per day, given in divided doses. Treatment should be continued for at least four weeks and once a remission has occurred the drug can be reduced and continued at a maintenance level for at least a further three months.

If a patient fails to respond to the above and and E.C.G. shows no evidence of bundle branch block, imipramine (Tofranil) or amitriptyline (Tryptizol) may be tried in low doses − e.g. 10 mg t.d.s. Amitriptyline has sedative properties which are useful when anxiety or restlessness is part of the clinical picture; imipramine has stimulative properties which can be helpful if the patient is withdrawn or apathetic, but it can aggravate pre-existing tension or anxiety. Anticholinergic side-effects − e.g. dry mouth, constipation, blurred vision, dizziness, difficulty in micturition and drowsiness − may be troublesome and these drugs should not be given to patients with urinary retention or glaucoma.

With all antidepressants the patient and his relatives should be advised that improvement is not to be expected until the drug has been taken for ten to twenty-one days. The patient should be encouraged to persist with any specific drug for four weeks before assessing its effectiveness. Antidepressant medication should be continued for three months after maximum benefit has occurred and thereafter gradually withdrawn over a period of a few weeks.

Monoamineoxidase inhibitors (M.A.O.I.s) have the potential of causing serious side-effects and are not the drugs of first choice in the treatment of depression. Phenelzine (Nardil) has been shown to be less effective than imipramine in the treatment of the severe endogenous type of depressive illness (British Medical Journal, 1965), but appears to be effective in some cases of neurotic depression.

Lithium is a potentially very toxic drug, the use of which requires regular monitoring of serum lithium levels and it is therefore best given under specialist supervision. Patients with recurrent depressive illnesses may be advised to take lithium on a long-term basis because of its proven prophylactic value in reducing the frequency and duration of further episodes of manic-depressive illness (Angst *et al.*, 1969). Common side-effects are nausea, vertigo and hand tremor. Polyuria and polydipsia in association with a nephrogenic diabetes insipidus and hypothyroidism may also occur. Particular care in control is required with patients with cardiac arrhythmias (British Medical Journal, 1977).

The value of electro-convulsive therapy (E.C.T.) as a means of treatment has lately been the subject of a detailed survey by The Royal College of Psychiatrists (1977), who concluded that there is incontrovertible evidence that this is an effective treatment in severe depressive illness. It is particularly effective in the endogenous type of depression and exerts its effects more rapidly than anti-depressant medications. The assistance of an anaesthetist is required in its administration and hence it is given in hospital, usually after the patient's admission, although with less-severely-ill patients it may be given on an out-patient basis, the patient returning home under supervision a few hours after treatment. Elderly patients are particularly prone to complain of subjective memory impairment following E.C.T. but this is transient. Treatment is usually given once or twice weekly and often six to eight treatments are required. E.C.T. is contra-indicated in the presence of cardiac failure, or a recent coronary thrombosis or cerebro-vascular accident.

Psychosurgery may be offered to patients who have failed to respond to adequate exposure to all other appropriate forms of treatment and who remain severely distressed. Recent large studies, with follow-up, on patients subject to procedures using stereotactic techniques have shown good results in 68 per cent of chronically-ill patients, with a very low incidence of undesirable side-effects (Goktepe *et al.*, 1975).

The immediate results of treatment in providing relief of symptoms are very encouraging in the majority of elderly depressives but there is a considerable tendency for further affective illness to occur. The prognosis is not closely related to the type of clinical picture and, whilst there are many exceptions, the factors which make for a good prognosis include severe symptoms, extravert personality, onset before the age of 70, recovery from an earlier attack before the age of 50, and a positive family history of affective disorder. In contrast, patients with definite evidence of dementia or other brain damage rarely make a good recovery from the depression (Post, 1962).

Hypomania and mania

The essential features of these illnesses are a mood of elation with increased self-confidence and assertiveness, pressure of talk and over-activity in association with easy distractability. These symptoms are developed to a pathological degree. Judgment is disturbed and insight almost wholly lost. The successful conduct of business and private affairs is jeopardised because of a lowering of moral standards, extravagance and generally irresponsible behaviour resulting from disinhibition. If the patient's relatives or general practitioner have had previous experience of him in a hypomanic phase they will have no doubt when the illness is returning, but in the earlier stages it is often very difficult to institute treatment because of the patient's inability to see himself as ill. Great tact is required in handling such patients, particularly because of their irritability, but if a good relationship can be established in the early stages this will enable the patient to be kept under observation and admitted to hospital as soon as this is required, thereby avoiding the patient's behaviour complicating his life unnecessarily.

In hospital the excitement and over-activity are usually most rapidly and effectively controlled by haloperidol. This belongs to the butyrophenone group of neuroleptic drugs, but phenothiazines may also be used. For the acutely disturbed physically fit patient of average physique 5 mg haloperidol can be given intramuscularly and repeated six-hourly until the excitement is under control, whereupon a switch to oral medication should be made, e.g. 3 mg four times a day. Extrapyramidal symptoms are a common side-effect and usually respond to anti-parkinsonian drugs. Alternatively, chlorpromazine, 100 mg or more, three times daily according to the clinical response, may be given. Provided the patient's renal function and circulation are satisfactory a lithium salt, e.g. lithium carbonate (Priadel), may be prescribed although the combination of baloperidol and lithium should be avoided. Lithium is normally less rapidly effective than the phenothiazines or butyrophenones, but often begins to show its effectiveness after one or two days. Because of its potential toxicity careful and continuing supervision of patients on lithium is necessary. Sometimes electro-convulsive therapy will be advised, since this is rapidly effective in reducing the excitement. Hypnotics may also be required for a short period to ensure adequate sleep and chlorpromazine, 100 mg orally, may be given at night. The patient should be encouraged to lead a quiet life but with the minimum of restrictions. Unnecessary or prolonged visiting should be discouraged when the patient is very disturbed.

When the patient has been discharged from hospital, the haloperidol will have been discontinued or reduced to a dosage which, in the continuing absence of symptoms, will be further reduced and eventually discontinued under out-patient supervision. If there is a history of previous manic or depressive illnesses the patient can be expected to be on lithium prophylactically. Most hospitals now have organised lithium clinics, but if not, monitoring can be carried out in the normal psychiatric out-patient clinic.

Blood samples will be taken at regular intervals to ensure that the serum lithium remains within the effective range of 0.6 to 1.5 mEq/L. Once stabilised, these may be taken at two or three monthly intervals. If, in between hospital visits, the patient shows further evidence of excitement or depression or intercurrent illness, additional serum levels should be obtained because of the risk of intoxication. It is important to impress on such patients the need for regular medication without which the likelihood of relapse is significantly greater. Once out of hospital, the patient should not be allowed to resume business activity until he has shown himself to be symptom-free and otherwise back to his normal pattern of living for a number of weeks. The hypomanic patient is not accessible to psychotherapy in the acute phase, but as his illness subsides some useful discussion of the patient, his life style and the psychological precipitants of his illness will be possible.

Late paraphrenia

This term refers to patients who in later life develop paranoid delusions in clear consciousness. The delusions are often, though not invariably, well-systematised and frequently associated with auditory hallucinations. A striking feature is the good preservation of personality. There is no generalised emotional blunting or thought disorder. The psychotic experiences seem fairly circumscribed and in matters not involving them there is no obvious interference with the patient's daily life. However, prior to the onset of the illness, these patients have often been known for their sensitive nature and their tendency to lead a relatively isolated life. The illness occurs more commonly in women and is accompanied in many patients by defects in seeing or hearing. In making the diagnosis an underlying depressive or organic psychiatric illness requires to be excluded. Anti-psychotic drugs cause the disappearance of, or reduce, the intensity of delusions and distress caused by the hallucinatory experiences, thereby reducing the possibility of socially unacceptable behaviour. Whenever possible, the patient should be encouraged to continue living at home. If the patient is willing, it may be helpful for him to attend for day hospital care. For those whose co-operation with oral medication is doubtful or absent long-acting anti-psychotic drugs should be considered, e.g. fluphenazine decanoate (Modecate), flupenthixol decanoate (Depixol) or fluspirilene (Redeptin). Injections are required at intervals of one week to one month depending on the drug and the clinical response. Oral anti-parkinsonian drugs are often required to minimise extrapyramidal side-effects. Such patients also benefit from regular supervision, not only to monitor the effectiveness of drug therapy and to add or discontinue anti-parkinsonian agents as necessary, but also to support the patient and to discourage any tendencies he may have to become more socially withdrawn or neglectful of himself.

Chronic schizophrenia

Within the past two decades, there has been an increasing movement to reduce the number of long-stay beds in mental hospitals and this has been effected to a variable degree in different parts of the country. Sometimes this has been achieved by requiring elderly chronic schizophrenics with residual symptoms, after many years in hospital, to go and live in an environment which is less suitable for their needs. The eccentricities, deteriorated appearance and behaviour, and the social withdrawal of such patients, may lead to anxiety within society and, in a small percentage, petty crime may become a problem (Rollin, 1963).

Chronic schizophrenic patients should only be discharged from hospital if they are moving to a residential situation which will be to their advantage and this necessitates taking into account the subtle but significant limitations imposed upon them by their illness. A positive policy of community care will keep such patients and their anti-psychotic medication under supervision — usually through an out-patient department and community nursing service. Hostels and group homes providing for such patients should have some arrangement for regular visitation by a member of a psychiatric team. This will normally enable the speedy transfer back to hospital of those patients for whom the move away has not been advantageous, or who have relapsed. It is important for those patients living away from hospital to be in a tolerant, supportive environment, with opportunities and encouragement to meet with others socially as they would in hospital. Despite having reached retirement age, often these patients will benefit from continued attendance at work or at a day hospital, even if only two or three times each week.

As a prelude to the possible discharge from hospital, relatives will usually be approached asking for their co-operation in allowing the patient to return home for a trial period. Since many of these patients will have had an acute illness with symptoms of a bizarre and frightening nature and subsequently have spent a long period in hospital, the relatives may be apprehensive and require reassurance and encouragement before participating in such a venture. Relatives should have some understanding of the patient's illness gained during visits, either intuitively or by talking to staff, but this can be usefully supplemented at this stage by discussion with the social worker involved in the patient's care. It will be helpful for them to have some explanation of the limitations imposed by the patient's particular illness and advice should be given which will enable them to provide the returning patient with a welcoming and accepting environment. Anti-psychotic drugs must be continued since relapse is a common consequence of their discontinuation.

Commonly used drugs in schizophrenia in the elderly, in addition to the long-acting preparations already mentioned, include:

(a) thioridazine (Melleril) — 30 to 100 mg daily in divided doses. Associated with a low incidence of side-effects;

(b) pimozide (Orap) — 2 to 10 mg daily as a single dose. Moderate tendency to produce extrapyramidal symptoms;

(c) haloperidol (Serenace) — 1 to 10 mg daily in twice daily doses. Extrapyramidal symptoms common.

All anti-psychotic drugs may produce extrapyramidal symptoms (parkinsonism; dystonic reactions; restlessness). These may be controlled by reduction of the dosage or orphenadrine (Disipal) 50 to 100 mg morning and mid-day. Autonomic side-effects (dry mouth, nasal stuffiness, blurred vision, postural hypotension) are minimal with thioridazine.

Neuroses

Neurotic illnesses in the elderly are rarely seen in psychiatric out-patient departments. Such illnesses are unlikely to manifest themselves for the first time in the older age groups and, when this appears to be the case, more detailed history-taking will often reveal that the symptoms are the presenting features of an endogenous depressive illness. The patient with a true neurotic illness will have shown similar responses to difficulties in adjustment throughout his previous life and his current symptoms often may be seen as a consequence of recent psychological stress. The possibility of the patient's neurotic symptoms — most commonly anxiety, phobic symptoms, hypochondriacal concern, or depression with a fluctuating degree of anxiety — having become intensified or having reappeared as a consequence of some underlying physical illness, should also always be considered. Neurotic symptoms may interfere with the patient's ability to concentrate and cope with everyday tasks to such a degree as to give the impression of a dementing illness.

The establishment of a good relationship with the patient, on the basis of which simple supportive psychotherapy can be given, is an essential part of treatment. The general practitioner is normally in a uniquely advantageous position for giving such effective psychotherapy, for which the patient will be greatly appreciative. Time is required to gain a tolerant and sympathetic understanding of the patient and his problems and subsequently to have realistic and practical discussions as to possible solutions to current problems and to help the patient as he works through these. In supporting the patient it is necessary to accept uncritically the patient's personality limitations, as well as any mental or physical deficits, and to boost the patient's ego by making the most of his personality assets. Endeavours to change the patient's personality by overt criticism or perhaps by attempting to reveal the patient's true character to himself in a more subtle manner will not meet with lasting success, are likely to damage the doctor/patient relationship, and in this way may intensify the patient's illness. Some neurotic patients will become very dependent upon their doctor for continuing support for several weeks and sometimes for much longer, but the value of frequent visits and discussions should not be underrated. This supportive therapy may save many hypochondriacal patients from unnecessary investigations in various hospital departments, although many general practitioners will find that such care can only be given to a very small number of patients, because of the time involved. The psychiatric out-patient clinics will have more time at their disposal, but many elderly people are hesitant to attend such clinics, partly, no doubt, because of the physical difficulty in getting there, but also perhaps because they see in the out-patient department the threat that this may lead to permanent institutional placement.

In all neurotic illness anti-anxiety medications may be required to lessen the patient's distress, e.g. lorazepam (Ativan) 1 mg b-t.d.s.

A true obsessional neurosis of any severity is uncommon in the elderly and disabling obsessional symptoms in this age group will more frequently be part of a depressive illness. For the true neuroses of this type one, or a combination, of various types of behaviour therapy, e.g. response prevention, systematic desensitisation, confrontation, have been found effective, so that referral to a psychologist either directly or through a psychiatric out-patient department will be appropriate. Drugs may also have a useful contribution to make, e.g. small doses of phenothiazines or clomipramine (Anafranil) have been found to be particularly useful clinically.

The rare distressing obsessional symptoms which do not respond to the above measures may respond successfully to psychosurgery.

Personality disorders

People who have had a lifelong difficulty in interpersonal relationships, often with prominent traits of self-centredness, possessiveness, irritability and an over-critical attitude, may come to the attention of the medical profession for the first time in later life. Medical referral arises when those in daily contact with such an individual reject him because they find his behaviour unacceptable. This will often arise shortly after the individual moves to new surroundings, e.g. a residential home, or after the death of a long-suffering relative. The individuals in the new environment will be unable to accept, at any rate initially, the antagonism caused by the arrival of the aberrant personality. At all ages, such individuals are the despair of all with whom they come into contact, although a recognition of their personality limitations as such, and allowance for them, makes life much more tolerable for all concerned. Such people are not ill and it is unrealistic to expect that they should become any more the responsibility of hospitals than of other agencies.

EMERGENCY SITUATIONS

Elderly patients may present as a psychiatric emergency because of their acutely disturbed behaviour or because of a considered need for immediate specialised psychiatric help.

The acutely agitated or excited patient

The majority of elderly patients constituting an emergency will be in an acutely restless and disturbed condition. Such behaviour may result from a variety of psychiatric illnesses and the most appropriate management, as in any situation, will be dependent upon an accurate diagnosis. The conditions most likely to be responsible will be:

(1) acute confusional state;
(2) hysteria;
(3) depression;
(4) schizophrenia; or
(5) mania.

Alcohol intoxication with its disinhibiting effects will often intensify the presentation of the patient's distress.

In a small percentage of patients it will be impossible for anyone to quieten the patient or establish effective contact. In such cases their agitated or destructive behaviour may require symptomatic treatment, e.g. by the administration of chlorpromazine, 50 to 100 mg intramuscularly (to a patient of good physique and in good health), repeated after an hour if necessary. On rare occasions, when the patient is behaving in a dangerous manner, it may be necessary to ask for the assistance of the police in restraining him. In the majority of cases, however, such anti-social or aggressive behaviour will not be present, the patient clearly suffering far more than those about him, and it will be possible to make some assessment of the underlying cause.

The entrance of a kindly, unhurried and competent medical attendant will in itself often have a pronounced calming effect. Initially attention should be paid to the patient rather than to the relatives, although they may have a valuable contribution to make towards a correct diagnosis at a later stage. The patient should be seen alone and, if possible, removed from surroundings and individuals who have been possible precipitants or excitants. With minimal prompting the patient should be encouraged to talk about the crisis situation as he sees it and encouraged to express any paranoid feelings or aggression at his own pace and without criticism. Particular enquiry will be required to decide whether there is evidence of any clouding of consciousness denoting an acute confusional state. Specific questions should be asked with regard to recent medication or other drugs the patient may have been taking, including alcohol, his recent health and any current physical symptoms. If there is any question of physical illness a physical examination will be necessary.

Pointers to the various possible basic psychiatric conditions will be as follows.

1. *Acute confusional state*
Reduced grasp and awareness will result in rambling speech. Delusions and hallucinations may be present but will be transitory. Memory for recent events will be absent or inaccurate and orientation for time and place and possibly also for person will be impaired. Often the fluctuating level of the patient's awareness of his surroundings will impress the examiner, the patient answering appropriately one minute and wholly inappropriately the next. It will be relevant to enquire from relatives whether these symptoms are a wholly new development or whether forgetfulness and confusion have been a slowly increasing problem over the past few months or years, in which case the confusion is likely to be part of a senile or arteriosclerotic dementing process.

Management. Patients with an acute confusional state require admission for further investigation. This should be to a general hospital, geriatric assessment or psychiatric unit, assuming that the necessary facilities and expertise will be available.

In a small number of patients investigation will reveal no obvious cause and symptomatic treatment only will be appropriate. Wherever possible this should involve some degree of acceptance of the symptoms by the patient and his relatives, together with an occupational and social programme, if the patient is sufficiently well to be able to co-operate in this, rather than undue reliance on sedation.

The severely restless or confused patient will require medication as a matter of urgency, e.g. chlorpromazine, 50 to 100 mg intramuscularly, or diazepam, 5 to 10 mg intramuscularly, repeated after one hour if necessary. Less severe cases may be given lorazepam, 1 mg orally, up to three times daily.

2. Hysteria

Faced with some unexpected or overwhelming catastrophe or blow to self-esteem an elderly person, with an ever-decreasing hold on his environment, may fairly readily exhibit an hysterical state of panic or acute distress. The attention-seeking nature of the symptoms will often be fairly clear to others although the patient's distress may have communicated itself to relatives and friends, who may become almost as disturbed as the patient. The arrival of the doctor or some other unemotionally involved authoritarian figure, carrying implications of help, will often cause a dramatic drop in the level of tension created and the insults which may have been the precipitating factors will often emerge fairly soon in the course of the interview.

Management. The hysterical patient will usually be greatly helped by being able to ventilate his anxieties or causes of concern to an interested and sympathetic listener. Discussion of the patient's current life situation and encouraging him to think how his difficulties might be met in a practical way could be useful, although often such considerations will be more appropriate at a subsequent interview. Of more immediate therapeutic value will be the patient's need for interest, understanding and reassurance as to his ability to surmount the present difficulties and continuing support if necessary. It will often be useful to prescribe a single dose of a sedative such as diazepam, 5 mg.

3. Depression

The severely agitated and depressed patient's behaviour will not alter significantly coincidental with the doctor's arrival. The psychotic features — for example, overwhelming feelings of guilt or impending disaster — will preoccupy the patient's attention and will be little influenced by external events. Symptoms of a depressive illness often with depressive delusions and suicidal ideas will usually be obvious. (*See below* for action to be taken.)

4. Schizophrenia

Agitation in the setting of a late paraphrenic illness is likely to be associated with the patient's paranoid delusions and threatening auditory hallucinations. The bizarre quality of the patient's symptoms, the inability of the observer to understand such in terms of a primary disturbance of mood and the absence of clouded consciousness will suggest the diagnosis. (*See below* for management.)

5. Mania

The patient's excitement, over-talkativeness, over-activity and disinhibited behaviour will all be comprehensible as stemming from a mood of extreme optimism.

Management for depression, schizophrenia and mania. The call for medical intervention in the agitated depressive, depressed, excited schizophrenic or manic patient will usually be an indication that community support has temporarily broken down and admission to a psychiatric unit or hospital should be sought. This will be particularly necessary if there is a danger of suicide. Whilst transfer to hospital is being arranged the patient should be kept under continuous observation. Further restlessness, excitement or panic should be treated with chlorpromazine, 50 to 100 mg intramuscularly, repeated after one hour if necessary. Where admission is not considered necessary arrangements should be made for early referral to a psychiatric clinic.

The parasuicidal patient (self-poisoning or self-injury)

Whilst the highest rate of parasuicides is in those below the age of 30, such incidents also occur in the older age groups amongst whom are the highest rates of successful suicide.

If the patient has been recently in psychiatric care for a psychotic or depressive illness, admission to a psychiatric unit or hospital will be appropriate and may be arranged immediately the patient is no longer in physical danger.

If the suicidal attempt itself serves to reunite the patient with friends he felt he had lost, or to elicit meaningful apologies or other expressions of concern, the crisis will usually have been resolved and further parasuicidal attempts are unlikely, at any rate in the immediate future.

In other patients there may be doubt as to what is the appropriate disposal and, for such cases, admission to a short-stay observation ward of a psychiatric unit will be useful if it is available. If not, adequate sedation and the provision of a bed overnight in a general hospital may tide the patient over until psychiatric and social referral can be made the following day.

It has been official Department of Health policy for some years that *all* self-injury and self-poisoning cases should be seen for psychiatric assessment (Central and Scottish Health Services Councils, 1968). However, a recent prospective study of such patients failed to show a significant difference over the following years, as measured by repetition of the act or successful suicide, between those assessed initially by junior non-psychiatric medical staff and those assessed by psychiatrists (Gardner *et al.*, 1977). These results were obtained by junior staff who were specifically instructed in the principles of psychiatric assessment and who were clearly in sympathy with such a task, but when such training and interest are lacking it would seem wisest for such patients to be referred for psychiatric opinion. At the present time the very large number of such patients and the psychiatric manpower situation in many parts of the country are such as to make full psychiatric evaluation in all cases very difficult. Nevertheless all such patients ought to be taken seriously.

The demented patient
Patients with acknowledged dementia may present as an emergency because of some additional illness or injury, e.g. bronchopneumonia or a fractured femur. Whilst treatment obviously must be directed primarily at this additional disability, it is important to involve social workers at an early stage. A discreet assessment of the patient's ability to live independently requires to be made and, by making and maintaining contact with relatives and friends, encouragement given for them to resume their supportive role once the patient is ready for discharge. The social worker may be able to suggest ways in which additional support may be given.

Assessment
The more time and care that can be given in the initial stages of these emergencies, the less the likelihood of making an inappropriate disposal. Careful evaluation is required in assessing the patient's motivation. This may be difficult and should involve discussion with relatives and other close associates. Assessment can be complicated by the patient's realisation of the possible consequences of his act. Some patients will seek to pass off the incident as an accident, but such an excuse should be tempered by one's awareness that healthy people pay particular concern that they do not overdose or injure themselves. A patient's awareness that his action may result in considerable embarrassment may cause him to deny symptoms of psychiatric illness as well as his intentions of taking his life. Another difficulty in evaluation is that a suicidal attempt can have a cathartic effect leading to genuine, but often only temporary, feelings of betterment.

Severely depressed patients may dissimulate symptoms in order to secure their release from medical care, thus allowing them to make a further and possibly more successful attempt. The majority of those who injure or poison themselves, however, are not motivated by the firm resolution to end their own life. Some will injure themselves as a means of escape from unendurable tension, some to get their own back on others by giving them cause to feel guilty because of the patient's life-threatening behaviour.

In most patients, however, the incident is an impulsive act, often based on very transient feelings after an argument with someone to whom they are closely attached, frequently effected under the disinhibiting influence of alcohol, and it should be regarded as a "cry for help".

Management. If it is considered that there was a genuine bid for self-extinction, then a search for and removal of any potentially injurious instrument or drugs should be undertaken and thereafter arrangements made for continuing close observation in the immediate future, with every practical safeguard to ensure that the patient does not make further attempts at self-injury, even perhaps in some different way. It will be advantageous to have such a patient in bed and to have him adequately sedated, e.g. with chlor-promazine, 100 mg intramuscularly, repeated after one hour if necessary. Additional medication should be given very cautiously, however, if the problem is that of self-poisoning, and the synergistic effect of most psychotropic drugs with alcohol should also be taken into account. Where there is a clear risk of suicide there will be no problem in admitting the patient to hospital, if necessary on a compulsory basis.

If the patient's physical state is a cause of concern, e.g. because of the degree of drug intoxication or because of underlying physical illness, the patient should be admitted to a general hospital ward because of the particular need in the early stages for the expertise of physician or surgeon and possibly also for resuscitative procedures. Once such essential first aid has been completed, transfer to psychiatric care may then be considered.

Some demented patients present acute problems because of a sudden intensification of their confusion and consequent deterioration in their behaviour. The cause (*see* p. 434) will emerge as a result of history-taking (from the relatives) and physical examination and most commonly will be attributable to the toxic effects of drugs, an intercurrent infection or cardiac decompensation. Investigation and treatment will usually require temporary admission to a medical or geriatric unit with social work involvement as previously.

Other demented patients will present as an emergency because of some temporary breakdown in their own individual support services, e.g. the ill-health or some other preoccupation of the spouse or caring relative may have allowed the patient to wander or lose their way and fall into the hands of the police; or the home help or night nurse may be unexpectedly absent without replacement, because of illness or holiday. These are essentially social crises and their solution is with the social services.

The admission to long-term psychogeriatric care of patients presenting as an emergency with dementia should be discouraged. The national shortage of beds for this age group necessitates a judicious admission policy. The increasing tendency to appoint consultants with a special interest in the care of the elderly mentally ill (psychogeriatricians) and the policy of assessment of all cases prior to admission have been useful developments in recent years, attempting to ensure that within any community the most deserving cases gain admission as beds become available.

The alcoholic patient

An attraction to alcohol may lead to an emergency situation either because of acute intoxication or, in the alcohol-dependent, because of the development of withdrawal symptoms (delirium tremens). Alcoholism and alcoholic psychosis accounted for 9 per cent of all male admissions aged 65 and over to mental hospitals and psychiatric units in Scotland in 1979. Elderly patients, and particularly those with some degree of brain damage, may become intoxicated after drinking relatively small amounts and their aggressive behaviour which constitutes the emergency may be directed towards themselves or others. Often their behaviour will excite the attention of others who will attempt to restrain the patient, but often this simply makes the patient more aggressive. It is usually more constructive to encourage the intoxicated patient to sleep, or talk in an uncritical atmosphere (away from other people). Gastric lavage will often be helpful and admission to a detoxication unit for twenty-four to forty-eight hours will be more positively therapeutic than to a prison cell.

Delirium tremens

This withdrawal syndrome occurs when alcohol-dependent individuals are suddenly deprived of their usual intake, e.g. on admission to hospital or prison. Management is best carried out in hospital, where the immediate treatment is that of an acute confusional state (*see* p. 453) together with a multi-vitamin preparation, such as Parentrovite, 7 ml intramuscularly for seven days. Further treatment should be by referral to a psychiatric out-patient department or preferably to a specialised service for alcoholics where group therapy aimed at altering basic behaviour and attitudes to drink may be available.

LEGAL ASPECTS
(*see also* Chapter Six by H.R. Rollin)

Admission to hospital

One of the principles embodied in the Mental Health Act 1959, and the Mental Health (Scotland) Act 1960, is that the administrative and legal distinctions between mental disorder and other forms of illness should be abolished as much as is possible, and since their introduction the number of compulsorily detained patients has fallen dramatically. Nowadays, the majority of patients requiring psychiatric care as an in-patient are admitted without any legal formality whatsoever, in just the same way as are patients requiring general hospital care for physical illness, and these are referred to as "informal" patients.

Compulsory powers of admission will continue to be necessary if proper care is to be provided for some patients (e.g. those whose mental illness makes them unable to appreciate their need for care, or makes them positively unwilling to receive it), especially when their illness makes them a danger to themselves or others. Wherever possible, however, suitable care is to be provided for mentally disordered patients on an "informal" basis, i.e. with no more restriction of liberty or legal formality than for other types of patient. Compulsory detention is applicable to those who suffer from mental disorder which is of a nature or degree which warrants detention and where the interests of the patient's health or safety or the protection of other people cannot be secured except by detention, provided that, if the patient is over 21, the grounds are not on the basis of subnormality or psychopathic disorder. In Scotland, the term "psychopathic disorder" is not used, but the Scottish Act refers to some individuals whose mental disorder is a persistent one "manifested only by abnormally aggressive or seriously irresponsible conduct", and such individuals cannot normally be admitted for detention after the age of 21.

Informal admission
The "informal" admission of patients suffering from mental disorder is authorised by section 5 of the English Act and section 23 of the Scottish Act. Informal admissions include not only those patients who have expressed a wish to enter hospital but also those whose mental state makes them unable to consider the situation and give full and valid consent (e.g. patients with dementia), provided their relatives are not in disagreement and provided such care is considered appropriate medically.

An informal patient must normally be allowed to discharge himself from hospital at any time if he insists on doing so. An exception is made when the condition of the patient who proposes to leave is clearly such that he requires to be in hospital for the protection of himself or others, and in these circumstances the detention of the patient may be effected by providing an emergency application or emergency recommendation (*see below*). However, the principle is, that certification in this way will be carried out only exceptionally and in cases of real emergency.

Compulsory admissions — England and Wales

Emergency application. In cases of urgent necessity, an application for admission for observation may be made in terms of section 29. The application is made by any relative of the patient, or by a social service officer (known as the mental welfare officer or warrant-holder) and must include a statement to the effect that it is necessary for the patient to be admitted and detained as a matter of urgency. This procedure is to avoid unnecessary delay in getting the patient to hospital. Only one supporting medical recommendation is required and this must verify the urgency of the situation and state that compliance with the ordinary procedure for compulsory admission for observation (section 25) would involve undesirable delay. Once completed, such a certificate is the authority for the applicant, or anyone authorised by him, to remove the patient to hospital within the next three days beginning with the date of the examination by the doctor giving the recommendation or the date of the application, whichever is the earlier. The patient may be detained for no more than seventy-two hours, but if a second medical recommendation is provided within that time detention is authorised for a period of up to twenty-eight days.

Admission for observation. An application under section 25 of the Mental Health Act for admission of a patient for observation must be on the prescribed form by a relative or the social services warrant-holder and it requires the written recommendation of two medical practitioners each of whom agrees that the nature and degree of the mental disorder from which the patient suffers warrants detention in hospital and that such detention is necessary for the protection of others or the interests of the patient's health or safety. Admitted in this way, a patient may be detained for not more than twenty-eight days commencing on the day of admission. The term "admission for observation" is perhaps misleading since this will usually and quite legitimately include treatment.

Admission for treatment. An application for admission for treatment is made in terms of section 26. This also requires two written medical recommendations on the prescribed form each of which must state that the nature and degree of the mental disorder from which the patient suffers warrants detention in hospital and that such detention is necessary for the protection of others or the interests of the patient's health or safety. In addition, the reasons for these opinions must be given in language understandable to an intelligent layman and an indication must be given as to whether other methods of dealing with the patient are available, and if so, why they are not appropriate.

Once completed, an application for admission for observation or admission for treatment is the authority for the patient to be taken to the hospital within fourteen days of the date of the last medical examination and recommendation. Compulsorily detained patients may appeal against this detention to a Mental Health Review Tribunal within six months of the day of admission.

Medical Recommendations. Section 28 indicates the necessary requirements of the two medical recommendations. One must be given by a doctor recognised by the local health authority as having special experience in the diagnosis or treatment of mental disorder and, preferably, the other recommendation will be given by a doctor who has previous acquaintance with the patient. The two examinations of the patient must not be more than seven days apart and must be signed before the application. The applicant, his partner or assistant, may not make a medical recommendation. The two practitioners giving the recommendation must not be in partnership, must not have a financial interest in the maintenance of the patient, and must not be on the staff of a private hospital if this is where the patient is to be accommodated. The medical recommendations must also not be given by relatives of the patient or relatives of the other recommending doctor.

Remands for medical report. Courts in England and Wales requiring a medical report on a defendant may obtain this on an out-patient basis or, if this is inappropriate, by granting bail with a condition of hospital residence, or by remanding to prison.

Compulsory admissions: Scotland
Of patients admitted to mental hospitals and psychiatric units in Scotland for the treatment of mental disorder 90 per cent are admitted on an informal basis (Scottish Health Service, 1979). The majority of compulsory admissions are by an emergency recommendation in the first instance and only about 10 per cent of such patients proceed to full compulsory detention.

Emergency recommendations. An emergency recommendation may be completed in terms of section 31 of the Mental Health (Scotland) Act 1960, in cases of urgent necessity by any general practitioner. The consent of any relative or mental health officer must be obtained or, alternatively, reasons for failure to obtain such consent must be stated. The doctor must have personally examined the patient on the day on which he signs the recommendation and must state that by reason of mental disorder it is urgently necessary for the patient to be admitted in pursuance of an application under section 24. Once completed, such a statement authorises the removal of the patient within three days and his detention in hospital for a period not exceeding seven days. No prescribed form is necessary and any written or typed recommendation will be valid provided it complies with these requirements.

Compulsory admission. In addition to an application for admission made by the *nearest* relative or a mental health officer and two medical recommendations similar in content to those required by the English Act, in Scotland the Sheriff's approval is also required. The person making the application must have seen the patient within fourteen days of the date when the application is submitted to the Sheriff, and the application must be submitted for approval within seven days of the last date of the second medical recommendation. In considering the application and medical recommendations the Sheriff can make further enquiries from the patient and others, if necessary. The application, once approved, is the authority for the removal of the patient to the hospital named at any time within seven days of that date. The Mental Welfare Commission, which exercises general protective functions over the mentally disordered, is automatically informed of all compulsory admissions. The two medical recommendations must state the form of mental disorder, whether mental illness or mental deficiency or both, which necessitates the patient's detention, and the two certificates require to be in agreement about this for the application to be legally valid. The application and medical recommendations must be made on the prescribed forms which are available from the Records Office of any mental hospital.

Absence from hospital of compulsorily detained patients
Both the English and Scottish Mental Health Acts permit patients liable to be detained in hospital to be granted leave of absence as their mental condition improves. Should the mental state of such patients deteriorate whilst they are away from hospital the Responsible Medical Officer, on the authority of the current compulsory detention documents, may recall the patient to hospital if he feels this is appropriate in the interests of the patient's health or safety, or for the protection of other people.

Compulsory admission of mentally abnormal offenders
In Scotland, the Criminal Procedure (Scotland) Act 1975 enables a court to remand in hospital any person who is charged with an offence who also appears to be suffering from mental disorder: 6 per cent of men admitted in this way are over the age of 60. The purpose is for psychiatric examination and report by the Responsible Medical Officer and the essential concern is whether or not the accused is suffering from mental disorder which warrants admission and detention in terms of the Mental Health (Scotland) Act (section 24). Before an accused person can be committed in this way a doctor's recommendation is required and this is usually provided by the police surgeon.

The English Mental Health Act contains no identical provision, although the Butler Report on Mentally Abnormal Offenders recommended that legislation should be enacted to make remand to hospital for medical report or care possible (Butler, 1975).

Safeguarding of property and affairs

If, as a result of mental disorder, a person is unable to manage his affairs it is important that a disinterested party be appointed to safeguard his interests. This will usually be the situation with patients suffering from a dementing illness. The procedure is the same whether the patient is of informal or compulsorily detained status and whether the patient is in or out of hospital.

England and Wales: appointment of receiver

Application may be made by a hospital, the local authority, the doctor or anyone who becomes aware of the patient's incapability, and is made to the Court of Protection, 25 Store Street, London. Medical evidence is required to the effect that the person is "incapable by reason of mental disorder of managing or administering his property and affairs". The judge may appoint a Receiver to discharge the necessary responsibilities which involve administering the affairs and making provision for the patient, his family and others, in a manner that the patient might have been expected to do himself if he had not been mentally disordered. The Receiver will be discharged if satisfactory evidence is produced that the person has recovered his capabilities, or when the patient dies.

Scotland: appointment of curator bonis

In Scotland, a *curator bonis* will be appointed in similar circumstances. A petition by the patient's relative or other interested body is required supported by two medical certificates to the effect that the person is incapable by reason of mental disorder of managing or administering his property and affairs. The petition will be served upon the patient unless an opinion is added to the medical certificates that it is considered that doing so would adversely affect the patient's health. The curator acts under the supervision of the court accountant, makes an inventory of the estate and renders annual accounts.

Testamentary capacity

Relatives understandably concern themselves with the way in which an elderly person's estate may come to be divided. If no Will exists when the patient shows signs of mental illness, the relatives often act hastily in efforts to ensure that a Will is drawn up, sometimes also trying to exert influence in their own favour. If a person is known to have a mental disorder this will normally raise doubts as to the validity of any Will he makes, but the law allows a mentally-disordered patient to make a Will if his mind is clear in this respect at the time. Testamentary capacity is assessed quite independently of whether the patient is in or out of hospital, or whether the patient is compulsorily detained or not, and is best assessed by referral to a psychiatrist.

The patient should always be examined alone; relatives, friends, business associates and the lawyer should be questioned to ascertain the extent of the patient's property and to check the veracity of his statements; detailed verbatim notes should be made and preserved. The examiner's questions should be directed to ascertaining the following points.

(a) Does the patient understand the nature of making a Will and its effects?

(b) Has he a reasonable knowledge of the extent of his property?

(c) Does he know and appreciate the claims to which he ought to give effect?

(d) Is there any evidence of mental disorder which poisons his affections, perverts his sense of right, or clouds his judgment in any way?

If delusions or evidence of dementia, delirium or defectiveness are present, the patient's ability to make a valid Will should be regarded with great mistrust and every presumption made against it in the first instance.

Divorce

The Divorce Acts of England and Wales and Scotland are now similar in that the only grounds for divorce are that the marriage has broken down irretrievably. This can be established when there has been no cohabitation for two years and the defender consents to the granting of the decree of divorce. It may also be established where there has been no cohabitation for five years without such consent. A medical opinion as to whether the defender is capable of deciding whether or not to give consent to the granting of divorce will be required in the former and in Scotland will be sought by the Court through the Mental Welfare Commission. Special arrangements are made regarding financial provisions where the defender is undergoing treatment for mental disorder in hospital.

CARE OF THE DYING

The elderly mentally ill, especially those with functional illness, share common needs with those of good mental health from their medical attendants and show a variety of ways of coping with terminal physical illness, such as cancer. Patients with emotional discomfort, as with pain, require a sense of security by knowing that relief can be obtained whenever necessary, if not by the doctor's presence, at least through the agency of medication that he has prescribed. At all times those giving practical help should remind themselves of the need to show compassion and a feeling that they are trying to understand the patient and his predicament. This is perhaps particularly so in long-stay hospitals for the elderly, where terminal care is commonplace and where an attitude of seeming indifference may develop.

The dying patient's level of anxiety will be raised unnecessarily if emotional discomfort or pain is not appropriately relieved. Many will prefer to be nursed, particularly in the early stages, by their relatives. Visiting nurses and other professionals should be encouraged to overcome any natural hesitation in acquainting relatives with elementary procedures which they themselves cannot continuously provide, but which may be valuable to the patient. The doctor may need to give the relatives emotional support, particularly if they have had no previous firsthand experience of a similar situation. Like every human, the dying patient needs to feel wanted and loved, and the visiting of congenial friends and relatives should rarely be discouraged. If long-standing family disputes are resolved as members come to the patient's bedside, not only may this be a comfort to the patient, but it is also likely to minimise the intensity of subsequent bereavement reactions in those who have felt an obligation to visit.

Many with terminal illness will seek to deny its existence and in this way will be able to continue with a happier and more meaningful life longer than would otherwise be possible. However, it is important to satisfy oneself by gentle probing that the patient is coping with his situation by denial and not, as may happen, by suppressing conscious fears and anxieties about his illness and his future, which may have been built on what he has already been told or overheard, but not fully understood. Most patients will have problems, e.g. finances, visitors, pain, which they will discuss with benefit when they feel they have an interested listener. The impression that patients and relatives may have — that doctors do not want to know about the incurably ill — is, unfortunately, often correct and associated with a lack of education of the medical profession in counselling the critically ill, which in turn is part of society's general avoidance of this uncomfortable area. Once the patient has been diagnosed as critically ill, it is important for the doctor to maintain contact with the patient by visiting him regularly, talking on everyday matters, listening to his symptoms and generally creating an atmosphere in which he feels he can open up if he wishes.

The right of patients not to have the true facts thrust unwillingly upon them should be upheld. Only if he indicates his desire and is emotionally ready to hear about his illness, and perhaps prognosis, should he be sympathetically informed in a manner tinged with hope and with reassurance as to the doctor's continuing attendance and help. In this way the patient will work through the stages of anger and depression which often result from knowledge of the nature of his illness and will come to a relatively contented acceptance of the true state of affairs. Without such discussion the patient may remain bitter, possibly increasing his distress by blaming further symptoms on the treatment prescribed and, as a consequence, resisting further medical attention.

Should a patient die suddenly and unexpectedly, consideration should be given to the relatives who are likely to be particularly distressed because of the necessary medico-legal investigations and coroner's inquest. Such relatives can be greatly helped if the general practitioner can support the coroner's pathologist by explaining the cause of death in simple terms and by answering any other relevant questions as they arise. The emotional shock of unexpected death often prevents even the most intelligent relatives from absorbing the details at first hearing: without such follow-up and explanation, misunderstanding, unnecessary bitterness and secondary distress can so easily arise.

PROPHYLAXIS

Some degree of prevention of mental illness in the elderly can be attained by consideration of the various contributory factors.

Psychological factors
Whilst age is unescapable and the normal decline of intellectual processes is probably primarily dependent upon genetic factors, clinical observation, which is supported by some animal experiments, suggests that ageing may be accelerated by stress. Thus unnecessary psychological stress should be avoided. Whilst certain situations are inevitably stressful, e.g. death of a loved one or unexpected financial difficulties, it must be emphasised that less obvious situations may be stressful for an individual, depending

upon his own personal vulnerability, which only knowledge of that individual patient will reveal. Where emotional stress is present some environmental readjustments should be considered as a possible way of helping to alleviate this.

Social factors

Courses in preparation for retirement are now a common feature of Local Authority Further Education classes and pre-retirement involvement should be encouraged. Particular encouragement requires to be given to those most in need of these, e.g. those personalities with few interests or social contacts.

The natural tendency for the elderly person to become isolated should be given no encouragement. The unnecessary breaking of emotional and social ties, e.g. by moving house, should be discouraged and at the same time the maintenance or further development of friendships through social clubs, the church etc., should be fostered. The visiting of the elderly by relatives, friends and voluntary organisations is important to combat the development of a sense of rejection and isolation, and social agencies (home helps, meals on wheels, domiciliary chiropody, etc.) can give valuable assistance here, too. Sheltered houses will often be invaluable, particularly if they strive to give support, to safeguard the privacy and independence of the individual and sense of personal identity, and to arrange some sort of social life, e.g. by providing a common room and facilities for reading and social evenings. Future building programmes should ensure that local authority housing and social work departments, the hospital service and voluntary agencies co-operate in planning to meet such needs.

Physical factors

The patient's physical health should be kept at the optimum, with expert attention to any disabilities that arise, to ensure that maximum function is retained. Much anxiety and despondency can be prevented by giving patients who are physically ill an adequate explanation regarding their illness, its origin, any necessary investigations and the aims of treatment.

It is important to ensure that as the diet is reduced quantitively sub- or malnourishment does not result. The question of vulnerability to nutritional deficiency should be considered by appraisal of the physical health, mobility and dietary interests, and with an awareness that the housebound are particularly at risk (Exton-Smith et al., 1972). If an adequate diet is not to be achieved by the patient's own endeavours, then the help of relatives, neighbours, friends, home helps, meals on wheels should be enlisted, and the diet supplemented if necessary by additional vitamins.

It is especially important for the elderly that no drug should be prescribed without good reason, and as few drugs as possible should be given at any one time. Hypnotics are best avoided unless the patient persistently complains of insomnia or there is evidence of recent deterioration in sleeping habit, along with other symptoms indicative of a depressive illness. Possible explanations should be sought — the patient's routine may be at fault, e.g. long afternoon naps or stimulating drinks in the evening; physical symptoms may be responsible, e.g. breathlessness; or other medication may be causing confusion and associated sleeplessness, e.g. tricyclic anti-depressants or digoxin. Some explanation as to what are considered the normal sleeping habits of people in this age group may be of guidance to those with whom the aged person has recently come to stay. All effective hypnotics run the risk of causing dependency, so that it is preferable to give advice rather than medication. When all else fails, suitable hypnotics for the elderly are chlor-methiazole (Heminevrin) or dichloralphenazone (Welldorm), both of which are available in tablet and syrup form (*see* p. 444).

The occurrence of psychiatric emergencies should be minimised by the regular follow-up of certain patients. Severely neurotic patients often find it impossible to cope without continuing regular supportive out-patient psychotherapy. Schizophrenic patients on regular medication, including depot drugs, require to be followed up and encouraged to continue with their medication. Manic depressive patients on prophylactic lithium require regular super-vision and monitoring of serum lithium levels. The mentally frail within any community should be known to medical and social agencies through "At Risk" registers and thereby provided with regular supervision and maximum appropriate support.

Finally, the attitude of the doctor and all health and social service personnel to the elderly patient with chronic disabilities is of major importance. All should see their role as the management of such patients in a sympathetic and positive manner so as to ensure minimum disability and maximum contentment with life.

REFERENCES

Angst, J., Grof, P. and Schou, M. (1969): "Lithium", *Lancet,* i, 1097.

British Medical Journal, (1977): "Adverse effects of lithium treatment", *Brit. Med. J.,* ii, 346.

Central and Scottish Health Services Councils (1968): *Hospital Treatment of Acute Poisoning,* H.M.S.O., London.

Charatan, F. B. and Brierly, J. B. (1956): "Mental disorder associated with primary lung carcinoma", *Brit. Med. J.,* i, 765-8.

Clinical Psychiatry Committee of Medical Research Council (1965): "Clinical trial of the treatment of depressive illness", *Brit. Med. J.,* i, 881-6.

Cooper, A. F., Curry, A. R., Kay, D. W. K., Garside, R. F. and Roth, M. (1974): "Hearing loss in paranoid and affective psychoses of the elderly", *Lancet,* ii, 851.

Denmark, J. C. (1969): "Management of severe deafness in adults", *Proceedings of the Royal Society, 62, 965.*

Department of Health and Social Security (1972): *Nutrition of the Elderly,* H.M.S.O., London.

Department of Health and Social Security (1975): *Better Services for the Mentally Ill,* H.M.S.O., London.

Exton-Smith, A. N., Stanton, B. R. and Windsor, A. C. M. (1972): *Nutrition of Housebound Old People,* King Edward's Hospital Fund, London.

Gardner, R., Hanka, R., O'Brien, V.C., Page, A.J.F. and Rees, R. (1977): "Psychological and social evaluation in cases of deliberate self-poisoning admitted to a general hospital", *Brit. Med. J.,* ii, 1567-70.

Glassman, A.H. and Bigger, J.T. (1981): "Cardiovascular Effects of Therapeutic Doses of Tricyclic Antidepressants", *Archives of General Psychiatry, 37, 815-20.*

Goktepe, E. O., Young, L. B. and Bridges, P. K. (1975): "A further review of the results of stereotactic subcaudate tractotomy", *Brit. J. Psychiat., 126, 270-80.*

Kay, D. W. K., Beamish, P. and Roth, M. (1964): "Old age mental disorder in Newcastle Upon Tyne. Part I: A study in prevalence", *Brit. J. Psychiat., 110, 146-58.*

Kidd, C. B. (1962): "Misplacement of the elderly in hospitals", *Brit. Med. J.,* ii, 1941-5.

Learoyd, B. M. (1972): "Psychotropic drugs and the elderly patient", *Med. J. Aust., 1, 1131-3.*

Ley, P. (1977): "Patient compliance – a psychologist's viewpoint", *Prescribers Journal,* 17, No. 1, Elephant & Castle, London.

MacDonald, E. T., MacDonald, J. B. and Phoenix, M. (1977): "Improving drug compliance after hospital discharge", *Brit. Med. J.,* ii, 618-21.

McGovern, G. P., Miller, D. H. and Robertson, E. R. (1959): "A mental syndrome associated with lung carcinomas", *Arch. Neurol. Psychiat., 81, 341-7.*

Morris, J. B. and Beck, A. T. (1974): "The efficacy of antidepressant drugs", *Archives of General Psychiatry, 30, 667-74.*

Office of Population Census and Surveys (1977): *Population Projections 1976-2016,* H.M.S.O., London.

Parkes, C. M. (1964): "Recent bereavement as a cause of mental Illness", *Brit. J. Psychiat.*, **110**, 198-204.

Post, F. (1962): *The Significance of Affective Symptoms in Old Age*, Oxford University Press, London.

Post, F. (1965): *The Clinical Psychiatry of Later Life*, Pergamon Press, Oxford.

Robinson, R. A. (1975): *Modern Perspectives in the Psychiatry of Old Age*, Churchill Livingstone, Edinburgh and London.

Rollin, H. R. (1963): "Social and legal repercussions of the Mental Health Act 1959", *Brit. Med. J.*, i, 786-8.

Royal College of Psychiatrists, The (1977): "The Royal College of Psychiatrists' Memorandum on the use of electroconvulsive therapy", *Brit. J. Psychiat.*, **131**, 261-72.

Scottish Health Service (1979): *Scottish Mental Hospital In-Patient Statistics*, Scottish Health Service Information Services Division (Common Services Agency).

Scottish Health Services Council (1970): *Services for the Elderly with Mental Disorder*, H.M.S.O., Edinburgh.

Skegg, D. C. G., Doll, R. and Perry, J. (1977): "Use of medicines in general practice", *Brit. Med. J.*, i, 1561.

Stengel, E. (1965): *Psychiatric Disorders in the Aged*, Geigy (Manchester) for World Psychiatric Association.

Strachan, R. W. and Henderson, J. G. (1967): "Dementia and folate deficiency", *Quart. J. Med.*, **36**, 189-203.

FURTHER READING

Anderson, W. Ferguson and Judge, T. G. (Eds.), *Geriatric Medicine*, Academic Press, London and New York, 1974.

Howells, John G. (Ed.), *Modern Perspectives in the Psychiatry of Old Age*, Churchill Livingstone, Edinburgh and London, 1975.

Appendixes

Male/Female Sexual History Schedule*

(*See* Chapter Four)

Name:

Age:

Sex:

Occupation:

Marital status:

Religion and degree of devotion:

Puberty:

Age at puberty:

Signs of puberty:

Age of first ejaculation:

Age of growth of pubic hair:

Age of growth of facial hair:

Age of voice change:

Age of menarche:

Subsequent menstrual history:

Attitude about menstruation:

*Delete inappropriate items

Masturbation:

Age commenced:

Frequencies:

Maximum ever per week:

Mean frequency per week at time of referral:

Stimulative techniques employed:

Masturbation pattern throughout years:

Type of accompanying fantasy:

Homosexual:

Heterosexual:

Content of fantasy:

Subject's evaluation of effects on masturbation on:

Physical health:

Mental health:

Other:

Nocturnal sex dreams:

Frequency of dream with ⎫

⎬ orgasm:

Frequency of dream without ⎭

Content of dreams:

Pattern of spontaneous morning erections/vaginal lubrication:

Sex education:

Source of knowledge:

Formal sex education:

Age obtained:

Own view as to whether sexually knowledgeable or ignorant:

Interviewer's rating assessed on:

Knowledge of female/male sex anatomy:

Knowledge of female/male sex physiology:

Knowledge of female/male psychology:

Knowledge relating to coital techniques etc.:

Heterosexual history:

Age of first experience:

Type of experience:

Subject's evaluation:

Subsequent heterosexual outlets:

Ages involved:

Number of companions:

Kissing:

Fondling:

Mutual masturbation:

Coitus:

Other experiences:

Subject's evaluation as to whether sexually experienced or inexperienced:

Rater's assessment as to whether sexually experienced or inexperienced:

Attitude to premarital coitus:

Source of restraint:
Moral:
Lack of opportunity:
Lack of interest:
Fear of pregnancy:
Fear of V.D.:
Fear of social disapproval:
Desire for virginity in spouse:
Others:

Premarital coitus:
Age of first experience:
Age of partner:
Circumstances of coitus:
Successful or not:

Subsequent premarital coitus:
Assessed total number of partners:
Assessed total number of intercourses:
Emotionally/physically satisfying: (or not)

Sexual variation, i.e. homosexuality, autoeroticism, etc.:
Type:
Age of first experience:
Duration of disorder:
Facultative or permanent:

Attitude towards females/males:
Own attitude about orientation:

Marital intercourse:
Age at marriage:
Virginity or otherwise of spouse:
Lapse between time of marriage and consummation:
Satisfactory or otherwise:
Additional information:

Subsequent marital coitus:
Maximum performance ever:
Mean frequency of coitus in first year of marriage:
Degree of physical and/or emotional satisfaction:
Resumé of sexual activity till present:

Precoital sex play:
Type of stimulation practised:
Fantasies, etc.:
Duration:

Sexual inhibition:
Present or absent:
Type of sexual practice desired:
Subject's reason for his restraint:

Contraceptive history:
Type used:

Effect on performance:

Religious or moral view:

History relating to sexual disorder:

Time and circumstances of intial failure:

Type of disorder:

Time of onset:

Early (i.e. primary):

Late (i.e. secondary):

Type of onset:

Insidious:

Acute:

Presence of precipitating factors:

Psychological:

Physical:

Others:

Subsequent coital history:

Intermittent type of disorder:

Persistent type of disorder:

Presence or absence of sexual desire in coital situation:

Strongly desirous:

Moderately desirous:

Mildly desirous:

No desire:

Other feelings:

Emotional feelings towards sexual partner:

Loves partner:

Does not love partner:

Presence or absence of anxiety, anger/disgust etc. in coital situation:

Marital happiness:

Positively happy: Satisfactory: Unsatisfactory: Positively unhappy:

Reason for marital unhappiness:

Subject's explanation of sexual failure:

Subject's feelings about failure:

Partner's attitude:

Explicit:

Implicit:

Is partner contributing to disorder?

Alternative sexual outlet:

Masturbation:

Others:

Extra-marital relations:

If yes — frequency and type of experience:

Subject's reasons for conduct:

Previous treatment:

Type and duration:

Effects:

Subject's opinion:

Reasons for referral:

Route of referral i.e. G.P./self referral/etc.:

Relevant psychiatric history:

Past history and personal development:

Family and social history:

Physical examination:

Laboratory tests if indicated:

Rules for Compulsory Admission to Hospital

(reproduced from the Mental Health Act 1959
of England and Wales)

PROCEDURE FOR HOSPITAL ADMISSION

Section 25: Admission for observation
(1) A patient may be admitted to a hospital, and there detained for the period allowed by this section, in pursuance of an application (in this Act referred to as an application for admission for observation) made in accordance with the following provisions of this section.
(2) An application for admission for observation may be made in respect of a patient on the grounds —

(a) that he is suffering from mental disorder of a nature or degree which warrants the detention of the patient in a hospital under observation (with or without other medical treatment) for at least a limited period; and
(b) that he ought to be so detained in the interest of his own health or safety or with a view to the protection of other persons.

(3) An application for admission for observation shall be founded on the written recommendations in the prescribed form of two medical practitioners, including in each case a statement that in the opinion of the practitioner the conditions set out in paragraphs (a) and (b) of subsection (2) of this section are complied with.
(4) Subject to the provisions of section fifty-two of this Act (in a case where an application is made under that section for transferring the functions of the nearest relative of the patient) a patient admitted to hospital in pursuance of an application for admission for observation may be detained for a period not exceeding twenty-eight days beginning with the day on which he is admitted, but shall not be detained thereafter unless, before the expiration of that period, he has become liable to be detained by virtue of a subsequent application, order or direction under any of the following provisions of this Act.

Section 26: Admission for treatment
(1) A patient may be admitted to a hospital and there detained for the period allowed by the following provisions of this Act, in pursuance of an application (in this Act referred to as an application for admission for treatment) made in accordance with the following provisions of this section.
(2) An application for admission for treatment may be made in respect of a patient on the grounds —

(a) that he is suffering from mental disorder, being —

(i) in the case of a patient of any age, mental illness or severe subnormality;
(ii) in the case of a patient under the age of twenty-one years, psychopathic disorder or subnormality; and that the said disorder is of a nature or

481

degree which warrants the detention of the patient in a hospital for medical treatment under this section; and

(b) that it is necessary in the interest of the patient's health and safety or for the protection of other persons that the patient should be so detained.

(3) An application for admission for treatment shall be founded on the written recommendations in the prescribed form of two medical practitioners, including in each case a statement that in the opinion of the practitioner the conditions set out in paragraphs (a) and (b) of subsection (2) of this section are complied with; and each such recommendation shall include —

(a) such particulars as may be prescribed of the grounds for that opinion so far as it relates to the conditions set out in the said paragraph (a); and

(b) a statement of the reasons for that opinion so far as it relates to the conditions set out in the said paragraph (b), specifying whether other methods of dealing with the patient are available, and if so why they are not appropriate.

(4) An application for admission for treatment, and any recommendation given for the purposes of such an application, may describe the patient as suffering from more than one of the forms of mental disorder referred to in subsection (2) of this section; but the application shall be of no effect unless the patient is described in each of the recommendations as suffering from the same one of those forms of mental disorder, whether or not he is also described in either of those recommendations as suffering from another of those forms.

(5) An application for admission for treatment made on the ground that the patient is suffering from psychopathic disorder or subnormality, and no other form of mental disorder referred to in subsection (2) of this section, shall state the age of the patient or, if his exact age is not known to the applicant, shall state (if it be the fact) that the patient is believed to be under the age of twenty-one years.

Section 29: Admission for observation in case of emergency

(1) In any case of urgent necessity, an application for admission for observation may be made in respect of a patient in accordance with the following provisions of this section, and any application so made is in this Act referred to as an emergency application.

(2) An emergency application may be made either by a mental welfare officer or by any relative of the patient; and every such application shall include a statement (to be verified by the medical recommendation first referred to in subsection (3) of this section) that it is of urgent necessity for the patient to be admitted and detained under section twenty-five of this Act, and that compliance with the foregoing provisions of this Part of this Act relating to applications for admission for observation would involve undesirable delay.

(3) An emergency application shall be sufficient in the first instance if founded on one of the medical recommendations required by section twenty-five of this Act, given, if practicable, by a practitioner who has previous acquaintance with the patient and otherwise complying with the requirements of section twenty-eight of this Act so far as applicable to a single recommendation, but shall cease to have effect on the expiration of a period of seventy-two hours from the time when the patient is admitted to the hospital unless —

(a) the second medical recommendation required as aforesaid is given and received by the managers within that period; and

(b) that recommendation and the recommendation first referred to in this subsection together comply with all the requirements of the said section twenty-eight (other than the requirement as to the time of signature of the second recommendation).

Form 3A
(Hospital Code 90-543)

MENTAL HEALTH ACT 1959

Medical Recommendation for Admission for Observation (Section 25 or 29)

(1) Name and address of medical practitioner

1. I (¹) .... of ....
.... being a registered medical

(2) Name and address of patient

practitioner, recommend that (²)...

of ....

be admitted to a hospital for observation in accordance with Part IV of the Mental Health Act 1959.

2. I last examined this patient on .... 19.......... .

*Delete if not applicable

3. *(a)   I was acquainted with the patient previously to conducting that examination.

(3) Name of local health authority

*(b)   I have been approved by (³) .... under Section 28
of the Act as having special experience in the diagnosis or treatment of mental disorder.

4. I am of the opinion

(a)   that this patient is suffering from mental disorder of a nature or degree which warrants

his
—— detention in a hospital under observation for at least a limited period,
her

AND

(b)   that this patient ought to be so detained:
(i) in the interests of the patient's own health or safety,

Delete (i) or (ii) unless both apply

(ii) with a view to the protection of other persons,

AND

(c)   that informal admission is not appropriate in the circumstances of this case.

5. (*This section is to be deleted unless the medical recommendation is the first recommendation in support of an emergency application under Section 29.*)

In my opinion it is of urgent necessity for the patient to be admitted and detained under Section 25 of the Act and compliance with the requirements of the Act relating to applications for admission for observation other than emergency applications would involve undesirable delay.

Signed...

Date ....

RECORD OF RECEIPT (*This is not part of the recommendation, and is to be completed only if the medical recommendation is the second recommendation in support of an emergency application under Section 29.*)

(4) Insert time and date

This recommendation was received on behalf of the managers at (⁴).....................................

on..19.......... the patient having been admitted at (⁴)...................

on..19..........

Signed   ....
on behalf of the managers

Date   ....

Form 2

MENTAL HEALTH ACT 1959   (Hospital Code 90-542)

Emergency Application for Admission for Observation
(Section 29)

(1) Name and address
of hospital or mental
nursing home

TO THE MANAGERS OF (¹)...

(2) Name and address
of applicant

1. I (²)...of...

....hereby apply for the admission of

(3) Name and address
of patient

(³).. of ....

....to the above-named hospital for
observation in accordance with Part IV of the Mental Health Act 1959.

(4) State relationship
(see section 49
overleaf)

2. (a) I am a relative of the patient within the meaning of the Act, being the patient's (⁴)........

Delete (a) or (b)

OR

(5) Name of local
health authority

(b) I am an officer of (⁵)...
appointed to act as a mental welfare officer for the purposes of the Act.

3. I last saw the patient on...19.........

4. In my opinion it is of urgent necessity for the patient to be admitted and detained under Section 25 of the Act, and compliance with the requirements of the Act relating to applications for admission other than emergency applications would involve undesirable delay.

5. This application is founded on the medical recommendation forwarded herewith.

(6) If the medical
practitioner who has
made the
recommendation had no
previous acquaintance
with the patient, the
applicant should state
here why it is not
practicable to obtain a
recommendation from
a practitioner having
such acquaintance.

6. (⁶)..

....

....

Signed...

Date ....

RECORD OF ADMISSION (This is not part of the application, but is to be completed later at the hospital or mental home.)

(7) Name of patient

(a) (⁷)...was admitted to

(8) Name of hospital
or mental nursing home

(⁸) ....in pursuance of

this application at (⁹)...................................on...................19.........

Delete (a) or (b)

OR

(b) (⁷).. was already an in-patient

in (⁸)..

on the date of this application and the application was received by me on behalf of the managers

(9) Time and date

at (⁹).......................................on...................19.........

Signed..
on behalf of the managers

Date..

MENTAL HEALTH ACT 1959

Definition of Relative

Section 49.—(1) In this Part of this Act " relative ", means any of the following, that is to say:—

(*a*) husband or wife;

(*b*) son or daughter;

(*c*) father;

(*d*) mother;

(*e*) brother or sister;

(*f*) grandparent;

(*g*) grandchild;

(*h*) uncle or aunt;

(*i*) nephew or niece.

(2) In deducing relationships for the purposes of this section, an adopted person shall be treated as the child of the person or persons by whom he was adopted and not as the child of any other person; and subject as aforesaid, any relationship of the half-blood shall be treated as a relationship of the whole blood, and an illegitimate person shall be treated as the legitimate child of his mother.

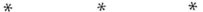

(5) In this section " adoption order " means an order for the adoption of any person made under Part I of the Adoption Act, 1958, or any previous enactment relating to the adoption of children or any corresponding enactment of the Parliament of Northern Ireland, and " court " includes a court in Scotland or Northern Ireland.

(6) In this section " husband " and " wife " include a person who is living with the patient as the patient's husband or wife, as the case may be (or, if the patient is for the time being an in-patient in a hospital, was so living until the patient was admitted), and has been or had been so living for a period of not less than six months; but a person shall not be treated by virtue of this subsection as the nearest relative of a married patient unless the husband or wife of the patient is disregarded by virtue of paragraph (*b*) of subsection (4) of this section.

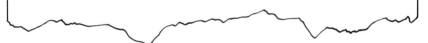

MENTAL HEALTH ACT, 1959

Joint Medical Recommendation for Admission for Treatment (Section 26)

(1) Names and addresses of both medical practitioners

1. We(1)..of ....

....and..

of.., being registered

(2) Name and address of patient

medical practitioners, recommend that (2)..

of...be admitted to a

hospital for treatment in accordance with Part IV of the Mental Health Act, 1959.

(3) Name of first practitioner

2. I (3)...last examined this patient on

....19.........

*Delete if not applicable

*I was acquainted with the patient previously to conducting that examination.

(4) Name of local health authority

*I have been approved by (4)...under

Section 28 of the Act as having special experience in the diagnosis or treatment of mental disorder.

(5) Name of second practitioner

3. I (5)...last examined this patient on

....19.........

*Delete if not applicable

*I was acquainted with the patient previously to conducting that examination.

*I have been approved by (4)...under

Section 28 of the Act as having special experience in the diagnosis or treatment of mental disorder.

(6) Names of both practitioners

4. We (6)..and..are of

(7) Insert mental illness, severe subnormality, subnormality, and/or psychopathic disorder (see definitions overleaf)

opinion that this patient is suffering from (7)..

....of a nature or degree which warrants $\frac{his}{her}$ detention in a

hospital for medical treatment within the meaning of the Act. This opinion is founded on the following grounds:—(8)

(8) Clinical description of the patient's mental condition

5. We are of the opinion that it is necessary—

    (i) in the interests of this patient's health or safety

Delete (i) or (ii) unless both apply

    (ii) for the protection of other persons

(9) Reasons should indicate whether other methods of care or treatment (e.g., out-patient treatment or local authority services) are available and if so why they are not appropriate, and why informal admission is not suitable.

that$\frac{he}{she}$should be detained in hospital, and our reasons for this opinion are:—(9)

Signed ....

Date ....

Signed ....

Date ....

MENTAL HEALTH ACT, 1959

Definition and Classification of Mental Disorder

Section 4.—(1) In this Act " mental disorder " means mental illness, arrested or incomplete development of mind, psychopathic disorder, and any other disorder or disability of mind; and " mentally disordered " shall be construed accordingly.

(2) In this Act " severe subnormality " means a state of arrested or incomplete development of mind which includes subnormality of intelligence and is of such a nature or degree that the patient is incapable of living an independent life or of guarding himself against serious exploitation, or will be so incapable when of an age to do so.

(3) In this Act " subnormality " means a state of arrested or incomplete development of mind (not amounting to severe subnormality) which includes subnormality of intelligence and is of a nature or degree which requires or is susceptible to medical treatment or other special care or training of the patient.

(4) In this Act " psychopathic disorder " means a persistent disorder or disability of mind (whether or not including subnormality of intelligence) which results in abnormally aggressive or seriously irresponsible conduct on the part of the patient, and requires or is susceptible to medical treatment.

(5) Nothing in this section shall be construed as implying that a person may be dealt with under this Act as suffering from mental disorder, or from any form of mental disorder described in this section, by reason only of promiscuity or other immoral conduct.

Index

Index

Accidents, 285
  alcoholism and, 286
  "compensation neurosis" and,
   285
  depression and, 286
Adoption, 387-92
  age of applicants and, 361
  identity and, 389
  inheritance in, 393
  marital conflict in, 353
  social worker's role in, 391
Adreno-cortical response to illness, 270
Affective disorders (*see also*
  Depression; Hypomania;
  Mania; Manic depressive
  psychosis), 255,268
Aggression and violence, 253, 259
Agitation, 443
Alcohol, 245
  as cause of psychiatric illness,
   425, 428, 443
Alcoholic dementia:
  clinical features, 212
  treatment, 234
Alcoholic fugue states, 245
Alcoholic hallucinosis, 245, 266
Alcoholism:
  aetiology, 205
  classification of, 205
  clinical features, 203
  complications, 210
  development of, 207
  incidence of, 204
  treatment of, 232

Amphetamines, 245, 250, 253,
  266, 267
Amylobarbitone (Amytal), 267
Anaemia:
  as cause of confusional state,
   426
Anaesthesia, 286
Antabuse, 124
Antidepressants (*see also*
  M.A.O.I.s; Lithium) 116,
  251, 421-2, 436, 437
Anxiety (*see also* Behaviour
  therapy; Doctor; Patient),
  114
Arteriosclerosis, 425
Assessment Centres:
  in care of elderly psychiatric
   patients, 431
Attachment:
  adoption and, 352
  bereavement and, 351
  Bowlby on, 349-50
  hospital care and, 351, 354
  insecurity and, 351
  obstetrics in, 354
  working mothers and, 369-70
Attempted suicide, 448
Audit, 106, 112
Autism, 401-5
  differential diagnosis in, 405
  general practice and, 404
  intelligence and, 401
  language development
   and, 403
  neurological disorder in, 404

Balint, 107, 122
Barbituates (see also Amylobarbi-
    tone; Pentobarbitone;
    Quinalbarbitone), 246, 250,
    266
Behaviour therapy, 299
    anxiety management training,
        34-5, 38, 39
    anxiety relief conditioning, 35
    assertiveness training, 37-8, 48
    aversion therapy, 39-42
    behaviour modification, 51-61
    behavioural analysis, 21-7, 44-5,
        49, 54
    behavioural psychotherapy, 19,
        20, 21, 51
    biofeedback, 34, 57-61
    cognitive change methods, 35-7
    covert assertion, 44
    covert sensitisation, 42
    flooding, 33, 35
    implosive therapy, 32-3
    marital contract therapy, 48
    masturbatory fantasy retraining,
        50
    relaxation training, 28-31, 34,
        38
    ritual prevention, 43-4
    self control training, 44-5
    self-reinforcement training, 46,
        57
    social skills training, 48
    systematic desensitisation,
        27-32
    thought stopping, 44
Benzedrine, 245
Benzodiazepines — see Chlor-
    diazepoxide; Diazepam;
    Temazepam
Bereavement (see also Attach-
    ment), 419
Biofeedback, 299
Biopsy (brain):
    in investigation of dementia,
        429
Black bombers, 245
Brain damage, 252, 268

Cannabis (alternatively Indian
    hemp, marijuana or

hashish), 250, 267
Cardiac arrhythmias:
    behavioural treatment of, 60
Cardiac failure, 425
Cardio-vascular disease, 271
Care, patterns of, 412
Catastrophic reaction, 420
    patterns of, 412
Catastrophic reaction, 420
Cerebro-vascular disease:
    as cause of confusional state,
        425
    clinico-pathological features,
        428
Chemical intoxicants, 245, 265
Child psychiatry (see Chapter IX)
    autism and, 401-5
    classification in, 358
    drugs in, 409-14
    encopresis and, 401
    enuresis and, 398
    general practice and, 346-9,
        355, 359-62
    history of, 344-5
    hyperkinesis and, 413
Cholecystectomy, 284
Chlordiazepoxide (Librium), 266
Chlorpromazine (Largactil), 265,
        266, 267, 268
Chronic diseases, 267
Cocaine, 248, 249, 267
COHSE (Confederation of Health
    Service Employees), 263,
    269
Committee on Safety of Drugs, 110
Community care — see also
        Community psychiatric
        nurse; Day hospitals;
        Group homes; Health
        visitors; Social work
    of elderly psychiatric patients,
        430
Community psychiatric nurse,
    263, 268, 270
Compliance, 109
Compulsory admission (see also
        Emergency admission (Men-
        tal Health Act)), 262
    England and Wales, 451
    Scotland, 453

Computerised tomography (C.T. scan) — *see* E.M.I. scan

Conditioning:
  classical, 4-7, 16-17, 40-2
    backward conditioning, 7
    conditioned response, 5, 11, 17, 40
    conditioned stimulus, 4, 12, 17, 40
    delayed conditioning, 6
    extinction, 6, 11, 28
    higher order conditioning, 5, 10
    spontaneous recovery, 6
    stimulus generalisation, 6, 10, 17
    trace conditioning, 6
    unconditioned response, 5, 40
    unconditioned stimulus, 4, 11, 12, 17, 40
  operant conditioning, 7-9, 52-7
    avoidance learning, 7, 13
    escape learning, 8
    negative reinforcement, 7, 11, 16, 25
    positive reinforcement, 7, 16, 25, 46, 54
    punishment, 8, 25, 40, 56
    shaping, 8, 20, 30, 53
    stimulus control, 8, 24
    superstitious behaviour, 15

Confusional states (*see also* Delirium; Delirium tremens), 244, 265
  causes, 425
  definition, 424
  emergency as, 443
  treatment, 427

Consultation, 129

Coronary care units, 272

Coronary heart disease and personality, 271

Curator bonis, 455

Day hospitals for elderly psychiatric patients, 432, 440

Death, prevention of stress predisposing to, 270

Delirium (*see also* Confusional states), 244, 424

Delirium tremens, 245, 246, 425, 449
  clinical features, 211
  treatment, 232

Delusions, 247, 257

Dementia (*see also* Alcoholic dementia), 257, 258
  Alzheimer's disease, 428
  causes, 428
  definition, 424
  investigations, 428-9
  management, 429-33
  presenile, 428
  senile, 428
  types, 428

Dependency, serious illness and, 273

Depot injections, 123

Depression — *see also* Antidepressants; E.C.T.; Manic-depressive psychosis
  attempts to categorise, 9-10
  diagnosis, 433
  emergency as, 445
  involutional, 256
  learned helplessness model of, 14-16
  management, 117
  treatment, 434-6

Dexedrine, 245, 246

Diabetes, as cause of confusional state, 425

Dialysis, maintenance, 295

Diazepam (Valium), 251, 266, 267, 269

Dispareunia and pelvic pain, 178-80

Divorce, 456

Doctor:
  and patient relationship, 83, 300
  "as prescribed", 106
  his behaviour and patients, 301, 302
  psychotherapy and the, 77
  tolerating anxiety, 76
  training of, 86

Drug, 109

Drug dependence, 245, 266

Drug dependence (*contd.*)
  aetiology, 198
  characteristics of, 196
  clinical features, 215
  complications of, 224
  personality factors in, 198
  pharmacology of, 201
  physical features, 196
  pregnancy in, 226
  prognosis, 236
  psychological features, 197
  sociological factors, 200
  treatment:
    methods, 228
    principles of, 227
    specific management, 234
Drug intolerance, 267
Drugs, therapeutic for children
    (*see also* Antidepressants;
    Hypnotics; Tranquillisers),
    409-14
  antidepressants, 411
  antipsychotic agents, 410
  chlorpromazine, 410
  haloperidol, 413
  hyperkinesis in, 411-13
  lithium, 411
  methylphenidate (Ritalin), 410
Dying, care of the, 456
Dysmnestic syndrome (*see also*
    Korsakoff's psychosis),
    212, 433, 442

Ejaculative incompetence, 172-5
Electro-convulsive therapy
    (E.C.T.), 118, 268, 269, 435-6
Electroencephalogram (E.E.G.),
    61, 299, 438
Electrolyte balance, 426
Emergency admission — *see also*
    Mental Health Act
  England and Wales, 451
  Scotland, 453
E.M.I. scan (computerised tomo-
    graphy, C.T. scan), 438
Encephalins, 283
Endorphins, 283
Enuresis:
  alarms, 398-9
  clinical investigation in, 397

management of, 396-9
  prevalence of, 394
Epilepsy, 252, 267, 426
  behavioural treatment of, 59
Epileptic automatism, 252
  fugues, 252
  twilight states, 252

Family:
  conflict, 382-3
  general practice and, 347
  generation boundaries and,
    375, 382
  homeostatic mechanisms in,
    372
  myths, 374
  normal functioning of, 371, 377
  nuclear, 380
  psychosomatic, 405-9
  single parent, 383-7
  therapy, 369-75
  with working mothers, 379-81
Flashback, 248
French Blues, 245
Frigidity, 167-71

Gastrectomy, 273
General practitioner — *see also*
    Doctor
  prescribing psychotropic drugs,
    97
Glue sniffing, 223
Gout, 270
Grief, 290
  anticipatory, 291
  hypochondriasis and, 291
  morbid, 290
  selection for treatment and,
    292
  serious illness and, 290
Group homes, 440
Groups and physical illness, 301

Hallucinations, 247, 248, 257
  auditory, 247, 248
  tactile, 248
  visual, 247, 248
Hallucinogen dependency:
  clinical features, 222
  treatment, 235

Haloperidol (Serenace), 125, 269
Head injury, 426, 428
Health visitors, 414, 431
Hearing impairment:
  elderly, in, 417
  paraphrenia, in, 439
Hypertension, essential:
  behavioural treatment of, 59
Hypnosis and asthma, 274
Hypnotic drugs (see also Barbiturates; Sleep), 111, 425, 459
  dependency on:
    clinical features, 219
    treatment, 235
Hypochondriasis:
  depression, in, 443
  elderly, in, 417
  neuroses, in, 441
Hypomania, 438
Hypothermia, 426
Hypoxia, 244, 258
Hysterectomy, 284
Hysteria, 443, 445

Impotence, 162-7
Infection, 425
Informal admission (see also Mental Health Act), 261, 451
Insomnia (see also Hypnotic drugs), 459
Intelligence:
  definition of, 311-12
  distribution of, 312
  quotient, 313
  tests, 312, 315-16
Intensive care units, 287, 288
Interviewing technique, 420
  in psychiatric emergencies, 444
Isolation units, 289

Korsakoff's psychosis — see also Dysmnestic syndrome
  clinical features, 212
  treatment, 234

Learned helplessness, 14-16
Leukaemia and bacterial isolation, 289

Lithium, 124, 437, 438
Lysergic acid (LSD), 247, 248, 253, 262

Mainlining, 249
Mania, 438
Manic depressive psychosis (see also Depression; Hypomania; Mania), 255, 256
M.A.O.I.s (mono-amine oxidase inhibitors), 118, 436
Marinker, 128
Marital therapy:
  Institute of Marital Studies (Tavistock), 90
Mastectomy, 285
Medical model of psychiatric disorder:
  behaviour therapy, in relation to, 10, 51
  depression, in relation to, 9, 10
Medicine, art of, 267
Mental disorder — see also Affective disorders; Mental illness; Neuroses; Organic mental syndromes; Paranoid symptoms; Personality disorder; Schizophrenia; Severe subnormality; Sexual deviations; Subnormality
  categories of, 260
Mental handicap:
  clinical aspects of, 318
  concept of, 311
  coping with, 311
  management of, 323-38
  measurement of, 312
  nomenclature of, 317
  prevention of 319-22
  treatment of, 322
Mental Health Act:
  England and Wales:
    admission for observation, 452
    admission for treatment, 452
    emergency application, 451
    informal admission, 451
    medical recommendations, 452

Mental Health Act:
  England and Wales (*contd.*):
    remand for medical report,
      453
    safeguarding of property,
      454
    s. 4, 253, 260
    s. 25, 262
    s. 26, 262
    s. 28, 262
    s. 29, 262
    s. 40, 264
    s. 60, 242, 256
    s. 65, 242
    s. 147, 261
Mental illness, 261
Mental welfare officer, 262,
  268, 270
Meprobamate (Equanil), 251
Methedrine, 245
M.I.M.S. (Monthly Index of
  Medical Supplies), 107
Mind, theory of, 75
Misuse of Drugs Act 1971, 250
Modelling:
  behaviour modification in, 53
  genesis of depression and, 16
  genesis of phobias and, 12
  personal effectiveness, training
    in, 38
  vicarious learning and, 9
Mono-amine oxidase inhibitors –
  see M.A.O.I.s
Morbid jealousy:
  clinical features, 213
  treatment, 234
Multidisciplinary approach, 413
Multiple sclerosis, 294
Mutilating surgery, 276
Myocardial infarction and sex,
  184-6

Narcotic drug dependency:
  clinical features, 216
  treatment, 234
National Formulary, 111
Neoplasm, as cause of confusional
  state, 425
Neuroleptic drugs (*see also* Depot
  injections; Haloperidol;

Phenothiazines), 120
Neuroses (*see also* Anxiety;
  Depression; Hysteria;
  Obsessive-compulsive
  neuroses; Phobias), 259,
  269
  in elderly, 44
Neurosyphilis, as cause of
  dementia, 428
Non-compliance, 422
Nurses' role (*see also* Community
  psychiatric nurse), 413

Obsessional symptoms, in elderly
  depressed patients, 433
Obsessive compulsive neurosis:
  behaviour therapy for:
    covert sensitisation, 44
    ritual prevention, 43-4
  learning theory explanation, 13
  symptoms, 442
Occupational therapy, 414, 435
Opiates (*see also* Narcotic drug
  dependency), 249, 267
Organic mental syndromes – *see
  also* Confusional state;
  Dementia; Dysmnestic
  syndrome; Korsakoff's
  psychosis; Wernicke's
  encephalopathy
  causes, 425, 426
  definition, 424
Orphenadrine hydrochloride
  (Disipal), 267

Pain, 274, 275
  abdominal in children, 275
  endorphins and, 276
  intractable, 275
Paraldehyde, 265
Paranoid symptoms:
  in dementia, 431
  in elderly depressives, 433
  in paraphrenics, 439
Paraphrenia, 439, 446
Parasuicide, 446-8
Parents:
  counselling in adoption, 390
  counselling strategies, 363-8
  foster, 352, 378, 387-8

genetic counselling of, 393
in marital discord, 382-3, 386
in pregnancy, 353, 387-8
single, 383-7
Patient:
doctor relationship and, 83
tolerating anxiety, 76
Pentobarbitone sodium
(Nembutal), 266, 267
Peptic ulcer, 273
Peptides, 283
Personality disorder — see also
Psychopathic disorder
in elderly, 443
Phenothiazines (see also
Chlorpromazine; Depot
injections; Promazine;
Promethazine; Thiorida-
zine), 121
Phobias:
behaviour therapy for:
anxiety management
training, 34-5, 38, 49
anxiety relief conditioning,
35
cognitive change methods,
35-7
flooding, 33, 35
implosive therapy, 32-3
relaxation training, 28-31,
34, 38
systematic desensitisation,
27-32
learning theory explanation of:
conditioning, 10-13
incubation, 11
preparedness, 11
Physical characteristics of healthy
elderly, 417
Physical correlates of mental
state and mood changes, 269
Physical factors in prevention, 459
Police, 263, 268, 270
Political aspects of drug
prescribing, 102
Postgraduate education, 103
Premature ejaculation, 171-2
Prescribing for the elderly (see
also Drugs, therapeutic;
Repeat prescriptions), 421

Prevention of psychiatric illness in
elderly, 458
Promazine hydrochloride
(Sparine), 265
Promethazine hydrochloride
(Phenergan), 251
Property, safeguarding of, 454
Psychoanalysis, 127
Breuer and, 75, 76
Freud and, 75, 76, 87
hypnosis and, 76
hysteria and, 75
setting of, 87
Psychological characteristics of
healthy elderly, 416
Psychologist — see also Behaviour
therapy
in treatment of elderly, 416,
442
Psychopathic disorder, 258, 261
Psychopharmacology, 297
Psychosurgery, 437, 443
Psychotherapy — see also Chapter II
in various settings, 91
general physician and, 77

Quinalbarbitone sodium (Seconal
sodium), 246

Receiver, appointment of, 454
Referral, 123, 126
R.E.M. (Rapid Eye Movement)
sleep, 113
Repeat prescriptions, 107
Resistance in psychotherapy, 87
Respiratory disease, 274, 425

Schizophrenia (see also Neuroleptic drugs), 246, 253,
257, 268
catatonic, 254, 268
hebephrenic, 254
in elderly, 440, 441, 443, 446
paranoid, 255
Sedative dependency — see
Hypnotic drugs, dependency
on
Self-injury, 446-8
Self-poisoning, 446-8
Severe subnormality, 260

Sexual deviations:
  behaviour therapy for:
    aversion therapy, 41-2
    masturbatory fantasy
      retraining, 50
    self-reinforcement training,
      47
  learning theory explanations of:
    classical conditioning, 16-18
    incubation, 17
    preparedness, 17
Sexual dissonance, 175-8
Sexual inadequacy, 135-91
  biological factors, 152-4
    ageing, 154
  constitutional factors, 150-2
  organic causes, 138-41
    diabetes, 138-9
    side effects of drugs, 140-1
  prognostic factors, 186-8
  psychosocial causes, 142-9
    anxiety, 142-3
    depression, 149-50
    disgust, 144-5
    ignorance, 147-9
    inhibition, 146-7
    personality, 144-5
    sexual orientation, 149
  treatment, 155-61
    drugs, 159-60
    psychotherapy, 159
    relaxation, 155-6
    sensate focus activity, 156
    sexual aids, 160
    sexual education, 158-9
    squeeze technique, 160, 172
    vaginal dilatation, 160, 182
Sexual problems:
  encountered commonly in
    practice, 161-86
  in the elderly, 183-4
Sick role, 268, 273
Signe de Magnan, 248
Sleep, 111
  in elderly, 418
  physical illness and, 298
  Rapid Eye Movement (R.E.M.),
    113
Social characteristics of elderly,
  419

Social work:
  in dementia, 431
  in depression, 435
  in parasuicide, 448
  in psychiatric emergency, 448-9
  in schizophrenia, 441
  with elderly, 415
Soma, 115
Special hospitals, 253, 261
Spontaneous remission of
  neuroses, 2-3
Stimulant dependency — see also
  Amphetamines
  clinical features, 220
  treatment, 235
Subdural haematoma, 426, 428
Subnormality (see also
  Chapter VIII), 260
Suicide (see also Attempted
  suicide), 116, 256, 258
  in elderly, 433
Superstitious behaviour:
  learned helplessness and, 15
  obsessive-compulsive disorders
    and, 13
Surgery, mutilating, 284
Symptom substitution, 2

Talking treatments — see also
  Psychotherapy
  "Anna O.", 75, 76
  classification of, 86
  listening and, 76
  setting of, 81
  short interview, 85
  "talking cure" (the), 76
  techniques of, 80, 86, 87, 91
  timing of, 81
  verbalisation, 80
Temazepam (Euhypnos,
  Normison), 113
Tension headache, behavioural
  treatment of, 58-9
Terminal illness:
  environment and, 293
  psychotherapy for, 293
Testamentary capacity, 455
Thioridazine (Melleril), 265, 267
Thyroid disease, 425
Tranquillisers, 115, 251

major — *see* Neuroleptics

minor — *see* Benzodiazepines

Transference, 87

counter-transference and, 81

response to illness and, 268, 273

Treatment (*see also* Alcoholism; Antidepressants; Barbiturates; Behaviour therapy; Community care; Depot injections; Drugs; Electroconvulsive therapy; Lithium; Neuroleptic drugs; Prescribing; Psychoanalysis; Psychotherapy; Psychosurgery; Tranquillisers), 121

adherence to, 267

Unconscious, the, 75, 87, 88

Updating, 102

Uric acid, psychosocial factors in, 270

Vaginismus, 180-3

Violence — *see* Aggression

Visual impairment, 418

Vitamin deficiency, 426

Voodoo death, 270

Wernicke's encephalopathy, 212

Will, making of (testamentary capacity), 455